The Creation of Psychopharmacology

The
Creation of
Psychopharmacology

DAVID HEALY

HARVARD UNIVERSITY PRESS

CAMBRIDGE, MASSACHUSETTS

LONDON, ENGLAND

2002

The excerpt from the poem "On Being Numerous"
is from George Oppen, *Collected Poems*,
copyright © 1975 by George Oppen,
and is reprinted by permission of
New Directions Publishing Corporation

Library of Congress Cataloging-in-Publication Data

Healy, David, MRC Psych.
The creation of psychopharmacology / David Healy.
p. cm.
Includes bibliographical references and index.
ISBN 0-674-00619-4 (hardcover : alk. paper)
1. Psychopharmacology—History.
2. Psychotropic drugs—History.
3. Psychiatry—History. I. Title.
RM315 .H434 2001
616.89'18'09—dc21   2001039428

For Sarah
There will be no other words in the world
but those our children speak

Contents

From "On Being Numerous"

We are pressed, pressed on each other,
We will be told at once
Of anything that happens

And the discovery of fact bursts
In a paroxysm of emotion
Now as always. Crusoe

We say was
"Rescued."
So we have chosen

Obsessed, bewildered

By the shipwreck
Of the singular

We have chosen the meaning
Of being numerous.

George Oppen

Introduction

This book is about drugs, insanity, and society and about how changes in the relationship between them cause changes in the ways we experience our selves. Insanity has always been a source or expression of disorder in society and individuals. Drugs have played a more ambiguous role; in the hands of healers they have often been seen as restoring order, but those same healers have by using drugs put themselves at risk of being persecuted as magicians or witches, and even executed as threats to the social order.

In the past, the use of drugs to treat insanity was sometimes denounced as futile. As Heinrich Neumann, an early German alienist, put it in 1818, "It is high time that we should cease the search for the herb or the salt or metal which in homeopathic or allopathic doses will cure mania, deterioration, delusions, or excitement. It will not be found any sooner than one will find pills that will make a great artist out of an ignorant lout or a well-behaved child out of a spoiled child."[1] This statement was regularly cited by other alienists throughout the nineteenth century, from Amariah Brigham, a founder of the American Psychiatric Association, to Emil Kraepelin, the icon of modern psychiatry. Neumann, Brigham, and others thought that cures for mental disease could not be achieved by administering pills. But these alienists were in fact a small group whose brief was to manage the fates of a few lunatics, and hardly anyone scrutinized the treatments they doled out.

This book is about a series of discoveries of medications for mania, delusions, and poorly behaved children, discoveries that stand among the greatest triumphs in modern medicine. The discovery of chlorpromazine, the first of the antipsychotics, brought in its wake the discovery of a host of other drugs. It led to the discovery of the antidepressants from imipramine to Prozac, which became a symbol of the 1990s, to Valium and Ritalin, which have had as great an impact on the culture of our times as on the treatment of our nervous disorders. The discovery of chlorpromazine, marketed as Thorazine and Largactil, led directly to the current changes in health care that have become one of the major political issues of our age.

In contrast to the methods used in the days of Neumann, the treatment of nervous problems with drug therapies has now moved out of the asylums and into the community, and what was once the concern of a small group of alienists is now an issue for all of us. What is being done to us and why? Whatever is being done has made pharmaceutical companies, which barely existed before World War II, into giant corporations and the darlings of Wall Street. It has created a medico-pharmaceutical complex that appears to have gradually shifted from discovering treatments for major diseases to medicalizing aspects of the human condition. We live in a Brave New World which is shaped not just by new drugs created in company laboratories, but by an almost Orwellian capacity to control the flow of information.

These developments are part of a change in our culture, and they mean that we now experience ourselves in ways that are radically different from the ways in which others experienced themselves before us. For example, where once fear of God was a good thing that helped maintain the social order, fear has been replaced by anxiety and that anxiety is seen as a bad thing—something to be treated. Such changes can be linked directly to the processes that chlorpromazine stemmed from and gave rise to. This book is not about a definition of the human self, but it is about a set of conditions that have all but preset the terms in which any debate about the nature of self can take place.

Our story opens with the emergence of the asylums and modern ideas about mental illnesses. It opens with figures like Jean-Jacques Rousseau and Karl Kahlbaum, one of the first great alienists of the nineteenth century. For some a history is simply a chronology, in which early chapters detailing more distant times and characters are usually less interesting. But Voltaire's quip that history is a trick the living play on the dead should alert everyone to the fact that if people and ideas are introduced and left "in the past," that has been done to convey a message about how much more advanced, rational, and scientific we are now. In contrast, this volume begins and ends with Rousseau and Kahlbaum and an unsolved set of problems—exhibitionism and catatonia.

Chapter 1 also discusses the initial confinement of insane patients. These patients, however, had a type of disorder that is no longer recognized as insanity—delirium. The dragnet that trawled in delirious patients also hauled in a catch of new unsuspected species of insanity—the psychoses. But nowhere among the catch were the patients that now give the greatest causes for concern—the personality disordered, a newly demonized group, thought to be responsible for social ills from substance abuse to pedophilia and serial killing. There has been a transit of madness through different social stations; what is driving it?

Now that many asylums have closed, the accounts of what happened within their walls typically look back at a history of failed treatments involving strange drugs that ultimately led to a series of barbarities and culminated in psychosurgery. The history of these physical treatments, for many, stands as a potent symbol of the irrationality from which we have been delivered by the benefits of modern science. Chapter 2 looks afresh at the treatment landscape before the first antipsychotics and antidepressants.

There is in fact a growing body of evidence that indicates a success rate and quota of therapeutic rationality per physician fifty years ago that are higher than those that characterize many current practices.

Setting down the triumphs of the past is an important part of the plot. But it risks obscuring the extraordinary nature of the discovery of chlorpromazine. This story, one of the seminal events of human history, is laid out in Chapter 3. For an event so important, the story remains surprisingly unknown to many laypeople and unscrutinized by academics. In part, the reason is that chlorpromazine's discovery has been shorn of all of the developments that came in its train, such as Prozac and Valium, as well as a string of evaluative methodologies that now shape health care in profound ways. Given all these consequences, the details of how chlorpromazine was discovered are as important as the details about Sigmund Freud's changes of mind on whether sexual abuse had in fact caused the problems afflicting the patients he was treating.

Arguments about chlorpromazine tend to focus on the narrow question of whether it was responsible for emptying the asylums or whether other factors played a more important part. Too close a focus on this question leads to a neglect of the fact that this drug completely eliminated the original form of insanity—delirium—while at the same time bringing into the psychiatric ambit all the neuroses and personality disorders that lie at the core of psychiatric practice today. Chlorpromazine brought onto the agenda questions about the social control of behavior and did so explosively; far from getting the Nobel Prize that might have been expected for such a major discovery, Jean Delay was forced into retirement. This is a story with the dimensions of a Greek tragedy.

The year, 1952, in which chlorpromazine was discovered is a key year in the modern calendar. Another is 1968, when the world turned upside down. Old hierarchies came tumbling down. Old heroes of psychiatry such as Kraepelin, Philippe Pinel, and Freud were questioned and revealed as oppressors rather than liberators. The drugs, which had a few years earlier been acclaimed as awakening the chronically psychotic from irretrievable madness, were now castigated as chemical straitjackets. In the few books on the revolutions of the late 1960s, there is almost no mention of psychiatry, even though the key thinking in the period came from an alliance of antipsychiatrists and philosophers using the treatment of madness as a metaphor for the problems of society. There is no mention that two departments of psychiatry were occupied by protesting student revolutionaries, that some of the senior figures of world psychiatry were forced out of their positions, and that psychiatric treatments of proven effectiveness were banned in many countries. Neither historians nor psychiatrists have confronted these issues.

The antipsychiatry whose development is outlined in Chapter 4 provides a watershed that dramatically divides the years before 1968 from those that came after. At this point, the dominant psychiatric languages changed from psychological to biological and an ad hoc clinical pragmatism gave way to practice shaped by guidelines and algorithms. Before 1968, there had been a great outpouring of antipsychotic drugs; after 1968 it was to be almost twenty years before another wave of drugs appeared. What happened?

No lectures today on the science of the new antipsychotics make any reference to this extraordinary hiatus. In an era of science, the temptation is to think that whatever happened in the past for whatever irrational reason is part of a past that did not have the benefit of modern science. In the past, the politics of class, ethnic group, or religious affiliation supposedly dictated the course of events, but the hope today is that we are now firmly embarked on a scientific course where matters of public policy and individual values alike will progressively submit to disinterested scientific examination and solution. One of the messages of this book is that we are becoming less rather than more rational. Far from our problems yielding to science, science has become something of a problem. Far from history coming under control, things may in fact be spinning further out of control.

At the turn of the millennium, psychiatry and culture in general is being viewed in biological terms in a way never seen before. The role that chlorpromazine and the antipsychotics played in these developments cannot be overestimated. This is a story about the final death of vitalism, the notion that there is something special about human biology, something added by God or aliens perhaps. Chlorpromazine in this sense confronts us with ourselves. It has become important that we appreciate the theories that swirl about the biology of these new drugs because these theories now reach out into popular culture and powerfully shape the ways in which we see ourselves. The background to the new biology is outlined in Chapter 5. This is a story of the discovery of receptors. These were to be the targets of the magic bullets of modern pharmacotherapy. But the receptor vision quickly developed beyond a theory about how some drugs might work into a philosophy of how all therapies should work. And now it is accompanied by exhortations to third-party payers not to reimburse therapies that do not work in this fashion.

The twenty-year dry period where no new drugs of any significance appeared has given way to a new era of drug development. Chapter 6 details the new compounds that have emerged and the emergence of a different kind of drug development. New drugs now come as part of a market-development package, which, almost unnoticed by psychiatrists, has developed to the point where it has the power to rewrite psychiatric textbooks. In this new world, psychiatric concepts have become products in a marketplace in a way that leaves the rise and fall of psychiatric theories subject to the vagaries of industrial regulation and patenting. The rhetoric of modern drug development is powerful enough to blind clinicians to preventable deaths and obscure the fact that the life expectancies of their patients are falling rather than rising.

Despite this, there is a perception that psychiatry has put its house in order. The very visible process of agreeing and publishing successive versions of the American Psychiatric Association's *Diagnostic and Statistical Manual of Mental Disorders* underpins this perception. The year in which DSM-III, the third edition of this manual, was published, 1980, is another key year, a year in which a new biomedical self was effectively born. Chapter 7 illustrates the scope of the changes by discussing how matters such as the evaluation of drug therapies and the use of psychotherapies to treat psychoses were handled before and after this divide. The key question is whether we have set myth aside and become more scientific, as is commonly claimed.

The final chapter takes stock. Where does chlorpromazine fit into the flow of history? What is the ultimate significance of its discovery and the subsequent development of psychopharmacology? This is a field full of agents that might not only treat our illnesses but also tell us more about our selves, but it is a field riven by social and political tensions, so that many of these agents are banned. We live in an era when it has become possible not only to treat diseases but to enhance human potential, yet the divide between therapy and human engineering has not been the subject of sufficient debate.

The pharmaceutical corporations created to produce drugs like chlorpromazine are the companies that will own the products of the human genome project. But the origins of these companies and the dynamics that drive their development and accordingly govern their influence on all of us remain shrouded in obscurity. Remarkably, there has been no history of psychopharmacology to date. The media are full of stories about powerful psychotropic drugs being given to preschool children, but no one seems to know how we got to this state of affairs. In this book I tell the stories that led us to just this position and chart the choices that lie ahead.

As biological organisms, we know that we will die, but for the greater part of our individual and collective histories we have probably striven to ignore the full implications of our mortality for our personal identities. As we age and our personalities change, how much of this change has to do with changing biology rather than the impact upon us of experiences, good or bad? These questions take an acute form when we are faced with individuals whose personalities differ radically from the norm and we are asked to consider whether their biologies make them less than responsible for their behavior. No one did more through his writings or his personal example than Rousseau did to raise this question for all of us. He opens and closes the book.

But we are social as well as biological beings, and from society and culture come experiences of oppression and liberation, abuse and healing, as well as the institutions and networks that give a scaffolding to our lives. Changes in our social arrangements color the internal life of our psyches. We can read about the internal agonies, transports of bliss, or musings on fate of the heroes and heroines of literature dating back centuries and cutting across cultures and think we understand them, but in fact our experiences now are radically different from, and often fundamentally at odds with, the ideas of the self that existed in the West up to the opening of the twentieth century.

In ordinary life we slip easily between biological, social, and psychological realms, fitting the effects of our hormones into a set of social obligations filtered through previous personal experiences. But this is not possible with mental illness. In the realm of mental illness internal experiences may overwhelm social norms, physical treatments may appear to slash a path through social and psychological complexity, and social arrangements may be at their most oppressive. The story of psychiatry is a story of tensions that have not yet played out. It is a history where what we decide is the truth regarding our past has immediate and profound implications for how we view ourselves and our futures and how we treat others when they are at their most vulnerable. It is a history that affects all of us, whatever our ethnic group, gender, class, or religion. It is a history of the intersection of drugs, madness, social order, and the experience of the self.

1

Strangers in a Strange Land

Jean-Jacques Rousseau, perhaps the West's leading philosopher and wordsmith, is crashing through a series of underground tunnels in the dark, trying to avoid detention by angry townspeople. He is being pursued for exposing his genitals. He is caught and it takes all his skills to extricate himself from the situation. At least this is how Rousseau tells the story in his *Confessions*.[1] Unlike Augustine, who wrote his *Confessions* more than a millennium earlier, Rousseau does not repent his sins or invoke God to explain the mysteries of human nature. Rather he confesses to behaviors beyond his control and to wonderment as to the origins of these behaviors. He was stepping beyond the categories of good and evil or sinfulness and adopting a more psychological or modern attitude to his "madness." But it was to be over a century before such attitudes became widely adopted or even remotely understood and before they adumbrated modern understandings of mental illness.

Rousseau was one of the leading figures of the Enlightenment, that extraordinary period of Western history between the Reformation and the French Revolution which gave rise to both political revolutions and a revolution in the care of madness and disease. In the midst of the French Revolution, Philippe Pinel, one of the first physicians to work in a lunatic asylum, unlocked the chains binding the lunatics in the Bicêtre. This act was once frequently cited as conveying the progressive spirit of the times. But in the 1960s antipsychiatrists pointed out that Pinel and his pupil and successor, Jean Etienne Dominique Esquirol, were among the leading advocates of nineteenth-century efforts to confine the insane and medicalize their management. The ambiguity between Pinel's unlocking of the chains and the attempts to lock up the insane lies at the heart of our story.

FROM INSANITY TO MENTAL DISORDER

Pinel and Esquirol were indeed the key French figures behind the move to provide asylums to house lunatics, culminating in an act in 1838, inspired by Esquirol, which mandated the provision of asylums and the committal of the insane.[2] Esquirol sought to treat a "madness" different from the kind that afflicted Rousseau. All societies at all times have recognized that some individuals are so grossly aberrant in their behavior that they merit the epithets insane or mad. A simple social creation of madness of this sort would seem impossible, if only because infections are now recognized to be among the leading causes of "mad" behavior of the type that led to admissions to asylums in the nineteenth century. Infections such as AIDS, tuberculosis, and tertiary syphilis, as well as encephalitis and other infections, produce delirium or raving madness. Social deprivation may make infections more likely but social factors have minimal effects on the shape that raving delirious behavior takes. Madness of this sort is not socially created.

By the start of the nineteenth century, the treatment of these delirious states had become an issue in Europe and the Americas. In some cases, troublesome, raving individuals were locked in outhouses or in jails for years in what would-be reformers described as appalling conditions. There were few institutions dedicated to the treatment of insanity. The institutions that did exist, except for the private ones, were often places where patients were chained up and were often brutalized by the wardens, who were former farm workers, retired soldiers, or ex-jailers.[3] The management style was almost certainly influenced by beliefs that too close contact with those who were out of their wits would lead their watchers to lose their own wits. Where not febrile, these patients often had a history of head injury or were epileptic. Many believed that the patients had lost their humanity and had been reduced to the status of wild beasts. They were treated accordingly. The loss of their humanity was, however, a mixed blessing: the same loss that led to their brutalization made possible, according to some, the eventual accession of these souls to heaven, a salvation that would not have been possible if their behavior was under their control.

The effort to improve the treatment of the insane was born from impulses common in the early nineteenth century rather than from a specific desire to ameliorate the condition of the mentally ill. These impulses led to the first modern hospitals, the result of a moral movement. Hospitals had been institutions where patients went to die. If they were not terminally ill on entry, the conditions in the hospital were likely to lead to terminal illness. Reformers wanted to transform these facilities into institutions aiming at healing the patients. Recovery was to be brought about by improved living conditions, better food, cleaner air, fresh bed linen, good sanitation, and discipline. The discipline consisted of regular rising and retiring, abstention from alcohol, the consumption of wholesome meals, and engagement in exercise. All this was to be supplemented by the moral example of healthy living provided by the staff.[4]

The same movement also led to the building of asylums, whose very architecture would be conducive to recovery and would minimize the need for chains. Asylum building began in the early years of the nineteenth century and continued throughout it.

Some institutions had medical involvement from the start, most notably those in France and Germany, but asylums in Britain and America began with a variety of other professionals in charge and only later "fell" under medical control. At first, the new asylums were not crowded. The hope was that lack of crowding would lead on to recoveries, and recovery rates of up to 50 percent were reported.[5] Such rates are comparable to those of psychiatric facilities today.[6]

One consequence of the creation of asylums was that for the first time several hundred lunatics could be found in one location. Observers soon realized that traditional views of the nature of insanity, views held for over two millennia, could no longer apply.

Until the nineteenth century, the dominant view of insanity, shaped by the very visible madness of raving delirium and contemporary views of the nature of the soul, was that the mad were wholly insane. This view stemmed in part from an understanding of human beings as embodied souls, so that souls were responsible for their behaviors. The soul was held to be an indivisible spiritual entity, and it was therefore inconceivable that part of it could be deranged. If an individual appeared deranged and the behavior stemmed from the soul, it followed logically that the whole soul must be deranged and the individual must be entirely mad. The example of delirium, in which all of an individual's faculties appear simultaneously deranged, strongly supported this interpretation. But in the face of the obvious differences between mad people collected in the new asylums, these older ideas began to crumble.

The challenge to older ideas of insanity from inside the asylum was amplified by changes happening outside the walls. The scientific revolution that came with the Enlightenment had begun to change perceptions. Experiments by Alessandro Volta showed that nerves conducted electricity. The dissection of the body laid the basis for the discovery of the reflex arc in 1823. René Descartes had first used the term reflexes, almost two centuries earlier, to describe movements such as the rapid withdrawal of one's hand from a hot plate or a fire. The wisdom of these movements indicated that the soul must have "reflected" on the process to produce such an appropriate outcome, even though no one was aware of reflecting in this manner. But the description of a reflex arc in 1823 by François Magendie and Marshall Hall opened up the prospect that some behaviors were automatic, that they occurred without reflection, without control from higher up in the nervous system.[7] If so, some behaviors could be dissociated from others. And if that was the case some of behaviors might be under faulty control whereas others were not.

It was at this point that people who would later be called neuroscientists began to say that ultimately the mysteries of consciousness would be explained by them rather than by philosophers. The unity of the soul was no longer sacrosanct. Philosophers were profoundly disturbed by this, and by examples reported from the medical literature of anencephalic babies, who could apparently move, breathe, and exhibit some capacity for sensation and who lived for hours or days following birth. What did this say about the location and nature of the soul? Similarly disturbing were experiments involving the removal of the brains of animals, which in some cases did not result in completely passive animals.[8]

A great deal of early neurophysiology research took place in Edinburgh. Scotland was also the site of another development: faculty psychology. This was the creation of philosophers, such as Thomas Reid, interested in testing the workings of the mind rather than theorizing about them.[9] For testing purposes, they split the soul into emotional, volitional, and cognitive faculties. Faculties became a fashionable analytic device; at one point, theorists postulated up to forty different faculties. These developments made possible the phrenology of Franz Gall and Joseph Spurzheim, who said that the protuberances and depressions on the skull were shaped by the activity of a variety of different faculties, dispositions, and aptitudes, which a skillful diagnostician could supposedly map.

This changing climate made it possible in the 1820s for an alienist such as Esquirol, when surveying the asylum population, to begin to catalogue the different forms of insanity. He distinguished between mania or complete insanity and monomania or partial insanity, which effectively involved a mania of one behavior or faculty. It became possible to talk about patients having dipsomania, kleptomania, pyromania, or nymphomania, the implication being that one behavior was deranged but other mental faculties were normal. The identification of manias such as kleptomania shows a recognition that patients could be in some sense mad without being delirious or deluded.

The previous hallmark of insanity had been raving madness—either raving in the sense that patients rave with a high fever or raving in the sense that patients who are deluded rave. The common origin of the words "delirium" and "delusion" reveals this earlier understanding. Throughout the nineteenth century there were comparatively few admissions to asylums of patients who were not deluded. But it became clear that among asylum patients there were some who were not deluded and some whose delusions were so restricted to a single focus that for the most part they appeared almost normal.

This fact led to the formulation of manie sans délire—madness without delusions, a concept put forward by Pinel and Esquirol. Manie sans délire and the concept of moral insanity advanced a few years later by the English alienist J. C. Prichard are commonly cited as forerunners of the modern concept of personality disorders.[10] But if one reads the original articles and explores the context in which these ideas arose, it becomes clear that Pinel, Esquirol, and Prichard were not talking about personality disorders. One good reason is that the concept of personalities did not exist until later in the nineteenth century. These authors instead were talking about the possibility of madness without gross delusions, which could be found for example in severe obsessive-compulsive disorder (OCD) or what would now be called mood disorders. The regularity with which modern psychiatry appeals to these early-nineteenth-century ideas as the origin of the notion of personality disorders, despite the evidence, points to a mystery that will need examination later.

Esquirol's efforts to catalogue the types of insanity produced a recognizably modern classification of mental disorders. This included the first descriptions of a range of conditions, such as obsessive-compulsive disorder. Previously, OCD would have been seen simply as a form of insanity that manifests itself in underactivity and would have been diagnosed as melancholia. Whereas melancholia today is seen as a mood disorder, in the nineteenth century it was viewed as an insanity where the patient presented with an inhibition of activity, in contrast to mania, where the patient was overactive and raving. There was no sense that melancholia and mania were polar opposites. Esquirol in fact introduced the notion of a mood disorder, as something quite distinct from mania and melancholia. He was the first to conceive of the possibility that a mood faculty could be disturbed separately, regardless of whatever else might be wrong with the patient. He called this new disorder lypemania (from the Greek "lypē," sadness).[11] This formulation laid the basis for the concept of a depressive disorder as we now understand it.[12]

FROM MENTAL DISORDER TO BIOMEDICAL BEDROCK

Even as Esquirol's clinical work gave rise to a new classification of the insanities, he was being undermined by a startling discovery made in 1822 by Auguste Bayle: he identified characteristic changes in the brains of individuals dying with general paralysis of the insane, dementia paralytica.[13] Bayle's work made it clear that this condition, whatever its cause might be, could underpin a number of different clinical presentations, pointing the way from disorders to diseases. Patients could appear at some stages melancholic, at others manic, and finally they might become demented.

Disorders and diseases were, therefore, not the same thing. A disorder such as kleptomania might or might not be part of a larger disease entity.

Bayle's work gave rise to the anatomo-clinical method, which entailed two lessons. One was that brain function was important to the manifestations of madness. Among the first alienists to realize this was Karl Ludwig Kahlbaum. Kahlbaum's work led at the turn of the nineteenth century to the foundation by Carl Wernicke of a brain localizing school in psychiatry. Wernicke's most notable twentieth-century followers were Karl Kleist and Karl Leonhard, but this is a school of thought that has largely been written out of psychiatry in English-speaking countries.[14]

The other lesson was that in the absence of knowledge about the etiology of a condition, supplementing a study of the symptoms of a disorder with a study of its longitudinal course might lead clinicians to real disease entities. This in turn might prove fruitful for studies of etiology and treatment. This approach also began with Kahlbaum, but it reached fruition in the work of Emil Kraepelin in 1899, with his descriptions of two major mental illnesses, manic-depressive illness and dementia praecox—schizophrenia as it was later termed. Kraepelin's work was to grow in importance for psychiatry through the twentieth century, eclipsing first the work of Wernicke and his successors in Germany, then that of Esquirol and his successors in France, and finally that of Freud, Carl Jung, and the dynamic psychotherapists in the United States in the 1980s.

In France, meanwhile, there was another challenge to Esquirol, which came from a clinical rather than a laboratory discovery. Almost simultaneously, Jean Pierre Falret and Jules Baillarger described a condition that Falret called folie circulaire and Baillarger called folie de double forme. These two Parisian psychiatrists, one university based and one asylum based, recognized that two of the monomanias described by Esquirol could be linked. There was an overactive, euphoric, and grandiose mania that in many patients appeared linked to Esquirol's lypemania, the sadness mania. Patients cycled from pole to pole of this disorder, it seemed.[15] Esquirol's classification had survived Bayle's work, which depended on postmortem findings for its confirmation. But the descriptions by Falret and Baillarger, pointing to a disease that could be diagnosed in the living, effectively brought an end to the monomania concept. The new idea of a bipolar disorder demonstrated the value of looking not just cross-sectionally at patients but looking at the entire course of their clinical history.

A second development, with enormous resonance for the twenty-first century, helped bring about the demise of Esquirol's monomania formulations. Since John Locke, legal systems had been prepared to contemplate an insanity defense—but only if the accused had what essentially was delirium. This kind of insanity defense poses no problem to this day. Esquirol, however, described circumscribed disorders of a rational faculty, which led to delusions without delirium, and he also described disorders of both mood and the will, among which were kleptomania, dipsomania, nymphomania, and others. Through the 1840s and 1850s, on the basis of Esquirol's formulations, alienists in legal settings argued that patients who were not raving might in fact be mad. But if they were partially insane, were they more responsible for their behavior than the patient who was completely insane? The legal system and the public had great difficulty in answering this question.[16] The problem was compounded by the difficulty psychiatrists had in coherently defending the position that the insane were not fully responsible. This problem that was never satisfactorily resolved has increasing contemporary resonance as we struggle with notions of genetic loading for criminality (see Chapter 8). In the 1860s it was something of a relief for alienists to retreat from what was then portrayed as a medicalization of social problems to a concern with disease entities, to pull back from notions of disorders and move toward a disease-based classification system. These were the first moves in a dance that was to take shape over the following hundred and fifty years, in which one step forward into social problems was followed by one step back to the supposed bedrock of biomedical certainty.

The identification of another disorder, démence précoce, at this time by the alienist Bénédict-Augustin Morel had little immediate impact, but later the importance of this identification and of the rest of Morel's thinking became clear. Morel's description of a condition, affecting young men primarily, from which they were unlikely ever to recover fully marks an emerging awareness that mental diseases could be chronic conditions.[17] It also is the first outline of a disorder that later, as described by Karl Kahlbaum and Emil Kraepelin in particular, was to become the cornerstone of modern psychiatry and was in due course to be called schizophrenia.[18] With this clinical syndrome, Morel introduced another idea of far-reaching importance for both psychiatry and society—the notion of degeneration. During the second half of the nineteenth century, the idea that certain individuals might have a biology that predisposed them to crime or other forms of antisocial behavior and that society might need to protect itself against the inheritance of these attributes was to become a major theme in the interplay between culture and science.[19]

The most significant figure in the development of the schizophrenia concept before Kraepelin was not Morel but Karl Kahlbaum, who from 1860 through 1880 described a number of syndromes—paranoia, catatonia, hebephrenia, cyclothymia, and dysthymia. Kahlbaum's work has, however, been neglected, eclipsed by the later work of Kraepelin.

Kahlbaum was born on 28 December 1828 in Prussia, the son of a wealthy family that was able to sponsor his education and subsequent work. Kahlbaum was a liberal Catholic in a conservative Protestant state, at a time when such things counted. His entry into the university establishment was blocked.[20] He moved instead to a sanatorium in Görlitz, near Dresden, which he subsequently bought and transformed from an institution mainly for epileptics to one catering to psychiatric patients. There he was joined by Ewald Hecker, another whose career path was blocked by the politics of the day and whose sister Kahlbaum later married at the age of fifty.[21] Between them, Kahlbaum and Hecker introduced a variety of reforms such as greater freedom for patients and the removal of restraints.

In addition, they described their patients in a new way. Central to their descriptions was a consideration of the full history of the patient's condition. This approach, Kahlbaum argued, should give rise to clinical entities, or syndromes.[22] When he first presented his ideas in an academic forum, he was ridiculed so harshly that he deferred publication of the discovery of a new syndrome: hebephrenia. Hecker later in 1871 published the first account of the condition and ensconced the term "hebephrenia" in the psychiatric literature, where it was to hold a key place for a century.[23] This was a disorder, affecting young men, that was characterized by severely disorganized behavior. The patients were often silly and fatuous or apparently unable to plan and execute behavior. Instead they might copy the actions of the examiner, repeating words and phrases or gestures. They might or might not have delusions or hallucinations. This condition had a very poor prognosis.

In 1874, Kahlbaum described another syndrome: catatonia, one of the most extraordinary conditions in psychiatry, which in its acute forms quite literally has to be seen to be believed.[24] In mild forms, the patients are stuporous, but in more severe forms, they often lie or stand motionless in odd, sometimes apparently physically impossible, postures for hours or days on end, defecating and micturating on the spot, inaccessible to human contact. Kahlbaum described an overactive and underactive form of the disorder, which he saw as a motility psychosis, a madness affecting the motor areas of the brain. These states were usually episodic, with the underactive forms lasting over a year on average and the overactive forms more likely to clear up in four to six months, but sometimes patients exhibited only one form.

While some catatonic patients spontaneously recovered, others became chronic. Most psychiatrists, up to the 1960s, had the experience of witnessing chronic patients, patients who had been mute and inaccessible residents of a hospital for decades. By that time, under the influence of Kraepelin, this syndrome had become known as catatonic schizophrenia and so the patients' failure to respond was not surprising—unless one knew that this was not the condition Kahlbaum had described. Catatonia was an extraordinary as well as fearsome condition that appeared to have vanished by the 1960s, so that today's clinicians may never have seen a case. Its disappearance is commonly attributed to effective early treatment with antipsychotics, even though, as will become clear, antipsychotics may cause rather than resolve it.

Kahlbaum also described two affective disorders. One was cyclothymia, a condition that led to swings of mood which fell short of frank mania or melancholia. The other was dysthymia, a state of chronic misery that did not involve the signs of disturbed appetite, sleep, diurnal rhythms, and anhedonia, and anergia typical of melancholic depressions, but did involve chronic unhappiness that seemed almost ingrained in the fabric of the patient's being. In the twentieth century these syndromes were reclassified as cyclothymic and depressive personality disorders.

Finally Kahlbaum described a condition he termed paranoia. Far from being raving mad and full of delusions, individuals with Kahlbaum's paranoia could appear perfectly normal. They were able to reason and argue logically on a wide range of issues until the questioner happened to touch on a sensitive point. Then the interviewer would become aware that on certain issues a consuming passion had engulfed the individual and there was no reasoning with him. Formerly, the term "paranoia" had been a synonym for insanity or mania, but Kahlbaum transformed it into a partial insanity. He noted that it emerged at vulnerable life points, for example after childbirth or following the menopause. This work anticipated the later work of Ernst Kretschmer, who called a number of such states sensitive psychoses.

The work of Kahlbaum on the one hand and Falret and Baillarger on the other laid the basis for the celebrated achievements of Emil Kraepelin in the 1890s. Kraepelin was born in 1856, the same year as Freud. He studied in Leipzig under Wilhelm Wundt, who is seen as the founder of modern psychology. In Wundt's laboratory, Kraepelin was interested in the effects of drugs on the psychological faculties and aptitudes that Wundt was mapping experimentally for the first time. He coined the term "pharmacopsychology" to designate this new area within psychology.[25] He moved through chairs in psychiatry from Dorpat to Heidelberg to Munich, where he established the first major research institute in psychiatry. It was at Heidelberg that he formulated the views for which he is now famous, views that caused him to replace Freud as the representative figure in world psychiatry.

Kraepelin took hebephrenia, catatonia, paranoia, bipolar disorder, dysthymia, and cyclothymia as the building blocks for a new classification, which treated these various disorders as manifestations of essentially two basic disease entities.[26] Without reference to Kahlbaum, although influenced by him, Kraepelin adopted the approach of tracking the clinical course of disorders to see whether they were disease entities. He recognized the existence of essentially two major classes of mental disease entities to stand alongside the disease entities of general paralysis of the insane, the dementias, and other conditions that had an established brain pathology.

These two diseases were manic-depressive insanity and dementia praecox. In the case of manic-depressive illness, he took the formulations of Falret and Baillarger and added to them Kahlbaum's dysthymia as well as cyclothymia and a range of recurrent depressive disorders, subsuming the lot under the heading of manic-depressive insanity. These different clinical presentations, he argued, were simply accidental manifestations determined by the physiology or constitution of the affected individual. They differed no more than tuberculosis of the brain differed from tuberculosis of the lung. Clinically, both forms of the same disease might present very differently but essentially they were the same disease.

In the case of dementia praecox, Kraepelin amalgamated catatonia, hebephrenia, and some paranoid psychoses. The rationale for subsuming these three very dissimilar conditions under the one disease heading was that in all cases the individual was unlikely to recover. All three conditions appeared to be progressive, deteriorating, and irreversible, unlike manic-depressive disease, where full recoveries were possible. The argument was that the downward course of the disorder trumped any brain localization factors.

Similar arguments for most of the twentieth century have classified all dementing patients as having Alzheimer's dementia, even though some present with memory disturbances only and others with delusions or hallucinations. The common element lies in the duration of the disorder from the time of onset to death or debility. A quicker progression to death in younger patients would lead to suspicions of a different disease, such as Creutzfeld-Jacob disease, even though the initial clinical features might be very similar to those of Alzheimer's.

This approach contrasted with that of Carl Wernicke, Kraepelin's great contemporary and rival. For Wernicke, the differences between hebephrenia, paranoia, and catatonia were so great that different brain mechanisms must be involved. Wernicke was a brain localizer. Kraepelin was not, although he accepted that many of the clinical features of dementia praecox suggested abnormalities of frontal lobe functioning.

In 1900, it was far from clear that Kraepelin's new formulation would triumph. In the 1890s, both Pierre Janet in France and Sigmund Freud in Austria had begun to make an impact with a new dynamic form of therapy. This held the potential to transform completely the understanding of mental disorders. Freud's disciple, Carl Jung, working with Eugen Bleuler, investigated the possibility that dynamic factors played a part in the genesis, maintenance, or clinical presentation of dementia praecox.[27] Bleuler, influenced by this work, reformulated dementia praecox as schizophrenia. He argued that schizophrenia was a group of disorders and stressed the role that dynamic factors played in the clinical presentation. In Bleuler's vision, the functional mechanism of splitting, which led to thought disorder, was more important diagnostically than the course of the disorder or any brain localizing signs. Some patients, he argued, could recover.[28]

In 1906, Kraepelin visited America as the guest of Adolph Meyer. Meyer had in 1892 come from Switzerland to the United States, where he began work as a pathologist in the Illinois Hospital for the Insane in Kankakee. This experience stimulated his interest in psychiatry and he moved from there to Clark University, then Cornell, finally ending taking a chair at Johns Hopkins University in 1910. Meyer is portrayed now as a foil to Kraepelin, as a man who was against psychiatric diagnosis and disease entities. But for the first fifty years of the century, he was more important in the Anglo-American world than Kraepelin.

Meyer was initially enthusiastic about the Kraepelinian synthesis but later pointed out its limitations. Meyer focused on the role of reaction patterns, in response to biological, social, or psychological insults. This was a more synthetic view than Kraepelin's. It left room for the inclusion of dynamic factors in the overall clinical formulation of a case. This became the dominant American position until the 1950s, when psychoanalysis supplanted Meyerian biopsychosocial psychiatry. It also became the dominant British position through the influence of Meyer on David Henderson in Edinburgh and Aubrey Lewis in London.[29]

Kraepelin's views had little impact in France, until a version of them was imported in the 1980s from the United States in the form of DSM-III and neo-Kraepelinism (see Chapter 7). Until then French classification systems continued to distinguish between a variety of psychoses that had been described in the last twenty years of the nineteenth century and the first twenty years of the twentieth.[30]

Even in Germany, Kraepelin's triumph came late and may have depended to a substantial extent on the untimely death in 1905 of Wernicke, killed in a cycling accident. Krapelin's success in Germany was secured in the 1920s by the emergence of an influential group in Heidelberg, including Karl Jaspers, Wilhelm Gruhle, Willi Mayer-Gross, and Kurt Schneider. This group took a phenomenological approach to mental illness, aimed at eliciting characteristic signs and symptoms of the mental state of patients. They described the features of vital or endogenous depression and the first-rank symptoms of schizophrenia. They strongly endorsed Kraepelin's notion of a clinical entity and dismissed a focus on brain localization as biomythology.

THE BIRTH OF THE PERSONALITY

In the final chapter, I will argue that the Enlightenment, which led among other things to the decapitation of monarchs, as a necessary consequence led to a need to discover new means for nations to govern themselves. This entailed over time a transformation in social relations between people. Since these relations were no longer determined by social hierarchy in the same way as before, there was a need for a new set of sciences to map the new terrain, the sciences of man, one of which was psychology. Wilhelm Wundt, who was appointed to the chair of psychology in Leipzig in 1875, is commonly seen as the first psychologist in this modern sense. While the word "psyche" can be traced back to the Greeks, it took on new meaning in the 1880s.[31] In its older meaning the psyche was a soul, or something close to it, whereas the modern word refers to mnemonic capacities and sets of attributes and aptitudes that are anatomizable and quantifiable, with no reference to the moral center of the individual.

It would seem almost impossible for modern Westerners to think that societies or individuals could function without concepts such as the psyche or personality, which we take for granted. In fact, though, until the twentieth century, human beings derived their identity from their place of birth and the network of relationships in which they were reared. And character was something more related to a person's spiritual being than personality now is; it was thought to hold relatively independently of the circumstances of a person's birth. Then industrialization and urbanization created a growing number of people who could not be as readily defined by place of origin and relational ties, people who interacted with a far larger number of others than had hitherto been the norm, people who needed a "self" to present to these many others and who began to define themselves in terms of their self-presentations. The notion of a personality as distinct to a character began to emerge. The idea that this personality might be subject to its own disorders erupted dramatically onto the late-nineteenth-century psychiatric scene with the appearance of multiple personality disorder. Clearly one could not have multiple characters in the same manner. Accordingly personality must be something quite distinct from character.

Before 1896, or thereabouts, humans clearly had rich inner lives, with latent as well as manifest emotions, just as they have now. Before this watershed, the heart might have had its reasons and the soul its depths, and after 1900 this was still the case. But another realm opened up, through which our behaviors traveled on their way from the depths of our souls to realization. Henceforth manifest behaviors would be scrutinized to ensure that they were not in fact being driven by a systematic bias stemming from this realm, resulting from unresolved conflicts, subconscious motives, or traumatic memories. The work of Freud, Janet, Ivan Pavlov, and Jung opened up a realm of psychic as distinct from moral functioning, where some of an individual's behaviors could be seen to lie outside his conscious control. This was the realm of personality, with its stream of consciousness, rather than that of character, with its set of moral values. The persona emerged on the stage of consciousness, with its dramas of hidden memories and motives, amenable to dynamic approaches.

The new "psychic" issues crystallized around the question of responses to traumatic events, in particular the trauma of sexual abuse of children. The idea that children might be abused sexually had first been put about in mid-nineteenth-century France. Accusations of sexual abuse and the possibility that these might be false were quickly linked to hysteria, the commonest form of nervous condition seen by physicians. As Paul Brouardel put it in the 1880s, "Hysteria plays a considerable role in the genesis of these false accusations, either because of genital hallucinations which stem from the great neurosis or because hysterics do not hesitate to invent mendacious stories for the sole purpose of attracting attention to themselves."[32]

The initial debates about sexual assault concerned its physical consequences. Jean-Martin Charcot, the foremost neurologist of the day, who was treating hysterics at the Salpêtrière, made a connection between traumatic episodes and hysterical dysfunctions that could be reversed by hypnosis. Pierre Janet, one of his pupils, perhaps the first neurologist to spend an entire career working on the psychoneuroses, took the process one step further in 1889 and proposed a traumatic origin for hysteria.[33] Janet described trauma-induced splits in consciousness and linked these to a psychosyndrome that had appeared in France in the previous twenty years: multiple personality disorder. His views and the new syndrome appeared to be particularly popular in America.[34] Although Janet was effectively the first psychodynamic psychiatrist, his formulations and therapeutic practice in contrast to Freud's were entirely compatible with the later work of Pavlov, so much so that later behavior therapists could trace a lineage for behavior therapy back to him.[35]

In 1893, Joseph Breuer and Sigmund Freud, employing Janet's approach to therapy, specifically linked the genesis of hysteria with sexual assault. A great part of Freud's rationale for so doing lay in the fact that his hysterical patients appeared not simply to remember episodes of abuse but to relive them. They reenacted the abuse in front of him, apparently with a reemergence of the physical stigmata of the assaults upon them, in a manner that Freud felt left no doubt about the reality of their memories.

Abuse had happened. Janet and Freud between them had discovered the dynamic psyche and psychotherapy.

A key aspect to Freud's thinking, which tracked closely with German medical thinking, was introduced by Robert Koch in the 1880s: the notion that for a specific disorder there must be a specific cause, which should ideally respond to a specific treatment and no other. Freud's seduction theory was Koch's bacterial theory of infection translated to another domain. Behind it was the same stimulus that led Kraepelin to specific disease models, rather than the syndromal models outlined by Kahlbaum and later Meyer. Unlike Kraepelin's, Freud's formulations pointed to a specific therapy: an abreaction and anamnesis for the traumatic events. When his patients failed to respond to his treatment as the new notions of specific diseases and specific therapies demanded, Freud lost faith in the seduction theory.

From the seduction theory, Freud moved to a new psychoanalytic interpretation of mental life, in which the management of constitutionally derived libidinous energies would shape personality development and give rise to the materials of human fantasies. Given the complexity of most psychiatric conditions, this switch to a constitutional focus had much to commend it. But Freud was not giving up on the idea of specificity. In place of the specific pathogen of sexual abuse, he erected a specific psychoanalytic theory, with treatment following as a logical consequence of the premises of the theory. This was a theory that could provide the basis for the emergence of a new profession.

This change of horses in midstream is a major discontinuity in Freud's thinking, not found in Janet's work. The differences between the two schools of thought can be seen in their approaches to the war neuroses. Behavioral disturbances had been recognized in battle situations since Herodotus's description of the case of Epizelus at the Battle of Marathon in 490 B.C.E. Similar problems arose in the American Civil War, the Franco-Prussian War of 1870, and the Boer Wars, giving rise to a variety of terms such as Da Costa syndrome. There were also a growing number of behavioral problems after train crashes, which were referred to as traumatic neuroses. In 1893 Ewald Hecker used the term "anxiety neurosis" for the first time to describe these conditions, and then in 1894 Carl Wernicke described them as anxiety psychoses. This profusion of names was to lead in the 1940s to the idea of operational criteria, which later formed the bedrock of DSM-III (see Chapter 7).

World War I produced more soldiers with behavioral disturbances than any previous war. The classic condition was called shell shock. Those advocating physical theories of the neuroses argued that the impact of shells produced a shock that led to minuscule tears in the spinal cord and that these tears were responsible for the dysphonias, aphasias, and pareses characteristic of shell-shocked soldiers. In contrast, the psychoanalysts argued that wartime conditions recreated an infantile situation, with commanding officers featuring as father figures or older brothers in a manner that aroused primal sadistic and homosexual impulses. Shell shock was merely the environmental trigger that brought about collapse: "[the] trauma that upset the entire economy of the mental energy also of necessity upsets the equilibrium between their [the soldiers'] repressed impulses and the repressing forces."[36] The horrific events that a soldier witnessed were incidental to the adequacy of his management of his primal impulses.

Janet took a third approach, arguing that shell shock involved dissociations of consciousness and the active repression of memories of terrible events. Certain personality types might be particularly likely to experience shell shock, but anyone could suffer from it. In extreme cases, the combination of personality type and trauma could lead to the emergence of multiple personalities. This conclusion dictated a therapeutic focus on getting the patient to remember what had happened. Mainstream clinical practice followed Janet's line in both world wars, with judicious recourse to both stimulants and sedatives.

World War I had a major impact on psychiatry. It and World War II led to a swing away from the genetic or hereditarian theories of mental illness that had dominated since Morel and toward theories of environmental causation. It put a premium on dynamic psychiatry that had dramatic consequences for all of psychiatry in the wake of World War II (see Chapter 4). It led to the first establishment of outpatient clinics to treat the returning victims of the war, a first hint that psychiatry might be possible outside the walls of the asylum. It put a focus as never before on the personality of the soldier. Would he crack under pressure?

This new figure on the psychological stage, the persona, might be alienated from his true self or maladjusted to society, in which case he would be more likely to crack under pressure. One of the jobs of therapy was to undo this alienation. This change in psychiatry was linked to a profound shift in how the average person viewed himself. Intellectuals such as Voltaire might have seen God as a convenient fiction, but for most people before 1900 the aim of life in some sense was to achieve holiness. After 1900, the goal increasingly was to be adjusted, or not alienated. Multiple personality disorder was the most dramatic symbol of the new order, but it was only one of a large number of conditions termed psychoneuroses. These formed the bread and butter of office practice for a new profession of psychological healers, who in the twentieth century progressively replaced the vicars and pastors of earlier centuries. Under the influence of dynamic theories, it became legitimate to ask whether the fasting or stigmata of saints might have stemmed from anorexia nervosa or hysteria. Where once alienation had been seen as a consequence of sin, it now became at least partly a matter of health. A quest for health began to compete with the quest for holiness. Once holiness had been seen as the pinnacle of authenticity, but now it was conceivable that those who sought it might be "sick" or might end up profoundly alienated.

An alternative view, first formulated by Karl Marx around 1850, introduced the biases that stem from class or other affiliations that confer social advantage, such as race, age, and sex. This tradition gave rise to notions that the commonly experienced self, the personality, was an introject of many social discourses that profoundly alienated the individual from his "true" self. From this perspective the psychodynamic vision was later scrutinized and criticized by social philosophers such as Herbert Marcuse, who accused the mental health establishment of psychologizing alienation and profiting from the business. Such critiques of psychodynamic psychiatry were a prominent feature of the student revolutions in 1968 (see Chapter 4).

Orthodox psychiatry in the early twentieth century stood far removed from both Freudianism and Marxism. The notion of personality did not affect psychiatry until 1925, when Kurt Schneider of the Heidelberg school produced the first clinically relevant categorization of personality disorders.[37] There had been little need for any consideration of personalities and their disorders for the first century of asylum psychiatry, because there were virtually no patients with such disorders within the walls of the asylum. When the psychoneuroses erupted onto the scene, they were initially considered disorders to be treated by neurologists and physicians with an interest in psychosomatic medicine.

The need for a psychiatry of personality grew when Kahlbaum defined paranoia in a manner that brought it close to being a disorder of the personality rather than a disease entity. Kahlbaum had furthermore, in contrast to Kraepelin, viewed dysthymia and cyclothymia as disorders affecting the whole fabric of the individual, not as the more discrete mood disturbances Esquirol and Kraepelin had taken them to be. Finally, by the 1920s, as the numbers of admissions to asylums for the mental consequences of physical illnesses began to fall, a process had begun of increasing rates of admissions for patients with psychopathic personalities, as Schneider called them.

Multiple personality disorder plays a striking role in the history of twentieth-century psychiatry. Janet made the concept popular in the first decades of the twentieth century, but with the triumph of Freudian and other analytic approaches over Janet's dynamic approaches, multiple personality disorder all but vanished, only to reappear (as we shall see in Chapter 7) on an epidemic scale in the 1980s, apparently the consequence of trauma or sexual abuse during childhood.[38] Many psychiatric patients who had been diagnosed as having schizophrenia were rediagnosed as having borderline or multiple personality disorders. Whatever this says about the nature of the syndromes, it clearly says something about the changing nature of psychiatry. In the early years of the century, these patients were seen in office practice by a group of therapists who were not alienists. By the end of the century, they were being seen by the descendants of the alienists, and if admitted, they went to general hospital psychiatric units, not to asylums. The engine that drove this change was chlorpromazine.

THE PSYCHIATRIC MATRIX: 1890–1914

The years around the turn of the century were extraordinary for medicine and psychiatry. In the 1880s, the first bacilli had been isolated, and Robert Koch had made what was then viewed as the radical proposal that many diseases, far from being disorders of the whole person, were specific diseases caused by specific pathogens.[39] His colleague Paul Ehrlich a few years later introduced the idea of a magic bullet, an agent targeted at a specific disease in a specific part of the body (see Chapter 2). In the first week of 1896, Wilhelm Roentgen startled the world with the first X-ray images of the human body. The skin was no longer the screen of the body; it had become one more organ as physicians looked as easily at the heart, lungs, and gut in action as they did at the skin that had formerly hidden them from view.[40]

In 1899, Kraepelin produced the sixth edition of his textbook on psychiatry, the first to launch his now celebrated distinctions between manic-depressive disease and schizophrenia. In 1895, Freud proposed the seduction theory of hysteria. In the years from 1896 through to 1900, he was in the throes of recanting and had begun to glimpse the outlines of a new psychoanalysis. In 1896, Gustav Le Bon published the first edition of his book *The Crowd*, in which he wrote about the revolutionary potential of the people, which had been seen in the European revolutions of 1789 and 1848 and again in the Paris Commune. This book was a direct ancestor of the social psychiatry that was to emerge in the course of World War II and group approaches to mental illness.[41]

Within the asylums, populations of patients had been rising through the century, leading to alarm at the apparently increasing incidence of insanity. Asylums that had originally been designed for 100 patients were now holding 600, 700, or 800. What features of modern life could produce such an increase were a regular feature on the programs of the meetings of asylum officers.[42] In addition to the inexorable rise in insanity, the asylum business had given rise to another gloomy discovery, that many of the patients that had been caught in the trawl for delirious states had chronic insanities.[43] An older idea that raving delirious states typically led to death or burned themselves out had given way to a recognition that some people might need to be committed for life. Moral treatment fostered the recovery of those delirious patients who did not die, but it did little for those who needed commitment for life. Later in the twentieth century, just before the advent of chlorpromazine, some American asylums had up to 16,000 patients and many European asylums held up to 4,000 or 5,000 patients. This state of affairs would have been unimaginable to the original asylum builders.

These developments gave rise to a traditional view that is deeply misleading. Relative to the increase in the population in the United Kingdom, for instance, the asylum population began to fall after 1915, forty years before the introduction of chlorpromazine.[44] This doesn't mean, however, that there was any decrease in the amount of "psychiatric business." Comparing rates of admission to psychiatric beds in 1896 and 1996 reveals a fifteen-fold greater rate of admission and a three-fold greater rate of detention in 1996.[45] By mid-century, as will become abundantly clear in succeeding chapters, the nature of psychiatric business was changing. An increasing proportion of patients had personality disorders and other forms of manie sans délire.

When chlorpromazine emerged in the 1950s, it was to be an engine that drove change, but there was an important institutional change that had taken place earlier in the century that was to critically shape how psychiatry would develop. This was the institution in 1914 in the United States of by-prescription-only arrangements for certain pharmaceuticals. The significance of this development escaped the attention of alienists of the time. And indeed it would have required an extraordinary degree of foresight to appreciate the consequences for their profession of a set of arrangements put in place to manage a social problem— drug abuse—which was at the time thought to be unrelated to mental illness. The fact that it has escaped the attentions of historians of mental illness is far more surprising. These have focused on legislation to restrict the liberties of the seriously mentally ill, from French laws in 1838 onward, not noticing that these restrictions affect an ever decreasing proportion of those who are being treated for nervous disorders, while other restrictions put in place in 1914 affect an ever growing proportion of the population. This scotoma extends into failures to notice the importance of drugs as a force that drives history and their role as commodities in twentieth- and twenty-first-century economies.

For some decades before 1914, there had been another war in progress, a war on drugs. The drugs of concern were the opiates and cocaine. This war was of no concern to psychiatry because neither substance abuse nor the abusers, who were thought to be at risk of becoming low-life addicts—who would later been seen as personality disordered—were then seen as psychiatric problems. Addiction was a social problem; after a variety of social approaches failed to resolve it, the Harrison's Narcotics Act aimed at trying to control it by introducing prescription-only status for opiates and cocaine.[46]

The problem would be managed by making these drugs legally available only through a medical practitioner. Previously, a prescription from a doctor was only one way for people to get the drugs they needed. A person with a prescription could bring it back to a pharmacist on numerous occasions for refills without further endorsement from the doctor. Or having once obtained a drug by prescription, people could revisit the pharmacist and ask for the same medicines again for either themselves or family members. The majority of medicines sold were, in fact, over-the-counter preparations of "patent" medicines, many of which contained a variety of opiates, alcohol, and other substances.

In 1906, a food and drugs act had been passed to regulate the marketplace for medicines, many of which were ineffective and others of which were dangerous. The act required the producers of medicines to state the contents of the product on the label. The hope was that this would provide consumers with the knowledge they needed to make an informed choice about what they bought.[47] The pharmaceutical industry lobbied hard against this act before it became law, but later many enterprising manufacturers found ways of making the labels work to their advantage, in some instances labeling their product "as approved by the Chemical Bureau."[48]

Because medicines, including opiates and later bromides, barbiturates, chloral hydrate, hyoscine, and other compounds, were available without a prescription from a physician or psychiatrist, there was a considerable recourse to pharmacotherapy in the management of community nervousness—the gamut of nervous conditions later treated in psychiatric clinics and offices or in primary care rather than in psychiatric hospitals. Just as with alcohol today, people could obtain these medicines without a therapy establishment constraining their liberty. People could treat themselves without having to be told that they were alienated from their true selves and without being alienated further by treatment. They remained far removed from orthodox psychiatry, which until the middle years of the twentieth century dealt almost exclusively with asylum patients suffering from psychoses.

The modern face of psychiatry owes a great deal to the fact that in 1951, just when the new medicines of the pharmaceutical revolution inaugurated by the antibiotics were coming onto the market, the Food and Drug Administration (FDA), in the Humphrey-Durham amendments to the 1938 Food, Drugs, and Cosmetics Act, declared that all new medicines would be available by prescription only.[49] There was vigorous, sustained, and widespread opposition to this move, with critics complaining that a system put in place for addicts was inappropriate for free citizens. This protest in fact contributed to the establishment of the Kefauver-Harris hearings aimed at reviewing pharmaceutical practices.

Senator Estes Kefauver noted that a unique characteristic of prescription drugs is the difference between the buyer and the orderer: "He who orders does not buy; and he who buys does not order." Hence the ability of the ordinary consumer to protect himself against the monopoly element inherent in trademarks is nonexistent. The consumer is captive to a degree not matched in any other industry.[50] As the Kefauver hearings tailed toward an inconclusive end, the thalidomide crisis occurred. It turned out that thalidomide had been available over the counter in many European countries. Even though the same thing could have happened had it been available by prescription only, one of the consequences of the crisis was to leave the patient a continuing captive of an emerging medico-pharmaceutical complex.

As a result of the Humphrey-Durham amendments, the new tranquilizers and antidepressants that became available in the 1950s all fell within the remit of psychiatry. Ironically, this owed something to the success of psychodynamic psychiatrists in persuading their medical brethren and the rest of the world that community nervousness was part of the business of psychiatry. Had psychoanalysis not had the impact it had, particularly in the United States, the bulk of neurotic, personality-based, and substance abuse problems would have remained in the hands of neurologists or physicians interested in psychosomatic medicine— as they have in countries such as Japan.

2

The Doctoring of Madness
before Chlorpromazine

The modern story of drugs and madness starts in 1950, with the synthesis of chlorpromazine, the first of the antipsychotics. But a deeper narrative began in 1828 when Frederick Wöhler demonstrated that urea, an organic molecule excreted in urine, could be synthesized in a laboratory.[1] For the first time a molecule associated with life had been synthesized. Neither Wöhler nor Justus Liebig, his collaborator, seems to have been surprised by the result. For others, though, this experiment became a key demonstration that there was nothing intrinsically special about human life. Making life did not require a divine or other mysterious intervention. This experiment is often cited as sounding a death knell for vitalism, a turning point in history.

History is made when events happen that change our understanding of ourselves. Until Wöhler, key happenings had been engineered by politicians or statesmen, often on battlefields. After Wöhler, they began increasingly to be experiments in laboratories rather than events on battlefields, with biology assuming an increasing role in human affairs. Those who celebrate Wöhler's contribution to the death of vitalism are celebrating a contribution to the growth of an ordered society shaped by scientific rationality. Other, more ambiguous aspects of the discovery are typically left unnoted.

Before 1828, drugs had been a powerful force in history, a force more likely to bring disorder than order. Drugs were a force against which religious and political establishments struggled. A convincing history now links the use of ergot and other agents to visions that led to the activities of witches—and their persecution—in seventeenth-century Europe, a series of "hysterias" affecting towns or peoples, and cults such as the mystery cults of ancient Greece.[2] Reactions to the writings of Samuel Taylor Coleridge and Thomas De Quincey in the nineteenth century, for example, portrayed the world of the drug-taking artist as degenerate, and declared that the West could triumph over other cultures by avoiding the use of opiates and other motivation-sapping drugs.[3] With the synthesis of urea the stage was set for the development of abilities to synthesize new agents that could either threaten or buttress the social order—new agents, moreover, that could be patented and would become market commodities and indeed would establish markets.

The pace in this narrative quickened in 1856, when William Perkin in London, distilling coal tars in an effort to produce quinine, accidentally produced an organic chemical that stained cloth. He had made a dye—aniline purple, later marketed as Mauveine. Other chemical experiments on coal tars had produced a range of colored dyes but they had not led to links between academic chemistry and industry. Perkin's willingness and efforts to capitalize on his discovery marked a milestone on the road to the growth of applied science.[4]

Perkin's work on dyes emerged just when the new science of organic chemistry had developed to the point where his findings could be exploited. Following Wöhler's discovery of urea, the 1850s saw the discovery of the chemical principles of isomerism and valency, by August Kékulé, Archibald Scott Couper, Liebig, and others, which made it possible to explain the structure of organic molecules.[5] The discovery of dyes gave commercial value to organic chemistry, laying the basis for the development of the chemical and later the petrochemical industries. The new science made it possible to manipulate carbon-based molecules systematically to produce soaps, detergents, plastics, resins, adhesives, preservatives, pesticides, cosmetics, textiles, dyes, and, above all, pharmaceuticals.[6] A host of companies, including the forerunners of some of the most famous modern corporations, were soon established, as it became clear that there was a substantial market for these products.[7] Following Liebig and Wöhler's early development of a chemical laboratory, German companies moved more quickly into this new market than any others.

In 1876, Heinrich Caro, working at the Badische Anilin und Soda-Fabrik (BASF) in Germany, synthesized a new dye, methylene blue, from p-aminodimethylaniline. Caro had a rival for any possible patent, however: Charles Lauth in England had in the same year used a similar process to produce Lauth's violet. It was important to understand the structures of these new compounds and the possible methods of producing them because the patent would be worth a considerable amount of money. So Caro paid Auguste Bernthsen, a Heidelberg chemist, to study the structures of the compounds. Bernthsen demonstrated that both compounds had the same core nucleus but differed in their side-chains. Bernthsen named the new nucleus the phenothiazine nucleus. Caro's immediate problem had been solved. Since the two compounds were different molecules, both Caro and Lauth could patent their compounds. Caro's new dye, methylene blue, was to play a significant role in the development of the biological sciences and was to be a direct ancestor of chlorpromazine, the drug that made modern psychiatry.[8]

The transition of dye-producing companies into a pharmaceutical industry began in the 1880s, when it was found that some of the new dyes could selectively stain different bacteria. Robert Koch had just proposed that specific bacteria might cause specific diseases but few accepted his claims. Even the demonstration of microorganisms under microscopes did not persuade some. Maybe what were being called different bacteria were all just the same and merely took slightly different shapes under different conditions.[9] A series of discoveries by Paul Ehrlich and Koch proved Koch was right. First Ehrlich noted that dyes reacted with tissues rather than just stained them. Methyl green stained the nuclei of cells green but the cytoplasm red. Methyl violet stained bacteria in a tissue sample without affecting the tissue itself. Following Ehrlich's lead, Koch used methylene blue to prove the distinctiveness of the mycobacterium that he claimed caused tuberculosis.

A new world was born, in which instead of there being a few diseases stemming from humors that were out of joint, there were soon to be thousands of specifically different diseases. But beyond this, the interaction of these dyes with living processes led Ehrlich to the concept of a magic bullet, an agent that would be useful in dealing with one disease and not with others. Magic bullets would cause no side effects because these dyes also selectively stained different cells in the body. This discovery made it possible to show not only that the heart was different from the liver but that both the heart and the liver contained lots of different types of tissues. Each of these tissues might go wrong in its own way, without anything being wrong with the rest of the organ. The treatments for the disorders affecting each of these tissues would, like the dyes, act only on the target tissue and not on others in the body.

Methylene blue turned out to be one of the most interesting of the new dyes. In addition to staining the mycobacterium responsible for tuberculosis, it stained the malaria parasite. And if it stained the parasite it was obviously acting chemically on the parasite. Ehrlich decided to try methylene blue as a treatment for malaria. The thinking was the same as that which later led to the successful use of trypan red in the treatment of trypanosomiasis, the parasite that causes sleeping sickness. Other researchers then demonstrated that many of these dyes, such as Congo red, gentian violet, and prontosil red—which forty years later was to give rise to the first magic bullet—had antiseptic and analgesic properties. Methylene blue had some general antiseptic properties, but it was less successful in the management of infections than either trypan red or prontosil red. Methylene blue was, however, to lead to treatments for madness in a way that no other dyes would.

TOOLS OF THE ALIENIST'S TRADE

One of the components of the trick that the living play on the dead that we call writing history is to paint a picture of progress. Nowhere in history is this seen more clearly than in the history of medicine, where former ages are portrayed as dark ages. Within the history of medicine, a special and particularly benighted place is kept for the realm of biological therapeutics in psychiatry before the advent of chlorpromazine and imipramine. Until recently, it has been all but unquestionable that nothing worked before the revolutionary breakthroughs of the 1950s. As a consequence, it is now widely thought that treatment with physical therapies before 1950 must have constituted some form of abuse because the treatments were never shown to work and yet they were forced on unwilling patients. Most commentators on the period are happy to portray the era as a deep dark age, from which the discovery of chlorpromazine emerged to lead us to the sunny uplands of modern psychopharmacotherapy.[10]

Even the best-known revisionist history, which argues that psychiatry was always biological and psychoanalysis was a strange lapse in judgment, Edward Shorter's *History of Psychiatry*, makes concessions to this point of view by talking of a First and Second Biological Psychiatry.[11] In the late 1990s, a challenge to these views has emerged from work on the history of physical therapies in psychiatry, in particular the history of psychosurgery.[12] This work has provided an increasing body of evidence that, for example, psychosurgery, far from being a mistake, was developed from cutting-edge scientific research, that its benefits in individual cases have probably been underestimated, and that it and other physical therapies made a contribution to improving the morale of asylum patients.

The psychosurgery story is a complex one that evokes deep-seated responses from almost everyone. Trying to understand what happened is akin to trying to understand and accept how the Nazis could have been the first to put in place measures to control smoking as well as a range of other enlightened health policies. It is difficult to accept that good and ill can coexist to this extent, a fact that must play some part in how we now view these physical therapies, since before imipramine (the first of the antidepressants), mood disorders were often treated with electroconvulsive therapy (ECT), a treatment that when properly used was much more effective than modern antidepressants. One of the major psychoses, general paralysis of the insane—dementia paralytica—which had accounted for between 5–20 percent of admissions in some places, had been cleared up completely with fever therapy and later penicillin. A case can also be made that in some countries the management of opiate addiction was more successful than it now is. Previous treatments were therefore often more successful than we now concede, and this seems as true of psychosurgery as it does of other treatments.

Whereas psychosurgery is taken as an example of the barbarity of former treatments, insulin coma therapy (ICT) is paraded as an example of how ludicrous previous therapies could be. Recent research, however, suggests that ICT might have been doing a lot more good than we now think. If so, the history of how we have viewed this treatment will be another story that tells us more about ourselves and our attitudes to treatments than it does about the treatment itself. Even more striking than the ICT story, though, is the story of the discovery of a cure for catatonia—a cure that has been written out of history. This I will explore later.

Besides these treatments for the psychoses, there were a host of treatments for "nerves." These developed with no input from alienists. Until the synthesis of chlorpromazine, the gap between nerves and lunacy was immense. Chlorpromazine and its off-spring liberated psychiatrists from their institutions and sent them out into the community. We need to survey the landscape they found in order to understand the full impact of this deinsti-tutionalization.

Within the Asylum

Within mental hospitals, the pressing need was for sedation. The initial agents used were opiates, hyoscine and digitalis. There are good indications that these drugs were used from about 1840 to deliver what amounted to sleep therapy, a therapy later formally "discovered" by Jacob Klaesi in the 1920s.[13] Liebig and Wöhler synthesized chloral in 1832. In 1869, Otto Liebrich discovered that chloral had more reliable sedative properties than any other drug of the time. Liebrich's discovery led rapidly to chloral's widespread use for sedation.[14] It replaced the opiates in many hospitals and digitalis in almost all. Chloral remained in use, in conjunction with or alongside paraldehyde, a range of barbi-turates, bromides, and anticholinergic agents, through the second half of the nineteenth and the first half of the twentieth cen-turies.[15] Paraldehyde was a related compound—a distinctively foul-smelling one. Its odor shaped the memories many older clin-icians had of the asylums in the 1950s. Before chlorpromazine, there was a foul stink that often lingered on clothes hours or days later. After chlorpromazine, the smell was gone.

Methylene Blue

Before chlorpromazine, the propaganda is that the management of the psychoses was not scientific, whereas afterward it was. Psy-chiatrists became proper doctors and even scientists, whereas be-fore they had been on the margins of the medical profession, looked down upon by all, with treatments that resembled nothing else in medicine. This view needs to be challenged. In addition to sedation, psychiatrists tried a range of other treatments in the hope of curing patients rather than merely sedating them. The examples of methylene blue and lithium may make this clear.

Exactly the same logic that led Ehrlich to try to cure malaria with methylene blue also led to its early use in the treatment of nervous disorders. Ehrlich was again the first to try. Finding that when it was injected into frogs, it selectively stained nerve cells, he tried it unsuccessfully as a cure for neuralgia. This work led to a widespread awareness of methylene blue's action on nerve cells, which following Ehrlich's lead provided a good reason to test its efficacy for psychiatric disorders. In 1899, Pietro Bodoni reported on its use to treat psychotic disturbances.[16] Bodoni's study makes three things clear. First he explained the rationale for its use: the prior demonstration that it acted on nerve cells. This may seem slapdash now, but it was a better foundation than those underpinning other approaches of the time. Second his report makes it clear that methylene blue effectively calmed psychotic agitation. Third he reported that many other physicians in the Genoa region had been using it.

Despite the availability of a better than average reason for its use and despite demonstrations that it worked, methylene blue nevertheless fell out of use. The main reason for its eclipse probably lay in the emergence in 1903 of the barbiturates. These were much more effective sedatives than methylene blue, an important finding at a time when the idea that an agent could do anything other than sedate lunatics lay fifty years in the future. The barbiturates were such effective sedatives that their use gave rise to sleep therapy, which involved putting patients into continuous sleep for several days or even weeks to give their nervous systems a chance to stabilize. A systematic form of therapy of this sort emerged in the years between 1900 and 1915.[17] In hospital settings, this approach clearly cured a number of acute illnesses, even fairly severe ones. Methylene blue, in contrast, did not sedate to the extent needed to allow this kind of therapy. Finally, in addition to the effects of sleep therapy in treating schizophrenia, clinicians saw that barbiturates actually cured one form of schizo-phrenia, catatonic schizophrenia. This forgotten discovery, dis-cussed further below, was written up in 1930, but it had almost certainly been noted widely before that.

Effective though they were, the barbiturates left many prob-lems unsolved. Other therapies, such as insulin coma and the shock therapies, emerged, and the use of methylene blue also reemerged. In the 1930s, the chemical process of oxidation be-came a focus of interest for treating a variety of diseases. Methyl-ene blue was an oxidative agent and might therefore be of benefit in treating toxic states. William Allexsaht reported that he used it explicitly for this reason in 1938, and found it clearly beneficial in treating certain dementia praecox states.[18] This report had even less impact that that of Bodoni. Allexsaht may have suffered from the same bad luck that Bodoni had in that another more dramatic discovery was made at just the same time—the discovery of the convulsive therapies.

The point here is not to rehabilitate methylene blue but rather to show that people thought much the same way before and after chlorpromazine. Yet another psychiatric discovery of methylene blue may bring this point home. It became clear in the 1970s that methylene blue could inhibit the transport of vana-dium across nerve cells. Given other work indicating abnormali-ties of vanadium transport in manic-depressive disorders, this discovery led to the idea that methylene blue would be useful in the management of manic-depressive disorder. It is. Grahame Naylor and his colleagues, in Dundee, demonstrated in a con-trolled study that it had a clear prophylactic effect on this condi-tion, reducing the number of manic-depressive episodes over two years.[19] Needless to say, no one uses methylene blue for this pur-pose today. The reason is not competing therapies, although there were many, but that patents had been obtained on newer agents and no drug company would market an old drug even if it worked. In all three instances, then, there were competing thera-pies or interest groups likely to make more money out of other

therapies than they would from methylene blue. In no case, however, was there any greater theoretical rationale for the use of
these other therapies.

The fact that methylene blue worked should not cause surprise. As will become clear in the next chapter, methylene blue is
the basic compound from which chlorpromazine and many other
antipsychotics are made.[20] It is very closely related to another dye,
imminodibenzyl, or summer blue, from which imipramine and
the tricyclic antidepressants, as well as carbamazepine and many
other anticonvulsants, also come.

Contrast these uses of methylene blue with the early use of
chlorpromazine, introduced in the 1950s. The pharmaceutical
company Rhône-Poulenc synthesized a number of phenothiazine
antihistamines in the 1940s. Some of these immediately found
their way into psychiatric practice, not for any sophisticated scientific reasons, but because they were effective sedatives. Chlorpromazine became established because of its obvious efficacy as a
sedative, linked shortly afterward with extraordinary commercial
support. Methylene blue and other antihistamines had proved to
have uses in addition to sedation, and chlorpromazine was to
make even more obvious these nonsedative benefits. These benefits, along with commercial support, in due course helped to
generate a theoretical rationale for the use of chlorpromazine: the
dopamine theory of schizophrenia.

But the theoretical rationale came later. Unlike methylene
blue, chlorpromazine was initially used without any theoretical
rationale. The early users of chlorpromazine were not doing science in greater accordance with conventional theories of how
science is supposed to operate than were Bodoni or Allexsaht.
The early experiments with methylene blue were much closer to
standard models of how science is supposed to operate. Furthermore, chlorpromazine was first used largely in asylums, whereas
methylene blue was originally used in university settings.[21] The
methylene blue story is not some unusual quirk of history. The

story of the rise and fall of lithium also echoes the methylene blue story.

Uric Acid and Lithium

In the nineteenth century, what was called the uric acid diathesis became one of the dominant concepts in medicine.[22] Uric acid, a breakdown product of urea, was thought to accumulate to excess in some patients and in so doing to cause a number of disorders, from gout and rheumatism to cardiac disorders and what were later recognized as manic-depressive disorders. This idea in fact led to the hypothesis that some manic disorders might be a form of gout—a form where uric acid affected the brain and the nerves.

To twenty-first-century thinking, this is clearly a strange idea. But it is important to remember that this idea developed before the advent of X-rays, blood tests, or other ways to assess internal physiology. Physicians were restricted to inspecting urine, feces, blood, and other bodily secretions. Since urates precipitate out in urine, once chemical capacities to analyze these precipitates emerged, it was all but inevitable that theories would form about their role in a variety of disorders. The discovery that lithium dissolves urate stones set the scene for its use for a wide range of conditions, in almost exactly the same way that the fact that methylene blue stained nerve cells provided a rationale to try it in the treatment of nervous disorders.

The effects of lithium on urates quickly gave rise to an industry in lithium waters in both the United States and Europe. Some famous drinks such as 7-UP began life as lithium beverages. Health spas specialized in these waters, which supposedly produced a sense of well-being. This widespread use of lithium led to the discovery by Carl Lange in the 1880s that it had prophylactic effects in manic-depressive disorders. Lange was the most famous Danish neurologist of the day, a co-proponent with William James of a major theory, the James-Lange theory of emotions. Between 1880 and 1900, Carl and his brother Frederick managed an asylum where they treated hundreds of patients with manic-depressive disorders using lithium and reported favorable results.[23] Their experience was not unique. William Hammond at Bellevue Hospital in New York also used it to treat mood disorders in the 1870s and reported good results.[24]

Yet the use of lithium died out by 1900, and had to be rediscovered in the 1950s. If it worked, why did its use die out? At the end of the century, the uric acid diathesis was discredited, and with it went the theoretical rationale that underpinned treatment with lithium. Despite the fact that it worked, with no rationale for its use medical practitioners lost confidence in it. As the uric acid diathesis became incredible, the treatment became incredible also, and people were left to wonder how they could have thought such a treatment would work. Clearly, there is a delicate balance between the effects a treatment has and the reasons practitioners give as to why it works. Exactly the same thinking was later to underpin the use of Prozac, as we shall see.

Lithium did, however, remain in use in many nations until the 1970s for the treatment of rheumatism. A number of British country asylums had large supplies of lithium in stock at the turn of the century, from where it appears to have migrated with medical staff to Australia, where it could be found in the pharmacies of mental hospitals during the 1940s.[25] It was in just such a setting that John Cade rediscovered lithium's psychotropic effects in 1949.

Cade had a hunch that manic patients were overproducing some substance that might be bound to urates. When Cade used lithium to dissolve the urates from the urine of manic patients and gave the resulting mixture to guinea pigs, he noted the appearance of a tranquilizing effect. He then gave lithium to manic patients, and in a number of cases it appeared to bring about miraculous recoveries—at least so Cade reported. In fact, the results were mixed. A number of Cade's patients died. Lithium was clearly toxic, and this toxicity had led to its withdrawal by the FDA in 1949, the same year that Cade was beginning to experiment with it. Other clinicians read Cade's reports. Some tried the treatment, particularly in France, but the results were disappointing.

It was the efforts of another Dane, Mogens Schou, that made the difference. Schou did one of the first randomized controlled trials in psychiatry to demonstrate that lithium worked.[26] He and his colleagues later worked on methods to determine safe blood levels of the drug. A series of bitter disputes between Michael Shepherd of the Institute of Psychiatry in London and Schou kept people aware of this treatment.[27] Without Schou, it is doubtful if lithium would have survived its rebirth. As with chlorpromazine, practitioners had only a certain amount of disputed evidence of successful use—there was then and still is now no theoretical basis for lithium's use, no rationale that could then or can now be used to sell it. As a result, the use of lithium will almost certainly end when Schou dies. Another agent, probably of lesser efficacy, will displace it by virtue of a marketing strategy that depends on offering a "biological rationale." Commercial support is often attracted to the artistic verisimilitude of a theoretical rationale, particularly when this is accompanied by patent possibilities. The candidate compounds are circling: lamotrigine, gabapentin, valproate, and others (see Chapter 7).

One of the most obvious differences between the science base of the physical therapies before 1950 and that of the modern day is the rise of neuroscience. Until the 1960s, even basic questions about the mechanism of neurotransmission had not been settled (Chapter 5). Yet as of the turn of the millennium, the direct impact of neuroscience on therapeutics remains aspirational rather than of clinical utility (see Chapter 8). But neuroscience has functioned to provide updates on the uric acid diathesis. The emergence of the antidepressants, for instance, led very quickly to the development of "biochemical" theories to account for their effectiveness. But just as with lithium in the 1850s, these theories all stemmed from visible effects of the antidepressants on components of blood, urine, and other bodily fluids. As a direct consequence of these effects, it was proposed, in the 1960s, that mood disorders, for example, stemmed from lesions of mono-amine systems, just as it was once proposed that manic-depressive disorder stemmed from a problem with uric acid metabolism. In the case of Prozac, which works on the serotonin system, it was said that there must be something wrong with the serotonin system in people with depression. This is an idea that has never had any more evidence to support it than the uric acid diathesis had.

So, in conclusion, far from there being a difference between the kind of science practiced by clinicians before and after chlor-promazine, the lithium story illustrates a striking continuity. And it is far from true that older treatments were abusive because they were unscientific; once antipsychotic therapy became theory driven, when it was linked to the dopamine hypothesis of schizo-phrenia, the theory probably helped legitimize therapeutic abuse. It was theory that drove crippling megadose regimens of antipsy-chotics (see Chapter 6), just as theories from the best scientific centers in the world had previously driven psychosurgery.

Insulin Coma Therapy

Manfred Sakel trained in psychiatry in Vienna before moving to Berlin in 1927, where in a private clinic he first used insulin to treat morphine addicts.[28] Banting and Best had isolated insulin in 1922.[29] Three quarters of a century later, when its use is so well established and its connection with diabetes is so clear, it is diffi-cult to recapture the mind-set of the late 1920s. How could it ever have been used to treat psychoses? But as is almost invariably the case, a new agent, whether a hormone like melatonin or a drug like chlorpromazine, is initially pressed into a wide variety of uses because no one at that point knows what its full range of uses might be.

Insulin stimulates appetite, and this property almost immedi-ately led many psychiatrists to use it to treat agitated states. Fol-lowing this rationale, Sakel used it on opiate addicts. This early use of insulin was aimed at symptomatic relief. But when some patients accidentally went into hypoglycemic comas or had convulsions, Sakel noted that they did rather better. This finding led to efforts to produce comas or convulsions in patients with a variety of neurotic and psychopathic states. Sakel planned to effect a biological transformation of the person, a cure, by using insulin to influence the autonomic nervous system, which was widely seen at the time as linking the body and the mind. This thinking led to the creation of insulin coma therapy.

Sakel later claimed that his efforts to get his results published met with ridicule and that this reaction played a part in his decision to move back to the university clinic in Vienna in 1933. After he returned to Vienna, when he had recruited support from within the psychiatric clinic, he promulgated ICT as a means of treating psychosis.[30] In Vienna, ICT flourished. It was also in Vienna, in 1917, that Wagner von Jauregg had introduced malaria fever therapy for general paralysis of the insane, tertiary syphilis. It worked, and von Jauregg, rather than his distinguished colleague Sigmund Freud, got the Nobel Prize for psychiatry.

The impact of fever therapy in paving the way for ICT cannot be underestimated. Where before syphilitics were written off as morally degenerate, the possibility of treatment led, it seems, to a rediscovery of the humanity of these patients. A note of genuine therapeutic optimism was introduced to the asylums.[31] Just as ICT was to have several different uses, fever therapy was employed in more treatments than that for general paralysis of the insane. In some cases, it seemed to produce responses in other nonsyphilitic psychoses.[32] Against this background and particularly in Vienna, the home of both physical and psychodynamic therapies, practitioners came to believe that affecting the body and maybe the brain in some way could be curative.

But what were the early therapists doing? The dose of insulin that was given could vary hugely from one individual to the next. Moreover, the dose needed to produce a coma in one individual might differ from one week to the next. The therapy had to be given daily, sometimes for a month or two. It could not be given once or twice, like ECT, after which some improvement could guide further therapy. Finally, there was variability in the insulin preparations, which were initially bovine insulins. These differ from human insulin and accordingly it cannot be assumed that what these patients got was insulin and not in some sense another agent.

In addition, there was the problem of what constituted a coma. Some patients were unable to answer questions but yet could carry out actions in response to commands from the doctor. Were they in a coma? When did a coma start? There is in fact, even now, no clear point at which an individual can be said to be comatose. Patients slide from states of wakefulness through light sleep into deeper sleep and finally into coma. Conventionally it was said that when the patient did not respond to pressure on the eyeball, he was in a deep coma, and that failure to terminate the coma at that stage might lead to collapse and death.

The therapy was associated with fatalities, and therefore it required close medical and nursing supervision. It was only carried out in the premier hospitals of the day in wards dedicated to it. These wards had a much better staff/patient ratio than other wards. They were often purpose built, with new and clean facilities. Being able to offer such a therapy became a status symbol for many hospitals, just as being able to offer the latest high-cost drug or surgical technique is today. Accordingly, a considerable degree of enthusiasm and group morale must have built up in these units.

The treatment was anxiety provoking for the staff if not for patients. It is not clear what patients knew of the fatality rates. The staff knew, however, and they had to be ready with glucose to feed the patients rapidly or inject them if need be. Not only that, but the patients had to be monitored for the rest of the day because there were many cases in which an apparently restored patient collapsed into a coma some hours later.

In the course of treatment some patients had convulsions. Some hallucinated and displayed a variety of neurological complications such as jerks and tics. All of these reactions had to be managed. After the development of the convulsive therapies, these convulsions gave rise to the idea that ICT was another shock treatment, sometimes called insulin shock treatment, and the convulsions were regarded as a good thing. But the point to note is that all these neurological complications meant at the very least that far from working simply on blood sugar, insulin, whatever it was, was working on the brain.

The conventional story is that ICT never worked and that the advent of chlorpromazine led to its rapid replacement. If it worked at all, it is argued, it did so by virtue of improving the morale in the therapy units.[33] The patient expected the treatment to work, and therefore was not hopeless, as were most patients in psychiatric wards of the time. This is a very powerful explanation, but the traditional account is probably wrong.

ICT is actually quite mysterious. Clearly, it must somehow have changed glucose levels, and often patients appeared to come out of the coma in response to glucose infusions. But amyl nitrite or amphetamines could also restore patients. Glucose wasn't necessary. Furthermore, it is now known that insulin, far from being simply a treatment for diabetes, is present in the brain, where a number of insulin-like nerve growth factors function as neurotransmitters. Given that bovine insulin was at least as different from human insulin as estrogen is from testosterone, it is not inconceivable that it was acting on a range of receptors to produce neurological changes in patients. It was therefore working on the brain, but no one explored whether its neurological effects correlated with therapeutic benefits.

It should also be remembered that ICT was used for twenty years before the introduction of chlorpromazine. A therapy that did not produce some good would surely have faded away, given the intense amounts of labor involved and the risk of fatalities. The conventional wisdom is that ICT's reputation was finally compromised by two trials which showed that it did not work, one run by Max Fink in New York, where ICT was compared to chlorpromazine,[34] and the other by Brian Ackner in London.[35]

In fact, however, Fink showed that chlorpromazine and ICT were equally effective. The differences between them lay in the greater ease of delivering chlorpromazine, which led to a greater acceptability among nursing staff, and above all a lack of fatalities with the use of chlorpromazine. Ackner and Harris, comparing ICT to barbiturate coma therapy delivered in the same high-morale surroundings, found the same results for both approaches. Perhaps both worked. The standard claim, however, is that both barbiturate coma therapy and ICT produced placebo effects. In the case of ICT, it is suggested that ward morale created the psychosocial conditions that led to responses to ICT.

Placebos supposedly dupe patients. But leaving it at this neglects the fact that they may also dupe doctors, nursing staff, and others. We may often think of a placebo as a sugar pill, but what often end up being called placebos start off as treatments that, as far as both patients and staff are concerned, seem to be effective. Because of this perception they generate enthusiasm in medical, nursing, and other staff and patients may respond to that enthusiasm. In this sense, unquestionably there were placebo factors in ICT as there are in any therapy. But why should the medical and nursing staff have gotten excited?

Doctors and nurses often observed that patients treated with ICT emerged from a coma more accessible and open to psychotherapy than they had been beforehand. The confusion and delusions present as they went into a coma often seemed to be gone when they woke up. They appeared to relate more readily and warmly to the staff.[36] Patients showing responses of this kind have since been described simply as patients with a good prognosis. But something probably was going on in the patients that called forth placebo responses in the staff, a two-way and much more mysterious form of placebo than is usually dreamed of.

Insulin coma, of course, still happens today. Many people with diabetes taking insulin have hypoglycemic crises and go into a coma. And it is not uncommon to hear reports that as they slip into coma, even though matters are out of their control, far from feeling anxious they feel indifferent. On coming out of the coma they typically sweat profusely and feel cold. They may shake and tremble and have rigors. Human contact or anything that alleviates these rigors and warms them up again is embraced warmly and enthusiastically.

This pattern of responses fits a set of preprogrammed reflexes. Some of us have at some time experienced extreme fatigue or perhaps hypothermia, states where the person experiencing them ceases to feel anxiety.[37] This happens to people who have been swimming to the point of fatigue and then sink. In such situations people do not calculate that there is no point in going any further and then sink in panic. Fear appears to shut off and then they sink. Those who are saved often report that they were curiously, even blissfully, unafraid. The experience borders on a near-death experience. Exhilaration is not unusual.

ICT, at least in some patients, was probably tapping into reflex experiences of this kind. A mechanism of this sort can be expected to enable patients to begin to reorganize their resources and give direction to their lives. Sometimes this effect is portrayed in terms of physical therapies making psychotherapies possible. Rather than a psychotherapy that involves some preprogrammed set of instructions that one individual carries out on another, the insulin story suggests a kind of psychotherapy that happens when in some way a patient's psychological resources have been mobilized and the therapist, responding sensitively to the situation, helps channel these resources in fruitful directions.

ICT clearly worked in a number of senses, as the clinical trial evidence suggests. It worked in the sense that it had neurological effects. It worked in terms of generating enthusiasm in the staff. And it probably also worked for some "psychotic" conditions by providing some relief of anxiety and some opening up and mobilization of personal resources.

It disappeared, however, with extraordinary rapidity when chlorpromazine appeared, in contrast to psychosurgery, which continues to be practiced to the present day. ICT vanished like the memory of a former intimacy, never to return. Thus a former partner a man meets again after the passage of some months or years may seem almost like a complete stranger. He may introduce her to his new partner (who may also in turn become a stranger). What is being lost in these cases is the recognition that the first partner had been loved just as enthusiastically and as intimately at one point as another now is. By some psychological mechanism, she comes to be seen as part of a distant and mistaken life. From another perspective, however, the mistake may seem to lie in the repetition of the story rather than in the fact that the first partner was any less adequate than her successors. So it has been with ICT within psychiatry.

Before chlorpromazine Manfred Sakel and another famous proponent of ICT, Lothar Kalinowsky, and a few others had been the feted names of biological psychiatry, presenting the keynote speeches at psychiatric congresses. They haunted the psychiatric scene for many years after chlorpromazine's discovery, just like people attending a social event where their former partners are central figures. These former heroes in the psychiatric pantheon were looked down on by a new generation vastly less experienced than they, looked on as figures who suffered from a strange delusion and who were unable to let the past go. Their passing was unmourned and unhonored.

Outside the Walls

The most striking difference between the pre-chlorpromazine era and the turn of the millennium, fifty years later, is the group of drugs now called antidepressants. There were none before the discovery of chlorpromazine. There wasn't even the concept that there might be such a group of drugs. The word "antidepressant" was coined by Max Lurie in 1952, but the term took a while to take.[38] As late as 1966, *Webster's Third New International Dictionary* did not include this term, and other international dictionaries, such as *The Random House Dictionary of the English Language*

(1987), suggest the term "antidepressant" probably emerged in the mid 1960s. The early discoveries of imipramine (Tofranil) by Roland Kuhn, the first of what would now be called the tricyclic antidepressants, and iproniazid (Marsilid) by Nathan Kline, the first of the monoamine oxidase–inhibiting antidepressants, did not bring the term antidepressant immediately to the fore. Imipramine was initially called a thymoleptic and iproniazid a psychic energizer. The term antidepressant possibly took hold only because imipramine-like drugs appeared to be effective in treating hospital or melancholic depressions, and these drugs were not thought initially to be of particular benefit in treating the nervous disorders found in the community.[39]

Not only were there no antidepressants before chlorpromazine but depression, as we now understand it, did not exist. Depressive disorders, at least in Europe, were restricted to the melancholias, with or without delusions, and severe depressive personality disorders that led to admissions to the hospital at a rate of 50 to 100 per million of the population.[40] Current estimates for depressive disorders run at 100,000 per million, with 250,000 per million of the population having significant depressive symptoms. The only way to explain this shift is to assume that conditions currently described as primary care depressions and now thought to be in some way continuous with hospital depressions were before 1950 viewed as part of a general pool of community nervousness and were thought to be discontinuous with melancholia or hospital insanity.

"Nerves" and Salts

In fact, until the 1950s community nervousness was diagnosed as anxiety, or mixed anxiety depressive disorder, or "nerves" rather than depression. It is difficult to find out what people might have taken before the 1950s for their "nerves" and how often they took it, because whatever people were taking could be obtained without a prescription. As a result, there are few records to document the range of preparations in use or the frequency of their use.

Even hospital discharge summaries in that era often did not mention what drugs the patient was on because the patient could obtain the drugs himself. There was no need for the hospital doctor to tell the primary care physician about the patient's medications.

For "nerves" of this sort, there were in fact many treatments before imipramine and Valium. There is very clear evidence of a substantial use of opiates in the treatment of patients hospitalized with mood disorders, particularly in German-speaking countries, during the nineteenth century and the first half of the twentieth.[41] But this hospital use arose from a widespread community use of opiates, which can be traced back to the use of laudanum by Paracelsus during the sixteenth century. Before the 1914 Harrison Narcotics Act in the United States and subsequent acts in Europe, the widespread availability of opiates almost certainly led to their use in large amounts to treat nervous conditions. It was only when self-treatment or treatment by other family members failed that the patient would be brought first to his doctor and sometimes after that to the asylum.[42] In hospital settings, it is interesting to note, given the absence of modern ideas of magic bullets to cure specific diseases, practitioners did recognize that opiates were most effective in treating a set of conditions that were later called mood disorders.

Until the isolation of morphine, an alkaloid, or salt, from opium by Friedrich Sertürner in 1806, the active principles in plants were generally thought to be acidic. After the isolation of morphine many other alkaloids were isolated from plants during the mid-nineteenth century.[43] The most important of these for the treatment of nerves were hyoscine and hyoscyamine, which were extracted from henbane.[44] Not until almost a century later did scientists establish that hyoscine and mandragora from the mandrake root, which had been used for millennia for the management of "nerves," are anticholinergics, drugs that block the action of acetylcholine, a neurotransmitter. But the dividing line between therapy and wider effects on the social order is a fine one. Henbane, the plant from which hyoscine comes, had achieved perhaps its greatest fame as an ingredient in a witch's brew. It could supposedly cause a flight of the soul. It is now clear that in low doses anticholinergics can be euphoriants, while in higher doses they can cause out-of-body experiences and hallucinations and at very high doses delirium.

Hyoscine was initially used alone or in combination with camphor and lupulline in hospitals.[45] Then later it was used in hospitals, along with morphine and atropine, in a potent sedative cocktail called Hyoscine Co A.[46] In primary care and office practice in the first half of the twentieth century, it was used in combination with bromides and barbiturates.[47] The ready availability of all these agents also made them widely used by people who were medicating themselves.

A series of twentieth-century studies have proven that anticholinergic agents have antinervousness and antidepressant properties.[48] These studies make it reasonably certain that when nineteenth-century clinicians claimed that they saw beneficial effects from hyoscine, they were almost surely correct. And quite apart from clinical trial evidence, hyoscine was pleasant, sometimes bordering on euphoriant, and at the same time calming—characteristics that clearly would help in the management of nervous problems.

However, no modern pharmaceutical company has developed anticholinergics like hyoscine for the treatment of nervous problems. As popular awareness of the traditional origins of these drugs vanished, extraordinarily it became possible to call the anticholinergic effects side effects. This process culminated with SSRIs (selective serotonin reuptake inhibitors) like Prozac being sold on the basis that they were free of anticholinergic "side effects." The new situation is one in which some critics of pharmacotherapy have argued that antidepressants may in fact work only by virtue of their side effects.[49]

The idea that antidepressants might work through "useful side effects" seems almost impossible to comprehend now. Today side effects are what a clinician will be sued for. They are the unfortunate extras that accompany the specific effects of a magic bullet. But throughout most of human history, what are now called side effects have been taken as indicators that the drug was working. These "side effects" almost certainly contributed to what would now be called the placebo effect of former treatments. For example, in accordance with humoral models of disease, treatments were designed to mimic the body's own efforts at self-repair. Physicians administered treatments that caused diuresis, purging, vomiting, rashes, blistering, or fevers. Both patient and doctor were happy to see such evidence that the drug was working.[50]

Against this background, the use of hyoscine is particularly interesting. In the form of henbane, it was first used when physicians believed in a humoral model of disease, and its very obvious mental effects reassured physicians that it was working. But the combination of euphoria and sedation it produces also has face validity in modern terms since these effects are useful in the treatment of nervous conditions. This modern face validity underpinned the pragmatic use of hyoscine from the middle of the nineteenth to the middle of the twentieth century. Extraordinarily and paradoxically, with the emergence of empirical data to support this face validity, hyoscine and similar agents fell from grace. Hyoscine therefore sits Janus-faced looking back at an older mentality for administering psychotropic drugs and forward to modern confusions as to when drugs can be said to work. Does a drug work when it produces an obviously useful effect, such as the analgesia caused by morphine, or does it "work" only when controlled trials prove it does? (See Chapter 7.)

"Nerves" and Stimulants

The use of stimulants such as arsenic, strychnine, caffeine and camphor has a long history in general medicine for the treatment of a range of conditions, including nervous states. Coca leaves have also been used from antiquity. The first Spanish commentators on the use of coca in South America focused on its use to enhance normal functioning, to increase endurance, for example. The isolation of cocaine led to an exploration of its clinical uses from the 1880s on, and it was used as both a stimulant and an analgesic.[51]

The group of stimulants with the biggest influence on twentieth-century therapeutics has been the amphetamines. One reason for their development was the need to find compounds that would stimulate respiration to counteract the respiratory-depressing effects of the barbiturates, chloroform, and later halothane and other anesthetics. The Chinese herb ma huang, or *Ephedra vulgaris*, had been used in China for centuries to treat respiratory disorders. From this ephedrine was isolated, and it was found to have a clear chemical and physiological resemblance to adrenaline. From 1887 on, chemists at a number of German companies, including Merck, synthesized a series of related compounds that included amphetamine, methylamphetamine, methamphetamine, and MDMA (3,4-methylenedioxy-N-methylamphetamine), also known as Ecstasy.

World War I inhibited research on these compounds. Gordon Alles, working with Chauncey Leakey and Myron Prinzmetal in California, subsequently resynthesized them in the 1920s.[52] In Alles's studies, the most effective compound was phenylisopropyl-amine, or amphetamine, which he called Benzedrine. Smith Kline & French developed this as a nasal decongestant and treatment for asthma. Amphetamine came in two forms, a d and an l form. The d form, dexamphetamine (Dexedrine), when separated out was an unequivocal stimulant. Within two years of its production, Dexedrine had been used to treat a wide range of conditions and had been shown to be useful in the treatment of narcolepsy and effective as an appetite suppressant. The first placebo-controlled treatment trial in medicine involved its administration in 1939 to hospital patients in a cross-over study designed by Louis Dub and Louis Lurie, who found that it was effective in treating depression but not schizophrenia.[53]

Astonishingly, by 1937 amphetamine had also been shown to be an effective treatment for hyperactivity in children. Charles

Bradley gave Benzedrine to a group of severely disturbed children and reported beneficial effects: "to see a single dose of Benzedrine produce a greater improvement in school performance than the combined efforts of a capable staff working in a most favorable setting, would have been all but demoralizing to the teachers had not the improvement been so gratifying from a practical viewpoint."[54]

Another stimulant, methylphenidate (Ritalin) was first synthesized in 1944 by the pharmaceutical company Ciba; its pharmacology was described in 1954.[55] Later Leon Eisenberg used Ritalin in the first randomized controlled trial involving children, to test its effect on hyperactive states.[56] It was effective and its effectiveness led to the acceptance of the concept of minimal brain dysfunction, which in 1980 in DSM-III became attention deficit hyperactivity disorder (ADHD). Since then a growing, almost epidemic, use of Ritalin to treat this condition has become headline news.

Dexedrine and Ritalin are now conventionally thought of as stimulants rather than antidepressants. Following their introduction, they were used to treat nervous states in which fatigue was prominent. But, notwithstanding Dub and Lurie's study, they seemed less effective in treating the melancholic depressions found in hospitalized patients. The discovery of what are now called the antidepressants was notable precisely because these more sedative agents surprisingly led to a resolution of severe depressions where stimulants had not.

Although the "antidepressants" came into being as drugs that cured depression in hospital patients, the overwhelming majority of patients with depressive disorders now treated with antidepressants are not hospitalized. In these patients, it is clear that dexamphetamine and methylphenidate are as effective as the SSRI "antidepressants."[57] This finding was once widely accepted, and advertisements for methylphenidate as a treatment for depressive and fatigue states in outpatients appeared in mainstream journals, such as the *Archives of General Psychiatry*, until the mid-1970s.

Furthermore, the applications to the regulators for licensing as antidepressants a number of the better-known SSRIs did not contain a single study of depression in hospitalized patients because SSRIs could not be shown to work in these populations. Had the SSRIs been tested clinically in the 1950s, therefore, it is highly likely that they would never have been designated antidepressants.

The preceding discussion should make it clear that the seeming discontinuity between the pre-1950s and the present regarding the availability of "antidepressants" is more apparent than real. One of the few exceptions is the use of the SSRIs to treat obsessive-compulsive disorder (OCD), for which there were no clearly effective treatments before the 1960s. SSRIs are in fact more efficacious in treating OCD, social phobia, and even premature ejaculation than in treating depression. This suggests that these drugs ended up being termed antidepressants because of the prevailing market conditions around 1990 when they were launched rather than because of their effectiveness in treating depression.[58]

Some evidence that the apparent discontinuities between the pre- and post-1950s use of the antidepressants lies in our concepts about drugs rather than in what they actually do comes from the 1937 paper in which Bradley attempted to account for the efficacy of amphetamines in treating hyperactivity. There he referred to a body of work stemming from Pavlov's time on brain inhibitory and excitatory processes, according to which it might be possible to induce inhibition with a stimulant, depending on the constitutional type of the individual. In 1924, Pavlov's laboratory in Saint Petersburg flooded, and many of his laboratory dogs consequently became "nervous." Their nervousness seemed to depend on their temperament. Stimulants helped some. Sedatives helped others.

Studies stemming from this work found their fullest expression in the 1940s with the work of Hans Eysenck, a German émigré to Britain. At a time when psychology was about to become humanist, when nurture was about to triumph over nature,

Eysenck was a psychologist working on the biology of personality. He took the Jungian concepts of introversion and extraversion, as adapted by Pavlov, and anchored them in putative brain systems governing arousal and neuroticism—brain systems that he argued were genetically determined. In his system, those constitutionally prone to introversion were predisposed to OCD and phobic disorders while the extraverts under stress became hysterical or psychopathic.[59]

Eysenck devised a scale to measure these dimensions of personality, the Eysenck Personality Questionnaire (EPQ). Using this one can demonstrate the differential effects of stimulants and sedatives according to personality type. For example, answers to the EPQ indicate how much anesthesia will be required to anesthetize an individual for surgery. When the tricyclic antidepressants emerged in the late 1950s, they could not be slotted into this schema, and their apparent incompatibility with Eysenck's models led to the marginalizing of this body of thought. Depression, it was argued, was a categorical rather than a dimensional disorder.[60] From the 1960s onward, the dominant view of the tricyclic depressants, and of the psychostiumlants in the case of ADHD, was that treatments using them were correcting a lesion rather than modulating a constitution.

Today the failure of the tricyclic antidepressants to fit Eysenck's models looks as though it may have stemmed from the fact that, compared to the stimulants or sedatives, these are "dirty" drugs acting on multiple brain systems. The development of more selective antidepressants, such as the SSRIs, led to a reemergence of evidence that responses to such agents may depend more on the personality type of the patient than on the "disease." This idea resurfaced when Peter Kramer in *Listening to Prozac* claimed that some individuals could get "better than well" by taking Prozac. Far from appealing to drug companies, such a perspective unsettles them because it implies that there may be a right antidepressant and a wrong antidepressant for each individual, and if so drug markets would be fractured.

Company ambivalence may be a key factor in the continued eclipse of the thinking of Pavlov and Eysenck. But there are even deeper issues here. Treating a lesion or a disease involves the restoration of an original social order. Dimensional models of how stimulants work, in contrast, imply that it may be possible to modulate or enhance the normal—and therefore that the current social order is to some extent arbitrary. Despite the obvious utility of coca in enabling Peruvian Indians to work longer and harder, the conquering religious and social authorities banned its use. Early work on amphetamines showing enhanced performances in animals was also dismissed, on the basis that improving on the normal was simply not possible. A similar bias underpins the 1962 amendments to the Food, Drugs, and Cosmetics Act in the United States, which focused on developing drugs to treat a set of categorical disease states. The 1962 amendments aimed at producing a template for all of medicine without any consideration of whether this template would be appropriate for psychiatry. In 1965, a further piece of federal legislation restricted the availability of barbiturates and amphetamines.[61] The psychiatric management of nervous states was painted into a corner by these two pieces of legislation, and where practice has gone thinking has followed.

"Nerves" and Tonics

In addition to stimulants, before 1962 a range of tonics was in widespread use for the treatment of nerves. Tonics were agents that increased appetite, improved sleep, and generally promoted convalescence. Tonics had been used for centuries to treat symptoms of fatigue and nervousness, and a number of traditional tonics almost certainly have antidepressant effects. One of them, St.-John's-wort, outsells orthodox "antidepressants" in many countries.

In the 1950s, before the term "antidepressant" was coined, a number of companies produced tricyclic antihistamines. One of these, cyproheptadine, became widely used as a tonic and indeed earned a reputation as an appetite stimulant.[62] Cyproheptadine has since been shown in trials to be an antidepressant, and it is now clear that it has a receptor profile similar to those of many of the first generation of tricyclic antidepressants, as well as to those of mianserin, mirtazapine, trazodone, and nefazodone.[63] Other tricyclics, such as imipramine, which had similar tonic effects, became used as antidepressants. Indeed, the investigation of the tonic properties of isoniazid, used to treat tuberculosis, by Jean Delay in Paris and Max Lurie in Cincinnati, led to the discovery of the first antidepressant.[64]

Changes in regulatory requirements led to the eclipse of the tonics. Before 1962 it was possible to market nonspecific, multipurpose agents such as tonics. Before then, the market in tonics was much more appealing to pharmaceutical companies than a market in antidepressants. After 1962, the reverse was true.

There is a notable transcultural twist to the antidepressant story. Transcultural psychiatry is usually taken to refer to a variety of syndromes or practices not found in the West, with the implication that these reflect a primitive level of development. In the West, during the 1960s and 1970s, nervousness in nonhospitalized patients was generally seen in terms of anxiety, and minor tranquilizers were widely sold. In the 1980s, the problem of patients becoming dependent on the benzodiazepines led to the eclipse of the minor tranquilizers and to the virtual eclipse of the terms "anxiety" and "anxiolysis." That decade saw the birth of the notion that such nervousness was essentially mood based and that antidepressants were the drugs of choice in its treatment.

The replacement of the anxiolytics by antidepressants has, however, been an almost exclusively Western phenomenon. Benzodiazepines do not appear to produce comparable physical dependence in patients in Japan, for instance, where the minor tranquilizer market is vastly greater than the antidepressant market and where as of the year 2000 no SSRI had been marketed as an antidepressant. In addition, a recent survey by the World Health Organization of psychotropic drug use throughout the world found that patients with "mood disorders" were more likely to receive a prescription for a tranquilizer, while patients with anxiety were more likely to be given prescriptions for an agent that in the West would be called an antidepressant.[65]

Part of paradox in these findings begins to dissolve if the term "tonic" is substituted for "antidepressant." But what the findings indicate is that practices prevalent in the West before 1985 were in line with current practices worldwide, and the exception to the rule is the relatively odd set of practices that have grown up in the West in recent years. Is the West leading the way toward some biomedical truth or does this development tell us more about marketing truths? In other words has recent prescribing in the West been culture bound? The possibility that marketing now determines culture is at the heart of this book.

"Nerves" and Sedatives

Interpreting nervousness in nonhospitalized patients as anxiety based rather than mood based leads naturally to the idea of using what would now be called anxiolytics or tranquilizers. However, neither the anxiolytic nor the tranquilizer concepts were available during the first half of the twentieth century. The agents that were useful for treating "nerves" were seen as sedatives. It was not until the advent of meprobamate, in 1955, that the process of distinguishing anxiolytics from sedatives began. Meprobamate was developed by Frank Berger, from the propranediol group of drugs, which had been in use since 1905.[66] Berger realized that many of these compounds were muscle relaxants as well as sedatives, that these two effects could be dissociated, and that a nonsedative muscle relaxant would probably be anxiolytic.

Before meprobamate, the barbiturates and the bromides were the dominant sedatives. The first bromides were introduced in the 1860s. They were initially used in hospitals, where combined with henbane, digitalis, or cannabis they were effective sedatives.[67] By the turn of the century, the bromides had migrated into primary care practices. Some estimates say that by the 1920s and

1930s four out of ten prescriptions written by general practitioners were for bromides.[68] Enthusiasm for the bromides alone, or in
combination with other agents, prefigured the later reception of
Miltown, Valium, and Prozac.[69] There are clear similarities in the
rise and later fall of each of these agents. The bromides became so
widely known that their side effects made their way into literature
in the letters of Virginia Woolf, for example, and in Evelyn
Waugh's *Ordeal of Gilbert Penfold.*

The first barbiturates were produced in the 1860s.[70] They
came into wider use after the synthesis of Veronal by Emil Fischer
and Jacob von Mering in 1903. Fischer and von Mering discovered both the sedative effects of Veronal and a method of manipulating the core molecule to produce a series of barbiturate
derivatives.[71] That discovery made it possible to produce compounds with varying half-lives and other properties. It also made
it possible to introduce a series of "new" agents at regular inter-
vals, a fact that made these compounds appealing to the pharmaceutical industry.

In hospitals, the barbiturates became the most commonly
used sedatives and their use grounded the development of the
sleep therapies. Outside hospitals, the barbiturates were also used
extensively. A combination of dexamphetamine and amylobarbitone, sold by Smith Kline & French under the name of Dexamyl, became extremely popular in the 1950s.[72] Dexamyl has
extraordinary properties that have not yet been explained by
modern psychopharmacology. The idea behind the combination
of drugs had been to counteract the sedative effect of the barbiturate with a mild stimulant effect. But in fact the stimulant effect of
the combination greatly exceeded the effect of dexamphetamine
on its own. The combination of the two agents appeared to produce little dependence in patients and little toxicity, so that
patients were unhappy with the antidepressants that replaced
Dexamyl when the amphetamines fell from grace.[73] As we shall
see, it was only in the 1990s that efforts to explain how the
antipsychotics worked began to produce models that might ex-

plain why Dexamyl produced the extraordinary effects it did (see Chapter 5).

These sedatives, tonics, stimulants, and salts have now been largely left behind. We now view nervousness in nonhospitalized patients for what it supposedly really is—depression. And we have treatments rationally engineered to help. But in the last half century estimates of the frequency of depressive disorders have increased a thousand-fold, from 50 to 100 per million in the 1950s, to 100,000 per million now. There has been a shift from viewing certain conditions as problems of living, sometimes inappropriately treated with tranquilizers, to viewing them as diseases appropriately treated with antidepressants. The evidence that antidepressants cure these diseases, however, is meager. And since a diagnosis can be disabling, if the agents being used to treat the condition that has been diagnosed do not produce substantial benefits, it is less than clear than we are not sowing the seeds of a iatrogenic crisis on a grand scale.

CURES FOR CATATONIA

Perhaps the strangest story of the pre-chlorpromazine era concerns the discoveries of cures for catatonia. Under the influence of Kraepelin, this bizarre disorder, first described by Kahlbaum, became catatonic schizophrenia, a dreaded and untreatable form of the disease. Yet by 1952 and the discovery of chlorpromazine, supposedly the first treatment for schizophrenia, three different cures for catatonia had been discovered and the condition was rapidly vanishing from the asylums.

Rolv Gjessing's Contribution

The first cure is associated with the name of the Rolv Gjessing. Gjessing's early research was an anthropological study of

Laplanders in the north of Norway.[74] He then became the director of the Dikemark Sykehus, an asylum near Oslo, which served the north of the country. Patients from the Arctic were brought over a thousand miles in the guard's van of a train, heavily sedated with alcohol.

Faced with catatonic patients, Gjessing picked out the patients who had a periodic form of the disorder. He believed that they periodically retained too much nitrogen and that this caused their bodies to make a toxin that caused their schizophrenia. When bodily nitrogen got to a certain level, there should be a feedback mechanism, and this, he argued, was not working properly. The patients eventually recovered when the mechanism worked and got rid of the toxin. Gjessing thought that a biological clock underpinned the periodicity and if he could predict when a patient was going to become psychotic and then later recover, and if there were no social factors responsible for either, it would be a simple matter to find the clock. This was an early formulation outlining of what later came to be called circadian clocks and rhythms.[75]

Gjessing's work on periodic catatonia took place during World War II, which contributed to the course of his studies in several ways. First, when the Nazis ordered the liquidation of psychiatric patients, Gjessing refused to comply, thereby gaining the respect of his staff, who became eager to support his research. That research involved putting patients on fluid diets for months to monitor every detail of their intake and output to establish their nitrogen retention. If they refused the diet, the liquid was given forcefully by tube. By following this procedure, Gjessing may have unwittingly created the rhythms he found, since immobility in catatonic states does lead to muscle wasting and nitrogen loss, made worse by a constant diet of carbohydrates and fat.

These rhythms did, however, lead Gjessing to explore a recently synthesized hormone—thyroxin. Thyroid extracts, he suggested, would wash nitrogenous products out of the system. Giving massive doses of thyroid extracts in fact did bring patients out of their catatonic states. One explanation for this success is that these massive doses were a form of shock treatment.

World War II had another effect; it isolated Gjessing from the rest of the scientific community. Unable to write in English, he refused to write in German, and thus had difficulty in communicating his findings. This situation probably contributed to his failure to win a Nobel Prize, for which he would certainly have been nominated in normal times. Nobel Prize winners, such as Hans Krebs, and some of the leading skeptics of psychiatry, such as Aubrey Lewis, who was later to dismiss the antipsychotics, all agreed that Gjessing had worked out a cure for one form of schizophrenia. A wider recognition of his work might well have changed the course of the history of the antipsychotics.

The war had other effects. It hampered the spread of another cure for catatonia: the convulsive therapies. By the time chlorpromazine appeared a few years later, catatonia was a vanishing disorder. Whereas Gjessing had collected large numbers of periodic catatonics, and Kraepelin's textbook had put the figure at 13 percent of psychotic patients, catatonia had become an anomaly—a relic of former days.

Ladislav Meduna's Contribution

Electroconvulsive therapy is one of the most controversial treatments in psychiatry. Its origins lie in the mid-1920s and the research interests of Ladislav Meduna. Working in Budapest, Meduna followed a classic pathway in European psychiatry by first studying neuropathology, focusing on a set of brain cells called glial cells. He showed a number of changes in glial cells after brain insults—in rabies, encephalitis, fever, starvation, and pellagra.

In 1929, the claim was put forward that epilepsy and schizophrenia were mutually exclusive.[76] Several groups confirmed this finding. Hearing this, J. Nyiro and A. Jablonszky gave blood from schizophrenic patients to epileptics, hoping to reduce the frequency of their convulsions. Stimulated by this experiment, Meduna examined the brains of schizophrenics and epileptics and found that there were fewer glial cells in the brains of schizophrenics than normal and an excessive number in the brains of epileptics. Inducing convulsions in schizophrenics might therefore, he thought, help them. The obvious way to do this was to use a drug, but the most famous convulsant, strychnine, was lethal. Eventually he settled on camphor, which he later found had a history dating back several hundred years of producing recoveries in insanity—but usually only when it also induced convulsions.

When Meduna was working, the view was entrenched that schizophrenia was a hereditary and endogenous disease and therefore that "the fate of the patient was determined at the time of conception . . . and nothing could change that fate."[77] Even to think about treating a schizophrenic was presumptuous. Any response to treatment would have been interpreted as evidence that the patient did not have schizophrenia. Meduna therefore sought out a patient in the Budapest state hospital rather than one in the university hospital, where his colleagues might scrutinize him. The man selected had been in a catatonic stupor for four years. Meduna administered the camphor and he and the nursing staff waited forty-five minutes before a convulsion developed. Nothing much else happened, but they persevered. After five treatments, given over a series of days, the man's catatonia cleared and he was discharged.

The next five patients responded similarly. One of them went home after years of being away to find his wife living with another man, but even this shock did not cause a relapse. Nevertheless, the head of Meduna's hospital department, Karl Schaffer, accused him of sensation seeking and a venal desire to make money. Meduna continued to work, however, and reported on twenty-six more patients, of which half responded to treatment.[78] Meduna had by this time shifted from using camphor to using cardiazol. This more reliably induced convulsions but before doing so often caused profound anxiety. Then when Lucio Bini found in 1938 that convulsions could be induced electrically, even though he and many others found the treatment "barbaric and dangerous"— "in everyone's mind was the specter of the electric chair" many switched from inducing convulsions chemically to inducing them electrically.[79] Interestingly, Bini first tried his new therapy on catatonic patients.

Almost all histories of psychiatry now state that although the convulsive therapies were developed to treat schizophrenia, it soon became clear that they were ineffective in treating schizophrenia but were effective in treating mood disorders. This has made it possible for some of the critics of psychiatry to comment that if physicians were wrong about the efficacy of these therapies for treating schizophrenia, what guarantees were there that such therapies were useful in treating mood disorders? An alternative rhetorical jibe has been to ask how anyone could ever have thought this treatment would be useful for schizophrenia, unless he was blindly accepting an essentially crackpot theory.

The answer became clear only in the 1980s, when research reconfirmed that ECT is an effective treatment in up to 100 percent of cases of catatonia.[80] This research initially led to an argument about catatonia. If it was responsive to ECT, did this not mean that rather than being a form of schizophrenia, catatonia was really an affective disorder? Another possibility discussed was that catatonia is neither a form of schizophrenia nor a form of manic-depressive illness. Both Meduna and Bini had continued with their therapies because both for one reason or another had begun with a series of catatonic patients and had seen dramatic responses in these patients. But even by this time, catatonic patients were a disappearing breed in the asylums.

The Barbiturates

The dominant assumption now is that the advent of the antipsychotics led to the early detection and treatment of patients who were liable to develop catatonia and that therefore this form of schizophrenia simply does not develop any more. The fact that patients are supposedly less likely to be institutionalized now may be one factor that has contributed to the declining numbers of catatonics. Other factors may be an increase in the general health of patients and the availability of drugs like penicillin—retrospectively it has become clear that catatonia is often preceded by infections or fevers. But in recent studies, Max Fink and his colleagues at Hillside and Stony Brook Hospitals in New York have shown that in fact catatonia exists to the same extent as before—if one looks for it. The florid states of mute immobility lasting for months do not occur but the syndrome does exist.[81]

This research led Fink and his group to recognize that a cure for catatonia had been outlined in the 1930s.[82] In the 1940s and 1950s "catatonia" was used to describe a syndrome in which chronic patients could be resurrected from their state of immobility for hours by an infusion of barbiturates—hours during which the patients could converse and engage in other activities before sinking back into mute immobility. Continued barbiturate infusions, however, led to tolerance rather than a permanent cure. It was this problem that ECT overcame. What was lost sight of was that while the brief response to barbiturates did not permanently cure chronically catatonic patients, if patients with the syndrome were treated with barbiturates immediately after admission to the hospital, recovery and discharge were common. It had been routine practice for psychiatrists from the 1930s on to have barbiturate infusions available on wards. As a result, the only catatonic patients remaining in hospital in the 1940s and 1950s were the chronic patients, and it was these who later responded to ECT.

The syndrome probably does not evolve today as it did in the past, owing to an essentially accidental concomitant use of benzodiazepines as hypnotics or minor tranquilizers. Partly because of this clinicians miss important and obvious features of the mental states of many of their patients. They miss these features because of the power of a complex of ideas that has developed since the discovery of chlorpromazine, ideas which stress that chlorpromazine and its successors are antipsychotic and that catatonia is a form of schizophrenia. These ideas are part of a Kraepelinian synthesis that in 1980 transformed American and world psychiatry when it was enshrined in DSM-III. These ideas emphasize that we are now scientific about psychiatry whereas once we were not, and that accordingly there is no need to go back and examine the past. This is a complex of ideas that is not disturbed by a regular series of preventable patient deaths, as we shall see (Chapter 6).

3

Explorations in a New World

The 1930s brought explosive development in the field of pharmaceuticals. In Germany, I. G. Farben produced the first major magic bullet, sulfonamide, in 1935.[1] It was developed from prontosil red, which Gerald Domagk had found to have antiseptic properties. Sulfonamide was first used to treat Domagk's daughter, who rose from her deathbed cured of septicemia, which before that time had been fatal. Thousands of others were also successfully treated. The sulfonamides gave birth to the sulfonylureas, which were the first noninsulin treatments for diabetes. The sulfonylureas, in turn, gave rise to the thiazides, which became the first widely used antihypertensives.

Other antibiotics were needed, however, because many infections did not respond to the sulfa drugs. During World War II the U.S. government, pharmaceutical companies, and researchers worked together to capitalize on the antibiotic effects of penicillin and develop a mass-produced drug.[2] Streptomycin also became available toward the end of the war, along with atabrine, a synthetic substitute for quinine.

THE DISCOVERY OF CHLORPROMAZINE

The French pharmaceutical company Rhône-Poulenc was the world leader in the field of tropical infections. Its researchers were developing anti-helminthic agents to treat worms and other intestinal parasites. Since methylene blue showed promise of having an antiparasitic effect, the company's scientists put the phenothiazine nucleus through a series of protocols to see whether it had comparable effects. It did, but no greater than the effects of methylene blue.

Coincidentally, however, another division of the company was working on antihistamines. In this research group were several leaders of the antihistamine field including Daniel Bovet, Bernard Halpern, René Ducrot, and others.[3] This group had already synthesized a number of antihistamines, beginning in 1933 when Bovet synthesized the first one. In 1942, Halpern and Ducrot made Antergan the first clinically useful compound. Neo-Antergan, Benadryl, and others followed.[4]

Because of this work, the company's scientists were interested in antihistamine effects and decided to profile the phenothiazines to see if they had antihistamine effects. Paul Charpentier made up a series of compounds and Halpern and Ducrot immediately found that the new agents were significantly antihistaminic. This discovery led directly to the production of a series of phenothiazine antihistamines; the first to come to prominence was promethazine (Phenergan), synthesized in 1947. These new antihistamines were more potent and had fewer side effects than their predecessors.[5]

The antihistamines are now viewed as over-the-counter remedies for minor ailments, such as allergies. It is difficult today to view them as one of the key breakthroughs in pharmacology and difficult to recapture the tremendous excitement and enthusiasm they generated in the 1940s and 1950s. A better appreciation of how this research was regarded in the 1950s can be gleaned from the fact that Bovet was awarded a Nobel Prize for his work on antihistamines. James Black was later awarded a Nobel Prize for his work in distinguishing between histamine receptors, research that led to the synthesis of selective H-2 blockers, such as the anti-ulcer drugs cimetidine and ranitidine, which earned vast amounts of money for the pharmaceutical industry. Almost all antidepressants, including the SSRIs, and the antipsychotics came from the antihistamines.

From a technical point of view, the development of the antihistamines marked a watershed in the development of drugs. Working with particular nuclei, companies had developed capacities to attach successively different side chains to the nucleus and systematically map the properties of the resulting compounds. In the process, it quickly became clear that some of the compounds in a series were very different from others, and these quite different compounds were explored in the effort to develop even more useful compounds. The basic building blocks for modern drug development were put in place at this time.[6]

In contrast to earlier agents, antihistamines, researchers found, could block the actions of a humor in the body thought to be involved in stress reactions. Histamine was known to be mobilized in response to hypothermia, wounds, allergies, and a range of other conditions. Using antihistamines to alter the effects of histamine offered the possibility of reversing pathological processes in the body in a more precise and rational manner than had been possible with methylene blue. In the late 1940s, there were hopes that an effective antihistamine could be used for the management of cardiovascular, gynecological, obstetrical, and neurological conditions, especially Parkinson's disease.[7]

One of the antihistamines, promethazine, also had sedative properties, and it began to be used in sleep therapy regimes almost immediately. In 1950, Paul Guiraud, a senior Parisian psychiatrist, reported on its beneficial effects in the management of schizophrenia and other agitated psychotic conditions.[8] This use of antihistamines in sleep therapy influenced the early use of chlorpromazine and scientific interpretations of how it worked.

Following the early reports on promethazine and chlorpromazine, other nonphenothiazine antihistamines were used effectively to treat psychoses in eastern Europe during the 1950s, which suggests that not everything is yet known about the antipsychotic properties of the antihistamines.[9]

The initial interest within Rhône-Poulenc, however, was not in possible treatments for nervous disorders. The company was interested in the likely usefulness of the antihistamines for surgical purposes, as part of what became known as a lytic cocktail. Pierre Huguenard and Henri Laborit invented the lytic cocktail. Huguenard was an anesthetist, working in Paris, who had a penchant for combining drugs. In 1948 he was faced with a problem when one of his nurses needed an operation on her nose. Clearly he could not put an anesthetic mask on her face. He would have to sedate her in some other way. Adding to the difficulty, this nurse was squeamish and nervous about surgery. Huguenard suggested to her that she drink a new cocktail he had begun using made of Diparcol and Dolossal, a combination of promethazine and pethidine. During the course of surgery, he was surprised to find his patient relaxed and almost totally indifferent.[10] He reported this striking result to a fellow surgeon, Henri Laborit.

Laborit was a military surgeon at a time when surgeons were often also responsible for anesthesia, and he was worried about stress during surgery. Clearly opening the body is a considerable stress, and even if the patient is asleep the body through the nervous system and endocrine system responds vigorously to that stress. Quite apart from the drop in blood pressure that may be caused by loss of blood, there may be dramatic increases or decreases in blood pressure in response to the insertion of a scalpel. As Laborit saw it, the body needed not only sedation but also stabilization, especially for the more ambitious open-heart operations being contemplated in the 1950s.

Since stress of this type involves multiple body systems, it made sense to combine different agents to combat its various manifestations. Laborit therefore was interested in Huguenard's cocktails. He used the Diparcol-Dolossal combination and found its effects impressive. He too noted the indifference that it produced, and he noticed something else. Laborit had a hunch that stabilization could be produced by putting the body into a state of artificial hibernation. When the body is made hypothermic, some components of the stress reaction can be prevented. But cooling the body is also stressful. The new antihistamines blocked compensatory responses to cooling. Their effectiveness in making both animal and human bodies poikilothermic led to a vogue for hibernotherapy.

The Synthesis of Chlorpromazine

Laborit suggested to Rhône-Poulenc that it optimize the stabilizing effects of the antihistamines on the central nervous system. This idea led Charpentier in December 1950 to synthesize a new series of phenothiazine compounds. In early 1951 Simone Courvoisier put these through a series of screening tests for antihistamine effects. In perhaps the first industrial use of a behavioral test to screen for pharmacological properties, Courvoisier used the rope climbing test, devised in 1915 by David Macht for his studies on opioid salts.[11] This test involved rats, a platform on which there was food, a rope tied to the platform, and a shock stimulus. While using tests like this, Macht had envisaged a possible use of drugs to dissect psychological functions, suggesting in 1921 a possible new discipline of "psychopharmacology."

In the ordinary course of events, rats could be conditioned to respond to certain stimuli for a food reward or could be trained to perform certain behaviors in order to avoid an aversive experience such as a shock. On the rope climbing test, animals given some of these new phenothiazines did not climb the rope to get the food the way untreated animals did, even when alerted to the imminence of a shock. They seemed indifferent to the shock.

Charpentier had chlorinated some of the new series of antihistamines, a process known to make a compound more potent but also more toxic. One of the new compounds, RP 4560, chlorinated promazine, or chlorpromazine, had surprising characteristics. It had an effect on the sympathetic system: it reversed epinephrine's effects. It had marked cardiovascular effects on animals. It was anticholinergic. It potentiated barbiturates. It was anti-emetic. And the lack of response on the rope test following administration of chlorpromazine was more clear cut than with any of the other compounds. It seemed that the rats failed to respond not because they were sedated and not because their coordination was impaired; rather their lack of response seemed to stem from an indifference of some sort.[12]

Promazine, sold as Sparine, was one of the most sedative of the phenothiazine antihistamines. It has been used since for sedative purposes in hospitals and nursing homes, particularly with the elderly. But it is not clearly antipsychotic. Simply chlorinating it had seemingly produced a completely different molecule.[13] Even before it was given to patients, Courvoisier had demonstrated that the new molecule was distinctively different from the other antihistamines.

In fact, it was a different molecule with clearer central effects. From Laborit's point of view, clearer central effects did not mean a cleaner compound. Quite the opposite, for his purposes the greater the capacity of the drug to interfere with the largest number of systems possible the better. In the terminology of the time he wanted a ganglioplegic agent—a ganglion paralyzing agent. Such an agent's action, it was hoped, might be useful in treating a range of medical conditions.[14] The wide range of actions envisaged underpinned the trade name given to the new compound in Europe—Largactil, a name that came from Laborit. The new drug opened up huge possibilities for surgeons and other physicians, and the first major research project in the United States with chlorpromazine was undertaken by Leonard Steen, at Maimonides Hospital in New York, who reported beneficial effects in cardiac surgery.[15]

Laborit thought that chlorpromazine marked a significant

advance on promethazine, particularly in causing indifference.[16] In addition to giving it to patients, he apparently also gave it on 9 November 1951 to a psychiatrist friend, Cornelia Quarti.[17] At the time researchers were taking new drugs that acted on the mind, such as LSD, and reporting extraordinary subjective effects. But aside from feeling faint, Quarti seems to have felt some indifference and possibly some restlessness but little else. Similar reports had come from taxi drivers and others, who said they did not notice red lights when they had taken antihistamines.[18]

This indifference showed up in other circumstances also. Laborit had recommended that chlorpromazine be used to manage stress reactions in battlefield situations. Following this recommendation chlorpromazine was included in the medical kits of U.S. soldiers in the Korean War. Some soldiers injured in battlefield became indifferent after taking it and did not react quickly to rescue opportunities. Some lives may have been lost as a consequence, and chlorpromazine's use for this purpose was short-lived.[19]

The indifference was striking enough to lead Laborit to mention it to Pierre Hamon, a psychiatrist at the Val de Grâce Military Hospital in Paris. It was all but inevitable that chlorpromazine would be used psychiatrically at some point, just as almost every other drug was. Laborit's suggestion was to use it along with artificial hibernation to stabilize the nervous system. Hamon, Jean Paraire, and Jean Velluz tried it but not initially as a means of inducing artificial hibernation.[20] The first known psychiatric patient to get chlorpromazine was Bernard P., a manic patient, who was given a combination of chlorpromazine, barbiturates, and other drugs. He apparently did well on this regime.

Who should get the credit for the discovery of the psychotropic effects of chlorpromazine? Laborit, and others on his behalf, claimed that his input was essential. This seems reasonable, but it has to be borne in mind that his primary interest was the anesthetic effects of the drug. In 1953, for instance, Rhône-Poulenc sent several scientists to the United States to demonstrate the effects of chlorpromazine. Laborit was one of them but his task was to demonstrate chlorpromazine's usefulness as part of a lytic cocktail to be used in anesthesia. Indeed, he never advocated its use as an agent likely to have antipsychotic effects, though it is fair to say that the idea of an antipsychotic was all but inconceivable at the time.[21] However, the rationale for Laborit's way of using chlorpromazine was literally to melt away some weeks later, as we shall see.

The story of chlorpromazine's spread to the United States provides some insights on how it was initially received. Rhône-Poulenc canvassed a number of U.S. pharmaceutical companies for possible interest in RP 4560. None was interested. In 1953, after the psychiatric uses of chlorpromazine had been discovered by Pierre Deniker, Rhône-Poulenc finally licensed the drug to Smith Kline & French. Despite Deniker's discovery, however, SK&F did not initially aim to develop a psychiatric drug. At that time SK&F was a company undergoing rapid expansion owing to its discovery of the beneficial effects of combining amphetamines and low-dose barbiturates into a compound called Dexamyl. This product sold in huge amounts. But the company also had a cardiovascular drug that caused nausea and vomiting, and it was looking for an anti-emetic. Rhône-Poulenc's RP 4560 was anti-emetic, and so SK&F finally accepted chlorpromazine after having rejected Rhône-Poulenc's early overtures.

In 1951, SK&F recruited its first pharmacologist, Leonard Cook, who had just graduated from a new program at Harvard that had been set up to train pharmacologists to discover drugs. This program was a remarkable development because institutions like Harvard at that time were not noted for their openness to applied science. They were committed to establishing scientific truth without regard to its commercial applications. From this perspective no branch of science looked much more compromised than the pharmaceutical industry. Scientists working in pharmaceutical companies were not even permitted to join scientific organizations such as the American Pharmacological Society.[22]

Employed to develop new sedatives, Cook had difficulty measuring sedation in animals that had been given barbiturates. A low dose made the animal active before there was a dramatic transition to complete sedation. One solution was to find a compound to potentiate the barbiturate, so that a low dose of the barbiturate would produce sleep. The information from France suggested that RP 4560 would do this. Cook tried the drug and found that RP 4560 had sedative effects in its own right and that, unlike the barbiturates or other sedatives, it blocked conditioned responses.

SK&F's screening program for anti-emetics involved giving apomorphine to dogs to make them vomit and then administering other agents to see whether any would reverse this effect. When dogs were trained on this test, they began to vomit almost as soon as they saw Ed Weidley, one of Cook's assistants, approaching with a tray of syringes. But, Weidley reported, if the dogs were given chlorpromazine they did not vomit at sight of him. Cook explained that chlorpromazine had an anticonditioning effect; the dogs, he said, had learned to associate Ed with getting sick but this association was now being blocked. Cook was wrong. The team went on to produce nausea and vomiting by many different means, such as putting the dogs into slings and rocking them back and forth until they vomited. There was no association to be blocked but still chlorpromazine prevented the vomiting.

Chlorpromazine was SK&F's new anti-emetic agent, and in 1955 the compound was licensed as SKF 2601. Since nausea and vomiting characterized many conditions, including morning sickness, there was potentially a big market for the drug. Some, however, were skeptical about SKF 2601. Edward Domino at the University of Chicago was asked to work on the compound by the head of his department, Klaus Unna. He found that chlorpromazine did indeed block apomorphine-induced vomiting, but at a cost—test animals became hypotensive and sedated. It didn't seem to Domino or Unna that this drug was worthy of further scientific pursuit.[23]

But despite these drawbacks, it was as an anti-emetic agent that chlorpromazine got its first license in the United States. Was this a clever strategy? Approaching the regulatory authorities with a request to license the drug to treat schizophrenia or psychosis might have led to failure to get the drug licensed as an antipsychotic. There never had been such a drug before, whereas regulators would understand the need for drugs to treat nausea and vomiting and would approve such agents if their safety had been demonstrated. And it had been proven safe: Massive overdoses of chlorpromazine did not kill any animals. No tumors grew.

Chlorpromazine at the Hôpital Sainte-Anne

But I am jumping ahead. In early 1952, news of chlorpromazine reached the Hôpital Sainte-Anne. Founded in 1863, the Sainte-Anne was the largest psychiatric hospital in Paris, and it housed the University of Paris's department of psychiatry within its grounds.

French psychiatry had just been through a troubled period. It was preeminent during the early nineteenth century, but German psychiatry had eclipsed it around the turn of the century. However, the leading French academics accepted neither the Kraepelinian synthesis nor the doctrines of Freud. They held to a more complex classificatory system of the psychoses.[24] And even though they were sympathetic to psychoanalysis because of the French origins of psychodynamic psychiatry, "German" psychoanalytic therapy essentially had to be reinvented by Jacques Lacan before it could prosper in France. In addition, World War II had seen a liquidation of psychiatric patients in areas occupied by the Nazis and the deportation in 1942 of Claude Levy-Valensi, the professor of psychiatry at the University of Paris.[25] Confirmation of his death in 1946 led to the need to appoint a successor.

The professorship was prestigious and there was vigorous lobbying.[26] Possible candidates included Henri Ey, an academic of unquestioned genius whose writings, a brilliant synthesis of organic and psychodynamic insights, were better known throughout the world than those of any other contemporary French psychiatrist.[27] In 1950, he organized and staged in Paris the First World Congress of Psychiatry, the first international psychiatric meeting following the war. This led to the founding of the World Psychiatric Association, of which Ey became the first general secretary.

Another candidate was Henri Baruk. His research involved a significant breakthrough, the experimental production of catatonia in animals. In the early 1930s, Baruk and Henk De Jong found that mescaline could freeze laboratory animals into cataleptic positions.[28] The inspiration for this work had come from a joint project in which Baruk and De Jong had produced experimental catatonia in pigeons by administering bulbocapnine.[29] Baruk drew attention to his discovery by walking around Charenton Hospital with a pigeon perched on his head. It was at just this time that Rolv Gjessing was claiming to have discovered cures for one form of catatonia and that the convulsive therapies were being developed to treat catatonic patients. Catatonia was the one condition in psychiatry where substantial breakthroughs seemed imminent, and Henri Baruk was one of the chief researchers in the field, although the significance of this work was eclipsed by the war.

Although oriented toward the physical therapies, Baruk was extremely hostile to ECT. This stance and the fact that he was Jewish may have cost him the post that his publications and record led him to expect.[30] Ey and Baruk were also disadvantaged because they were psychiatrists based in asylums rather than neurologists based at the Salpêtrière. From the first appointment to the professorship in the nineteenth century on, there had been a tradition of appointing neurologists rather than the foremost alienists of the day. Had Baruk been appointed, the story of chlorpromazine would have been entirely different because before Jean Delay or anyone else claimed this drug might help treat schizophrenia, Baruk and his colleagues had given it to animals and reported that it produced experimental catatonia—it caused rather than cured schizophrenia.[31]

The final candidate was Jean Delay. Born in Bayonne in 1907, he came from an established medical family with prominent Catholic connections.[32] He trained as a neurologist at the Salpêtrière before taking a psychology degree. An assistant in the department when Levy-Valensi was deported, he became the acting head. He was therefore perfectly placed to make a bid for the professorship and was appointed. Delay's background meant that the university department continued to be viewed as almost separate from the rest of French psychiatry. Delay was to continue this tradition, although he did allow Ey and Lacan to establish weekly seminars at Sainte-Anne. Delay's own work leaned more toward using physical agents, including drugs, both for therapeutic purposes and as tools in investigations of psychic functioning. This latter work involved developing psychometric instruments; it was spearheaded by Delay's assistant Pierre Pichot. Among the drugs Delay and Pichot investigated between 1950 and 1952 were the dinitriles, sodium succinate, and isoniazid.

The First World Congress of Psychiatry in Paris in 1950 celebrated the "new" shock therapies. Because of the war, Meduna's chemically induced convulsions and Bini and Ugo Cerletti's electroconvulsive therapy had not been properly presented in an international forum until this meeting. Information on insulin coma therapy and carbon dioxide inhalation therapy was also presented to the hundreds of delegates in attendance. Delay delivered the keynote address, clearly laying out the medical approach to the major psychoses, and his delivery was said to have been impressive.[33] The speech firmly established his name in the minds of his European contemporaries.

Within Delay's department at the University, there was a rigid hierarchical structure of a kind that is difficult to imagine now. Delay was at the apex of the pyramid, with his assistants Pierre Pichot and Pierre Deniker under him. Under them was a range of senior training positions, taken at various times by Jean Thuillier, Thérèse Lempérière, Bernard Sadoun, and later Pierre Simon. Below them were junior training slots taken by people whose names are on some of the most famous papers in psychopharmacology but who made no further contributions. The name of Jean-Marie Harl, an intern working with Delay and Deniker, appears on the first and most famous paper on chlorpromazine.[34] In 1952 Jean-François Buisson did research that demonstrated the effects of isoniazid in depression—a study that along with Max Lurie's of the same year with the same drug marks the discovery of the antidepressants.[35] Even lower in the ranks were the nursing attendants, whose contributions counted for nothing with Delay, even though in the departments in which the new psychotropic drugs were discovered their observations were often critical.

In those days people at the top of the hierarchy knew little if anything about those lower in the hierarchy.[36] Some years later, Pierre Simon was sent by the professor of pharmacology, Robert Boissier, to visit Delay. Delay sat him down and summoned Pichot and Deniker, who were considerably older and more senior than Simon, to stand on either side of his desk while Delay discussed matters with Simon for almost an hour. Pichot and Deniker's opinions were not solicited. But subordinates did not resent this treatment. Neither Pichot nor Deniker ever described Delay in other than warm terms, even though outsiders from less hierarchical set-ups perceived the atmosphere as stifling.[37]

In such circumstances, everything that happened within the department was seen as flowing from the head of department. Even if he was not actively making key observations, he made possible the conditions in which observations were made. Delay therefore had his name on all papers, usually in the first position, even when he knew little about the subject matter.[38] Clearly nothing could come out of his department that Delay did not allow out. If only for this reason, Delay is central to the chlorpromazine story.

At the time Sainte-Anne was a hospital of 4,000 patients with 1,000 nursing attendants, domestic staff, and medical staff.

Within the hospital the university department ran a male and female admission ward, as well as male and female long-stay wards, containing altogether about 200 psychotic patients.[39] The male wards were under the supervision of Pierre Deniker. He was an assistant professor in the department, having begun in 1939, when there were virtually no therapies. Neither insulin coma nor ECT came to France until after the war.[40]

Deniker had a brother-in-law who was an anesthetist and it was from him that he heard of chlorpromazine. Deniker then asked Rhône-Poulenc for a supply of the drug, and obtained it. The initial plan was to induce Laborit's artificial hibernation in Sainte-Anne. To this end the pharmacy supplied both the drug and icepacks, and on Deniker's locked ward patients were given chlorpromazine and then cooled down. The treatment appeared to calm the agitation of patients with delirium, mania, and psychosis even when chlorpromazine was administered without barbiturates or other agents. Deniker and Delay's claims for priority in the discovery of chlorpromazine rest heavily on their assertion that they were the people who gave chlorpromazine alone, rather than in a cocktail, and that therefore they were the ones to demonstrate its singular psychotropic effects.

While Deniker was managing the male locked ward, Jean Thuillier was helping on the male open ward. Deniker asked Thuillier to cover for him while he was on leave. Thuillier agreed and was surprised to find that the new treatment was being given without ice.[41] He berated the nurses, who said that the pharmacy could not supply ice fast enough and that the results with chlorpromazine were the same whether the patient got ice or not. On his return, Deniker investigated more closely and agreed—the artificial hibernation component of the treatment was not needed. So Deniker not only gave chlorpromazine alone but began to give it empirically—without theorizing about what it might be doing or why.

The effects of the new treatment were extraordinary. The first published reports were on the responsiveness of agitated, overactive, and manic states to chlorpromazine.[42] Standard psychiatric practice had been to avoid taking any clinical responsibility for such patients if possible. Many of Deniker's colleagues did not find out about the new discovery until his junior staff began to appear in the admission halls of the hospital, volunteering to take just these patients back to their ward.[43] Shortly thereafter the drop in noise levels was apparent even to members of the public living or working near the asylum.[44]

The conditions that responded best to chlorpromazine involved confusion and delirium. Later, other antipsychotics, especially haloperidol, were found to be effective in treating delirium. The discovery of this cure, however, is rarely celebrated, because the response of delirium to treatment took it away from psychiatry and into medicine and the trajectory of chlorpromazine took it away from traditional insanity into what had become the heartlands of twentieth-century psychiatry, the psychoses.

Not everything went well on Deniker's ward, however. Not surprisingly given its origins in anesthesia, chlorpromazine was initially given by intramuscular injection. These injections in doses of up to 50 milligrams often produced marked lowering of blood pressure, and it was regular practice for patients to be kept lying down to avoid problems with hypotension. Chlorpromazine was also sedative. Because of the combination of sedative and hypotensive effects and as part of a legacy of hibernation therapy, patients were often confined to bed during the first few days of treatment. The injections also caused phlebitis, and this combined with the effects of lying down led to thromboses.[45]

Severe dermatological reactions also occurred regularly, and affected both patients and staff. Staff members may have gotten such reactions from opening chlorpromazine capsules or vials to make up injections or to give the patients doses in their food. But there is no simple explanation that accounts for the frequency of the reactions or the fact that they occurred on both sides of the Iron Curtain in the mid-1950s and have not occurred since.[46] Whatever the cause of the allergic reactions, nurses became wary of handling chlorpromazine, a fact that almost certainly contributed to views that this was a very potent drug.

It quickly became clear that chlorpromazine was not sedating patients in the usual way. Sedatives usually put patients into a sleep from which they could be roused only with difficulty, and when they did wake up they would be groggy or drowsy. But patients on chlorpromazine although apparently asleep, responded rapidly to any approach, knew immediately where they were, and were able to react quickly. It was as though they had retreated from the outside world but could reengage if needed.

A number of patients appeared to wake up. Thuillier details the case of Phillippe Burg, a man who had been sunk in an inaccessible psychotic state for several years before the advent of chlorpromazine. No treatment had helped him. Everything had been tried but nothing worked. Over several weeks of treatment, he began to emerge from his torpor and communicate. Thereafter he progressed so rapidly that the staff allowed him to go out with his mother. They went to dinner at a famous haunt of Ernest Hemingway's, Closerie des Lilas.[47]

A typical example of how chlorpromazine helped psychosis is the case of a barber from Lyon who had been hospitalized for several years with a chronic psychosis and was unresponsive to his environment. When given chlorpromazine, he awoke from this stuporous state and told his doctor, Jean Perrin, that he now knew where he was and who he was, and that he wanted to go home and back to work. Perrin responded by challenging him to give him a shave. The open razor, water, and towels were produced and the patient set about doing his job perfectly. Either Perrin had considerable nerve or the transformations were truly extraordinary.[48]

In Bassens Hospital, Pierre Lambert was faced with a patient who had been psychotic for years, frozen in a series of postures. No one knew anything about him. He responded as dramatically as Perrin's barber to chlorpromazine, in one day. He greeted Lambert and the nursing staff on the ward round, asking them for some billiard balls, which he proceeded to juggle. He had been a juggler before ending up in the hospital. Another psychiatrist at Bassens filled a ward with chronically psychotic patients, pulled the curtains—it was still thought that chlorpromazine essentially delivered an improved form of sleep treatment—gave all patients chlorpromazine continually for months, and waited. A large proportion of these patients "woke up" as the weeks went on.[49]

A number of patients coming out of psychotic states in which they had been sunk for years were clearly surprised that prices were higher than they remembered them. It was as though time had stood still from the onset of their illness. Patients reported that the voices that they'd been hearing for years had gone. They were well and would like to go home. This result was as magical as the results achieved when penicillin was first used to treat patients with suppurating infections.

Delay and Deniker fired off articles to *Presse Médicale* and the *Annales Medico-Psychologiques*, getting their first paper published immediately before that of Hamon, Paraire, and Velluz, even though they had started their work later and had first communicated their findings only three months after beginning their work. This was academic gamesmanship of the highest order. They communicated the results in a variety of meetings. Coming from the department of psychiatry of the University of Paris, these reports, both verbal and written, carried considerable weight. Nevertheless, they received a skeptical response. Many thought treatment of psychosis was in principle impossible. This drug, they said, must simply be another sedative, albeit a somewhat more effective one. Henri Ey endorsed chlorpromazine as useful in the delivery of sleep therapies but would not go further. Even within the Sainte-Anne, the new treatment was not immediately adopted by everybody.[50] The younger generation tried it while the older alienists waited.

Nor was this use of chlorpromazine initially encouraged by Rhône-Poulenc; a psychiatric use for the drug was not what the company wanted since it was not clear that much money could be made from its use in psychiatry. There was no research basis for clinical trial work, and no experience of marketing to psychiatrists. Was it safe to dabble in this field, which other physicians did not view as real medicine? The efficient machinery that is in place today to ensure that clinicians hear rapidly about new developments—and the sweeteners that persuade them to try out the new drug on a few patients—did not exist within psychiatry at the time. Everything depended on the presentations of Deniker and Delay and their stature in the field, and on the lack of reports from other authorities that Deniker and Delay had got things wrong. No one could offer an explanation for what was happening, other than the extraordinary one that a treatment for psychosis had in fact been discovered.

The Spread of Chlorpromazine to Lyon and Basel

Clearly, the spread of chlorpromazine depended on the willingness of practitioners to try the new treatment. Some psychiatrists will always try new and unproven treatments, but they are usually mavericks whose opinions do not carry weight. Getting the mainstream to adopt a new treatment is another matter. In Paris, in clinics where the staff were younger, chlorpromazine met with enthusiasm, and every patient in the hospital might get it in a very short time regardless of diagnosis because nobody knew exactly what it did or which conditions it could help.

Outside Paris, psychiatrists in Lyon and Chambéry were the most influential in spreading the use of chlorpromazine. At Vinatier Hospital, in Lyon, Louis Revol, the professor of pharmacology, was an early advocate of chlorpromazine's use. This led Rhône-Poulenc in 1953 to send Paul Brouillot, its representative in Rhône-Alpes, to Vinatier to visit the hospital. At Vinatier Brouillot found an extraordinary atmosphere of enthusiasm and expectation and many successful cures, not the brutalities and awful sights and smells of the mental hospitals he remembered visiting in 1948. His interaction with the Vinatier psychiatrists led to the founding of a clinical research group, the Comité Lyonnais

Recherches et Thérapeutiques en Psychiatrie (CLRTP). The key members of the group were Pierre Lambert, the discoverer of the mood-stabilizing effects of Valpromide, Jean Guyotat, the first to describe an anti-obsessive effect of imipramine, Paul Broussolle, who, as we shall see, discovered a new group of antipsychotics, André Achaintre, Paul Balvet, and André Requet.

The members of this group were asylum psychiatrists, many of whom owed a primary allegiance to psychotherapy, and some of whom had antipsychiatric sympathies, who nevertheless collaborated to describe in detail the effects of chlorpromazine in over 600 patients. Their case histories provide the clearest descriptions of the impact of the new drug. They reported their findings at all the major psychiatry meetings from 1955 to 1960, meetings where the enthusiasm was sufficient to overcome even the antipathy between the French and the Germans. This was a discovery to rank with the discovery of penicillin, something that knew no frontiers.[51]

The Lyon group provided the first data on relapse. These psychiatrists were quick to let recovered patients go home. Many of these relapsed within days, and it became clear that ongoing treatment was needed. But ongoing medication required the cooperation of the patient's family doctor and local pharmacist. And some of them regarded these patients as dangerous lunatics, whom they had never expected to see again. Moreover, these patients were asking for supplies of a drug they knew nothing about. This state of affairs led to angry complaints from country doctors, who along with everyone else looked down on the asylum doctors.

There were also complaints from communities. Once word spread that patients were coming home from the asylums, petitions were drawn up protesting the discharge of these patients. Mayors and curates visited Vinatier and Bassens hospitals to plead with staff not to release patients. Warnings were issued that the patient's relatives and neighbors knew more about a patient's true nature than the doctors did.

The CLRTP group responded by sectorizing their services, so that teams of psychiatrists, nurses, and other therapists had responsibilities for managing the patients from specific areas. This approach very quickly led to a complete reorientation from mental illness to mental health—teams should look toward the mental health of a sector community rather than just after the needs of patients already diagnosed. The Lyon group and others found that rehabilitation methods and milieu therapy that had been in use before the advent of chlorpromazine helped resocialize institutionalized patients, as we will see in Chapter 4.

There was another key group in Basel. Almost immediately after Delay and Deniker's first reports on chlorpromazine, the professor of psychiatry in Basel, John Eugen Staehelin, sent Felix Labhardt to the Sainte-Anne to learn at first hand about the new treatment. When he returned to Basel, Labhardt introduced chlorpromazine therapy there. On 28 November 1953 Staehelin, Labhardt, and Paul Kielholz convened a conference at Friedmatt Hospital to which all Swiss psychiatrists were invited. There they outlined the benefits of chlorpromazine and explained how to do therapy with the new drug.[52]

In Basel, patients also woke up after being given chlorpromazine.[53] Two thirds of the psychotic patients either had a complete remission or a definite improvement. This success led Labhardt, Hans Steck, and others to increase the doses; they found that doses of 500 milligrams, doses considerably higher than those being used in Paris or Lyon, made a number of otherwise unresponsive chronic patients begin to respond. The average length of hospital stays halved.[54] The enthusiasm that infected Paris, and even more strikingly Lyon, gripped Basel too: doors were unlocked, staff morale increased, and the hospital was transformed.

But in many cases, the patients who responded faced problems. Some who had been hospitalized for years had no home to go to. Women were particularly affected because according to the

Swiss civil code chronic illness and hospitalization were grounds for divorce. The Basel group took the lead in establishing daytime and night-time facilities for patients. Some patients went to work from the hospital and returned at night. Others attended group and other activities in the hospital during the day but went home at night.[55] Nevertheless, in Basel as elsewhere, there were relapses. Nearly half of the responders relapsed, mostly after discontinuing treatment after discharge, but in a third of the cases patients relapsed despite ongoing treatment. Later Raymond Battegay and others established group therapies to minimize relapses, as we will see in Chapter 4.

The Spread of Chlorpromazine in the United States

As we have seen, chlorpromazine was slow to come to American psychiatry. Despite the work of Deniker and Delay, SK&F had only a limited interest in hospital psychiatry, where another drug, reserpine, was already making inroads. In the United States, office practice was where the money was to be made. Would the new drug, marketed as Thorazine, compete with the amphetamines or barbiturates or SK&F's own Dexamyl? In fact, had SK&F waited a few more months it might have given up on chlorpromazine because of the advent of another drug that swept the market in office psychiatry in 1956: Miltown.

But in 1953, SK&F asked several U.S. psychiatrists to test the new drug, and some agreed to do so. William Winkelman in Philadelphia used it in office practice to treat nervous conditions, concluding that Thorazine was helpful but not free of side effects.[56] Frank Ayd also used it in office practice and found that the new drug caused dystonias, jaundice, and a range of other problems. Vernon Kinross-Wright in Houston undertook a study and reported significant benefits, but he was treating hospitalized patients.[57]

A twist of fate shaped developments. Chlorpromazine was sold by Rhône-Poulenc in Canada. In 1953, one of its salesmen brought Delay and Deniker's articles to psychiatrists in Montreal. One day Heinz Lehmann, a German-Canadian who worked at the Verdun Hospital, read about chlorpromazine while taking a bath. The next day, he ordered supplies of the drug. He recruited a resident to help and gave chlorpromazine to seventy patients. He also gave it to some nurses to study how it worked. Many of the nurses suffered a severe drop in blood pressure but the patients began to respond. Astonished, Lehmann saw the awakening that psychiatrists in Paris, Lyon, and Basel had witnessed. As he later put it, if these patients or their relatives had been told that the price of these recoveries would be death in two years, they would have taken the two years of restored life.[58] These were unexpected transformations in patients who had previously had no prospect of recovery.

Lehmann raced to publish his results, worried that he might be scooped by someone in the United States.[59] His efforts led to his sharing the 1957 Lasker Prize with Laborit, Deniker, and Kline. He became a powerful advocate for chlorpromazine, and along with Fritz Freyhan and Herman Denber, he was a conduit for the exchange of North American and European experiences.

In the meantime, SK&F contacted Henry Brill at Pilgrim State Hospital in New York. As the commissioner for mental health in New York state, Brill was a key figure, and he all but instructed several of his colleagues to try out the new drug. Later he convened a meeting of New York State psychiatrists similar in importance to the one held by Staehelin in Basel. A range of asylum and office practitioners, such as Max Fink from Hillside Hospital, who came to hear about the new drug heard many reports of its benefits.[60] The SK&F representatives at the meeting were besieged with requests for samples.

State mental hospital doctors were so eager to use the drug that when chlorpromazine was finally launched as Thorazine, in 1955, even though the license application had been for an anti-emetic, the take-up in psychiatry was astonishing—SK&F reportedly took in $75 million the first year the drug was sold. To understand this figure, it needs to be appreciated that some of the American state asylums, such as Pilgrim State in New York, had up to 15,000 residents. Everyone got the new drug. Al Kurland, an early psychopharmacologist, was so impressed with the effects that he mortgaged his house to buy shares in SK&F.[61]

Like their counterparts in Europe, psychiatrists quickly realized that a new kind of psychiatry was needed, one with outpatient clinics to monitor the functioning of patients newly released from asylums. American psychiatrists quickly increased the dose of chlorpromazine much more than the Europeans had done, with Vernon Kinross-Wright, for instance, giving 2 grams of chlorpromazine per day and reporting if not benefits for every patient, then at least a lack of toxicity.

No consistently serious problems ensued from the drug's use, but there were a number of unwelcome side effects. An early problem that cropped up in the United States was jaundice, which had not appeared in European patients. Frank Ayd, for instance, found that two of his first three patients developed jaundice.[62] One woman's jaundice had persisted for some time before it came to his attention, but since she did not seem to be suffering unduly, he persisted with treatment, and in her case as in others, the jaundice disappeared.[63] Ayd later discovered the antipruritic properties of the phenothiazines by accident. His children were sick with chicken pox and he gave them another anti-emetic from SK&F, prochlorperazine (Compazine), and noted that their itching stopped.

In the United States, SK&F was faced with a challenge that did not develop elsewhere. The 1955 meeting of the American Psychiatric Association (APA) should have been dominated by Thorazine. But while Thorazine was on stage, the whispers in the wings were of an even newer drug, Miltown (meprobamate), which was launched in the second half of 1955. This was a drug for office practice. Only 20 percent of the membership of the APA were hospital psychiatrists at the time. No other Western country had this distribution of psychiatric power. By any reckoning, therefore, while Miltown might never have made a splash elsewhere, Thorazine's time at center stage in American psychiatry should have been short. The fact that it survived the inroads of Miltown and remained at the center of the scientific stage is compelling testimony to the recognition that chlorpromazine truly was a different drug.

Miltown's popularity did have one long-lasting influence on Thorazine. It made it into a major "tranquilizer." The term tranquilizer had first been used in 1953 by F. F. Yonkman, an employee of the Ciba pharmaceutical company, to describe another drug, reserpine. But the term had still not achieved currency, when Miltown's creator, Frank Berger, used it to keep people from thinking of his new drug as a sedative, like the barbiturates. The idea of sedation was not compatible with a treatment that would allow people to get on with their lives, so Miltown became a tranquilizer. And since Thorazine's profile overlapped that of reserpine, it too became known as a tranquilizer. But Thorazine and Miltown differed so much in their profiles of action that a distinction was very quickly established between the major tranquilizers, such as chlorpromazine and reserpine, and the minor tranquilizers, such as Miltown and later Librium and Valium.[64] Most American practitioners did not consider Thorazine an antipsychotic until many years later.[65] Meanwhile in Europe, chlorpromazine was on its way to becoming regarded as a neuroleptic. Not until the 1990s did practitioners worldwide come to regard both the major tranquilizers and the neuroleptics as antipsychotics.

The distinctive American contribution to the story of chlorpromazine was the effort to evaluate the new technologies. Confronted with the dominance of psychoanalysts within American psychiatry, the proponents of the new pharmacotherapies felt the need to justify use of drugs to a greater extent than did psychiatrists elsewhere. Accordingly, the Psychopharmacology Research Center was established within the National Institute of Mental Health (NIMH). Ralph Gerard and Jonathan Cole, the director of the new center, convened a meeting in September 1956 to look into means of evaluating the new agents.[66] Shortly thereafter, a series of studies was conducted that demonstrated beyond reasonable doubt that the new drugs had measurable effects.[67] This discovery of evaluative technologies, as will become clear, has done at least as much as the discovery of the new drugs to shape the modern era in psychiatry.

In other countries, the story was similar. In Germany, a younger generation, alerted to developments in France and eager to try the new drug, faced an older generation unwilling to do so. In Berlin, a trainee, Joachim Hiob, suggested giving it to a chronic patient, a woman with a paranoid hallucinatory disorder. The professor who was the chairman of his department argued against it, but Hiob secretly gave it to her. Two weeks later she had clearly improved. The professor pointed out to his residents, including Hiob and Hanns Hippius, that partial remissions of this sort could be seen in all sorts of patients. If they had tried chlorpromazine, he said, they would now mistakenly be attributing the change to it—and then Hiob confessed to what he had done. Around the country, juniors in the system—Bente in Erlangen, Schmidt in Heidelberg, Heindrich in Mainz, and Ingemeier in Munster—tried chlorpromazine and found that it worked.[68] The new drug was launched as Megaphen and it made these juniors the senior figures of a new psychiatry.

This scenario was repeated around the world, with one minor exception. The drug was made available directly by Rhône-Poulenc or under license from it in all countries except Japan. In Japan, Yoshitomi Pharmaceuticals had already, in the 1940s, developed the first chemotherapy for cancer—nitrogen mustard. But since it caused severe vomiting, the company looked for a suitable anti-emetic, and hearing about chlorpromazine, Yoshitomi synthesized its own. Rhône-Poulenc took the Japanese company to court, but Yoshitomi's chemists had made chlorpromazine by a method not covered by any of Rhône-Poulenc's use or process patents.[69] So in Japan, the drug was homegrown.

But the clinical experience was universal. Trainees like Michio Toru saw dramatic responses in patients with schizophrenia in university clinics or wards. These dramatic responses did not always prepare the trainees for life in the asylums. When Toru later moved to an asylum, he was so shocked at the failure of some patients to respond that he took the pharmacist to task for obviously providing something other than real chlorpromazine.[70]

In Britain, one of the first people to try the new drug was Joel Elkes, a professor of experimental psychiatry in Birmingham. Even before chlorpromazine, Birmingham was emerging as a center of excellence in the new neuroscientific era. Elkes and his wife, Charmian, organized a placebo-controlled cross-over trial to test the new drug, and concluded that in doses of 150–300 milligrams it did indeed produce significant benefits in chronically psychotic patients.[71] Meanwhile, Linford Rees in Cardiff randomized a hundred anxious patients to chlorpromazine or a placebo and found that chlorpromazine helped them, but at too high a cost in demotivation, Rees felt, for the drug to be useful in treating anyone with an executive job.[72]

In Britain, the high cost of chlorpromazine delayed its introduction to the National Health Service. Not only was it expensive but by 1954 it was competing with another antipsychotic, reserpine, that was cheaper. Not until 1957 or 1958 did many British hospitals use chlorpromazine more than reserpine.[73]

THE DISCOVERY OF RESERPINE

It is now almost completely overlooked that the discovery of the antipsychotic properties of chlorpromazine was paralleled by the discovery of another antipsychotic, reserpine. Indeed, in one sense the discovery of the antipsychotic properties of reserpine antedated the discovery of such properties in chlorpromazine.

Reserpine had been used in India since ancient times, when it was called sarpagandha.[74] Sarpagandha was a compound medicine whose most essential ingredients came from the plant *Rauwolfia serpentina benth*. This plant acquired its Western name in the sixteenth century, when Leonard Rauwolf included it in his classification of plants. The Portuguese explorers who established a base on the west coast of India at Goa referred to it as the "premium et laudatissimum remedium."[75] Thereafter it was included in many herbals for centuries.

Sarpagandha was traditionally used in India to treat a variety of ailments, including fever, vomiting, snake bite, insomnia, and insanity. It was also used to treat malaise consequent on illness. Its sedative effect led to its use in low doses to put children to sleep. In higher doses, it was used to sedate insane patients. It is impossible to know whether there was an Indian recognition of any distinctive, nonsedative, antipsychotic effect.

Then in 1931 G. Sen and K. C. Bose described the effects of *Rauwolfia* on blood pressure.[76] At the time hypertension and its complications had only recently been described in the West, and effective treatments were still lacking for this asymptomatic condition that can be diagnosed only with a stethoscope and the other accouterments of Western medicine. Sen and Bose were also using *Rauwolfia* by itself rather than as part of a mixture. That *Rauwolfia* might be useful in treating both hypertension and insanity did not pose a problem because distinctions between hypertension and nervous conditions were then far from clear cut. As late as the mid-1950s in the West, it was common for general physicians to accept that a possible origin of hypertension was anger or rage turned inward. A sedative drug could, therefore, conceivably be useful in treating hypertension. Other Indian researchers also reported the beneficial effects of *Rauwolfia* in treating hypertension.[77]

By the 1940s, Indian workers had begun to isolate alkaloids from the plant in an effort to find its active ingredients. This hunt attracted the interest of the major Western pharmaceutical companies, especially Ciba. The problem was that the plant contained numerous active substances, some of which antagonized the effect of others. Depending on the type of extraction methods used, a series of compounds could be isolated that had a profile of action entirely different from that of another series extracted under different conditions. The plant contained both substances that increased blood pressure and substances that lowered blood pressure, as well as both sedative and stimulant substances. Furthermore, plants from different parts of India differed in their alkaloid constituents, with samples from Bihar rich in one set of salts and samples from Dehradun rich in another set.

The need to isolate the antihypertensive properties of *Rauwolfia* was made more acute when Rustom Vakil published the results of his use of the plant in treating hypertensive patients in the *British Heart Journal* in 1949.[78] Hypertension was becoming a focus for medical intervention, and this study's results were sufficiently impressive to lead to trials of *Rauwolfia* in the United States. A study by Robert Wilkins presented at the New England Cardiovascular Society in 1952 demonstrated that this Indian cure also worked in Western patients.[79] The pharmaceutical companies increased their efforts to isolate the antihypertensive substance, because none of them could make money from the whole plant. Finally in mid-1952, Hugo Bein and his group at Ciba published the structure of reserpine, which they claimed was the most important active principle behind the actions of *Rauwolfia*.[80]

In treating hypertensives Wilkins noticed immediately that changes in mental state frequently accompanied the use of *Rauwolfia*. "Many patients become positively lyrical about their sense of well-being on the drug . . . with statements such as 'I've never felt as well', or 'I haven't felt this good for years' . . . 'Nothing bothers me any more.'"[81] These statements are reminiscent of those made about Prozac in the 1990s. A symposium was held in 1953, at the U.S. headquarters of Ciba in Summit, New Jersey, at which researchers grappled with the problem of the mixture of sedation and well-being produced by reserpine. It was in the course of this meeting that Yonkman used the term tranquilizer for the first time to capture this characteristic and distinguish it from sedation proper.[82]

The psychiatric actions of *Rauwolfia* came back to the forefront in March 1953, when the *New York Times* reported that a Dr. Hakim of Ahmedabad in India had received a gold medal for demonstrating the beneficial effects of Siledin in treating patients with schizophrenia.[83] Siledin contained *Rauwolfia* along with other plant materials. Unlike previous reports, which had praised *Rauwolfia*'s benefits in treating insanity, Hakim's findings reported response rates of 80 percent to the combination of drug treatment and ECT in 146 patients with manic depression or schizophrenia.

The stage was set to see whether Western psychiatric patients resembled Western hypertensive patients in responding to this Eastern medicine. In 1953 Ciba approached Nathan Kline, the director of a research institute at Rockland State Hospital, to undertake a study. Kline, who was soon to become one of the dominant figures of world psychopharmacology, had become a psychiatrist after earning a degree in psychology and philosophy. He had taken the job of research director at Rockland State Hospital shortly after qualifying as a psychiatrist. This was not a post linked to a university. The establishment of a research facility in Rockland was an attempt by New York state to boost morale at a problem hospital. Rockland was the hospital that featured in the famous movie *The Snake Pit*, which did much to fuel demands for change and improvement within American mental hospitals. The hospital was one that no one was keen to work in. Kline was young, dynamic, and well connected. He knew among others Mary Lasker, the main mover behind the Mary and Albert Lasker Foundation, a charitable foundation that supported medical research and awarded a coveted annual prize, the Lasker Prize.

Kline began by giving *Rauwolfia* to patients in Rockland, switching to reserpine when it became available. Altogether he gave one or the other to over 700 patients, while he worked out the appropriate dosage and which conditions the drug benefited. He was later to quip that he recognized that it was having some effect only when the hospital glazier remarked that he recently had had many fewer windows to replace on one of the wards. Kline realized that this was the ward on which reserpine was being used.[84] In 1954, he published his findings in the *Annals of the New York Academy of Sciences*, only weeks before Delay, Deniker, and Lempérière published similar findings.[85]

In 1953 Leo Hollister, a medical internist in California, was also given reserpine by the Ciba representative in his area. Although not a psychiatrist, he persuaded his psychiatric colleagues to send him patients from their wards. He assigned these patients to reserpine or a placebo without telling the referring physicians which patients got which. Within weeks it became clear that reserpine was working. Hollister's results were published in 1955.[86] His talk at the New York Academy of Sciences in 1954 and subsequent radio interviews attracted enormous public and media interest and did a great deal to create the impression that psychopharmacology was being born.

In many places, reserpine was available for some time before chlorpromazine in a variety of *Rauwolfia* preparations. As evidence for its usefulness in hypertension began to mount, psychiatrists could get it without waiting for the promotional push of a pharmaceutical company. By the end of the 1950s, there were twenty-six preparations containing reserpine on the market. Chlorpromazine, although available from 1954 on, was much more expensive, and its use accordingly spread more gradually. However, more hyperbole built up around chlorpromazine, since the companies licensing it could afford a dedicated sales force. In contrast, many of the companies selling reserpine did so without a large sales force, since with so many competitors vying for customers, sales were likely to go to a competitor.

In the case of reserpine, the key from a company point of view lay in working with the structure to come up with a new compound that could be patented, but this was difficult to do. The phenothiazine nucleus was almost infinitely manipulable, with a high proportion of the manipulations yielding psychotropic compounds. Closely related nuclei, for example, produced imipramine and amitriptyline, the first of the tricyclic antidepressants. The reserpine molecule was more complex and it was not clear which part of the molecule was responsible for the beneficial effects observed in patients. Eventually Hoffman La-Roche cracked the problem and produced tetrabenazine, a molecule with some usefulness to this day. But by then reserpine had run into other problems, as we shall see, and the phenothiazines had achieved a commanding position in the field that was challenged only in the late 1960s by haloperidol.

Throughout the 1950s, reserpine was far more frequently mentioned in the scientific literature than chlorpromazine.[87] One of the reasons for this was its use as an experimental tool. In 1955 Robert Bowman, working in Steve Brodie's laboratory in the National Institutes of Health (NIH), had invented the spectrophotofluorimeter. This device was the first to permit the detection of variations in the levels of chemicals known to exist in the brain in minute amounts, namely serotonin and norepinephrine (see Chapter 5). Aware of work linking LSD to the serotonin system, Brodie set about establishing whether the sedation in laboratory rabbits following the administration of reserpine correlated with the levels of serotonin in their brain. It did. The two-page paper published in 1955 in which Brodie and his colleagues outlined their findings is widely acknowledged as one of the landmark papers of neuroscience.[88]

For the first time a bridge had been built between behavior and neurochemistry. Investigators flocked to Brodie's laboratory to learn the new techniques.[89] His findings were widely replicated in other laboratories, and soon there arose a celebrated scientific struggle as Arvid Carlsson, one of Brodie's protégés, had the temerity to demonstrate that serotonin was irrelevant to what was happening—dopamine was the important neurotransmitter.[90] This dispute drew in a large number of researchers. Reserpine was at the center of these efforts to establish basic facts in neurochemistry. In contrast, chlorpromazine was still a total mystery.

No one knew how it acted at the biochemical level; only clinical results were available. In the records of the first International Neuropsychopharmacology meetings, in Rome in 1958, Basel in 1960, and Munich in 1962, reserpine is cited as often as chlorpromazine. Only later, when chlorpromazine began to yield its neurochemical secrets and reserpine began to disappear from clinical use, did the predominance of chlorpromazine become apparent in the scientific literature.

THE INSTITUTIONAL FRAMEWORK

With chlorpromazine and reserpine a new science was born. In 1950, news of the psychotomimetic effects of LSD had begun to leak from the Sandoz Pharmaceutical Company to selected investigators. In addition to treating mental illness, chlorpromazine cured the psychoses induced by LSD. The possibility abruptly opened up that psychiatry could become scientific. Models could be created of madness whose parameters could be manipulated as one would manipulate the parameters of models in any other area of science.

In the United States, Joseph Brady stumbled on an animal model of nervous disorders that showed how reserpine might work. His work, along with the work of Len Cook in SK&F and the reversal of the effects of LSD, made pharmaceutical companies think they could devise tests to screen the compounds on their shelves for candidate psychotropic drugs. They began to hire psychologists in Europe and behavioral psychologists in America to help with this work.[91]

The discovery by Giuseppi Morruzzi and Horace Magoun in 1949 of a reticular activating system in the brain was still hot news when Philip Bradley and his colleagues in Birmingham demonstrated that chlorpromazine had effects on this system that were distinctively different from those of the barbiturates.[92] This work led Bradley and Joel Elkes to develop the first clearly worked out speculations on the role of chemical neurotransmitters in mediating the effects of the new drugs.[93] All the elements—clinical, behavioral, and scientific—were in place for new interdisciplinary forums to develop.

One of the first meetings held around this time was a strictly clinical one. In 1955, Delay and Deniker convened a conference in Paris on chlorpromazine. Delegates came from North America, Europe, and elsewhere. Lehmann, Freyhan, and others attended, along with Willi Mayer-Gross from England, Lambert and his colleagues from Lyon, Labhardt and his colleagues from Basel, and Germans such as Hiob and Hippius. This was the first international meeting in psychiatry that the Germans had been able to attend after the war. Enthusiasm was boundless. The attendees heard glowing testimonies to the benefits of chlorpromazine, along with clear assessments of some of the problems associated with its use: relapses, extrapyramidal side effects, and others.

In 1956 in the United States, Ralph Gerard and Jonathan Cole convened a major conference on the Evaluation of psychotropic drugs. They invited experts in behavioral pharmacology, like Joseph Brady and Fred Skinner, experts in rating scales and clinical trial methods, like Louis Lasagna and Richard Wittenborn, electrophysiologists such as Edward Domino and Keith Killam, senior clinicians in the field. The meeting resulted in the publication of an astonishingly sophisticated 600-page volume.[94] The Americans opted for evaluation on a large scale through the institution of multicentered studies linking networks of hospitals, a decision that was to radically affect both world psychiatry and peri-millennial culture (see Chapter 7).

In 1957, Silvio Garattini organized a meeting in Milan that led to the formation of an international society, the Collegium Internationale Neuro-psychopharmacologium (CINP), whose first meeting was held in Rome the following year. Across Europe, the Czechs and the Scandinavians established national psychopharmacology groups in 1959,[95] with the Germans following suit in 1960.[96] In France, Delay's rival Henri Baruk set up the Société de Moreau de Tours, to meetings of which Delay was never invited.

Delay and Deniker had difficulty speaking on this new international stage. Delay never learned English; Deniker spoke in broken English from prepared texts and for some years was unable to answer questions. Herman Denber from New York initially acted as a go-between, shuttling backward and forward from the United States to Europe. The gap, however, was too great to bridge, and in 1961 the Americans established their own organization, the American College of Neuropsychopharmacology (ACNP).[97]

It went on in the next decade to become the leading organization in the field. These meetings provided forums in which scientists and clinicians from around the world could meet colleagues whose papers they had read or whom they knew by reputation. There was a cross-disciplinary fertilization, but the functions of many of these meetings were as much social and political as anything else. At other meetings, many of the participants from different disciplines had met with disdain from their colleagues. For example, pharmacologists were told that if they wished to present real science they should attend pharmacological meetings. The common perception was that the level of scientific debate would fall if pharmacologists attempted to present their findings to clinicians. ACNP was the one forum that rose above these jibes—but it took a decade before the scientific credentials of this or any of the other new forums were accepted.

THE IDEA OF A NEUROLEPTIC

Frank Ayd was one of several American clinicians asked by William Long of SK&F to test chlorpromazine before it was launched. He did so and found that when the dose was sufficiently high it produced a dystonic reaction.[98] In 1955 he shot a film of the first patient to become "twisted like a pretzel" and showed it to authorities at SK&F. Puzzled, the company sought the advice of a neurologist, who dismissed the reaction as hysterical. Ayd showed the film at a neurological meeting in New Jersey later that year; some attendees saw the reaction as hysterical and some did not. In the course of 1955, a variety of reactions appeared in patients being treated with chlorpromazine: dyskinesias, a strange restlessness now known as akathisia, lip-smacking movements, and Parkinsonian syndromes.

Clinicians from Europe and the United States observed similar reactions. They are now called the extrapyramidal side effects (EPS) of the antipsychotics. The motor division of the nervous system is divided into a pyramidal system, which takes the lead in willed or voluntary movements, and an extrapyramidal system, which provides the background tone that makes voluntary movements possible. The extrapyramidal effects of the antipsychotics soon captured the attention of neurologists and gave substance to the idea of neuropsychiatry.

These alarming reactions did not, however, sidetrack the chlorpromazine bandwagon. As regards the treatment of dystonias and Parkinsonism, it quickly became clear that anticholinergic drugs helped. In Paris, the staff in hospitals such as the Salpêtriêre, which had both neurological and psychiatric wings, was used to administering anticholinergic agents to treat Parkinson's disease. James Parkinson had described Parkinson's disease in 1812, and his is the description of the illness that is now classically appealed to, but his own work had little impact. It took the greatest neurologist of the nineteenth century, Jean-Martin Charcot, working in the Salpêtriêre from the 1860s through to the 1890s, to confirm the validity of Parkinson's observations and to bring the syndrome to wider attention.[99]

Charcot gave atropine, in the form of belladonna, to Parkinsonian patients. His demonstration that this motor disturbance was helped by atropine, an anticholinergic agent, while others were not was an important factor in confirming the validity of the diagnosis.[100] The tradition of using belladonna and later atropine almost certainly influenced clinicians in Paris faced with Parkinsonian conditions induced by the neuroleptics to turn quickly to atropine and other anticholinergic drugs to alleviate these conditions. Elsewhere a variety of treatments was tried, including the administration of coffee, before word spread of the benefits of the anticholinergics.[101]

In the United States Harold Himwich of the University of Chicago, one of the first animal experimenters to induce extrapyramidal syndromes with neuroleptics, was able to demonstrate that anticholinergic agents had a beneficial effect on them. Douglas Goldman of Cincinnati found the same effects in treating patients with Parkinson's disease who developed extrapyramidal syndromes.[102]

In France, the most dramatic extrapyramidal reactions occurred with the administration of another phenothiazine, prochlorperazine (variously marketed as Stemetil, Tementil, and Compazine). Given chlorpromazine's drawbacks as an anti-emetic, after it began to be used to treat psychiatric disorders, prochlorperazine, produced by Rhône-Poulenc, was developed as an anti-emetic and licensed to SK&F. Neither company had reason to think that it might be antipsychotic, largely because it was not sedative. It was given to French soldiers to alleviate seasickness during landing maneuvers carried out in choppy waters. Many soldiers ended up lying on the beach in spasms, indifferent to their environment—clearly a disaster. Military observers and their medical personnel called for help from Rhône-Poulenc in figuring out why the drug caused this odd effect. These military events were to contribute decisively to the crystallization of ideas about just what this group of drugs was doing.[103]

In April 1956, Rhône-Poulenc asked Paul Broussolle in Lyon to investigate the effects of prochlorperazine. Broussolle and his colleagues gave Tementil to twenty-eight patients and made a

surprising discovery. It was even more likely than chlorpromazine
to wake patients up. Mute patients who had been unresponsive to
chlorpromazine became active, almost overactive when given
prochlorperazine. This drug was clearly not a sedative but it did
seem to work as an antipsychotic. This discovery was a milestone
in the understanding of what prochlorperazine and similar drugs
could do. It led Broussolle to argue for the existence of a new
group of what he called incisive agents.

Prochlorperazine produced more clearly than chlorpromazine a set of reactions that were first termed excitomotor reactions but are now known as dyskinesias. Broussolle and the Lyon
group asked neurologists to advise them. It became clear that
some of the reactions intensified when attention was paid to them
and eased when no heed was paid to them. Thus there seemed to
be a suggestibility factor involved. The notion developed that in
some way the drug might predispose people to hysteria—might
"hystericize" the patient.

Several physicians in the south of France had also given
prochlorperazine to their pregnant wives to stop morning sickness. Reports began to come in of a number of bizarre effects.
Again, there was an element of suggestibility to them, and the fact
that the women were pregnant may have made it all too easy to
suggest that there was a hysterical component in these effects.

Many psychiatrists attempting to account for the effects of
prochlorperazine, chlorpromazine, and reserpine wondered if
they caused psychodynamic problems. This was still a Cartesian
world, in which for many practitioners the idea that the psychoses
could be neuropsychiatric disorders was still some way off. Linford
Rees in London, for example, faced with a patient with marked
tongue protrusion following administration of neuroleptics, had
it explained to him that the protrusion was a consequence of a
shock the patient had got after eating crackers with ants on
them.[104] This was an age when even frank neurological disorders
could be seen as deep-seated psychological problems. Parkinson's
disease, for example, was still seen in many quarters as resulting

from anger that an individual could not deal with, which had then been inhibited in a way that resulted in immobility.[105] Furthermore, although the anticonvulsants were beginning to change perceptions of epilepsy, only been a short time before convulsions had been thought to arise psychogenically.

Ideas about the impact of neuroleptics on the psychological organization of the personality can be most clearly seen in the case of akathisia, the most pernicious side effect of all. Descriptions of what retrospectively looks like akathisia have been recorded from as early as the seventeenth century. In 1861, a physician in the court of Louis Napoleon, graphically described a courtier who was unable to sit still. Since that condition was not one any courtier would desire, Trousseau was convinced that the problem was not a willed one.[106] At the turn of the century, Led Haskovec termed this phenomenon akathisia, literally meaning the inability to sit still. Akathisia reappeared with encephalitis lethargica in Europe following the great influenza epidemic of 1918. It was noticed then that while some encephalitis patients went into either vegetative or severe Parkinsonian states, others exhibited just the opposite syndrome: excessive motor restlessness.[107]

For thirty years thereafter, the phenomenon remained essentially unrecorded until the emergence of the neuroleptics. Chlorpromazine could cause it. Prochlorperazine was even more likely to cause it. But the drug most likely to cause it was reserpine. When given to treat hypertension, reserpine was noted to cause "increased tenseness, restlessness, insomnia and a feeling of being very uncomfortable."[108] In other cases "the first few doses frequently made them [patients] anxious and apprehensive . . . they reported increased feelings of strangeness, verbalized by statements such as 'I don't feel like myself' or 'I'm afraid of some of the unusual impulses that I have.'"[109] And in still another case on the "first day of treatment [the patient] reacted with marked anxiety and weeping and on the second day felt so terrible with such marked panic at night that the medication was cancelled."[110]

In response to such reactions to reserpine, Gerald Sarwer-Foner, for example, suggested that when caused by either chlorpromazine or reserpine, these problems involved stimulatory effects of the drugs that disturbed the psychological integration of particular patients. It was this disturbance of their integration that was the real problem, he claimed. The apparent anxiety that they were experiencing was not directly induced by the drug but rather stemmed from their worries about the emergence of repressed material. Such interpretations were not confined solely to those with a psychoanalytic bent. Hard-nosed biological psychiatrists like George Ashcroft of Edinburgh and Nathan Kline talked about the turbulent phase introduced by drugs such as reserpine or tetrabenazine.[111]

Faced with the tension, weeping, and anguish triggered by reserpine, for example, many clinicians interpreted these reactions as depression. Such interpretations led to the idea that reserpine caused depression, despite the availability from 1955 on of good trial evidence that it was as effective an antidepressant as Prozac.[112] Despite this evidence, the notion that reserpine caused depression took hold of clinical consciousness and appeared a decade later as the cornerstone of the amine theories of depression. These theories in turn gave rise to a host of drugs, such as the SSRIs, and popular ideas that depression involves a lowering of brain amines.[113]

Hans Steck of Lausanne and H.-J. Haase of Germany had a very different idea. Steck in late 1954 and Haase in early 1955 recognized that these reactions constituted the condition called akathisia after the encephalitis epidemic.[114] Steck and Staehelin had both trained with Eugen Bleuler at the Burghölzli in Zurich, a mecca for psychiatric training in the 1920s and 1930s. While there, he had seen the psychiatric consequences of the encephalitis lethargica epidemic. Many patients who had this encephalitis, especially those who were hyperactive, ended up in psychiatric wards. Impressed by the psychological effects of the brain disturbances caused in this condition, Constantin von Economo had written a monograph on the subject, in which he said: "Every psychiatrist who wishes to probe into the phenomena of disturbed motility and changes of character, the psychological mechanism of mental inaccessibility . . . must be thoroughly acquainted with . . . encephalitis lethargica. Every psychologist who attempts to deal with phenomena such as will, temperament and fundamentals of character such as self-consciousness, the ego, etc., and is not well acquainted with the appropriate observations on encephalitic patients . . . will build on sand."[115]

Von Economo's book ends with the statement "encephalitis lethargica can scarcely again be forgotten." But encephalitis lethargica was almost immediately forgotten by all except a few psychiatrists. Steck and Haase were among the handful of people who did not forget it. By the end of 1953, Steck and Staehelin, in Basel, were using higher doses of chlorpromazine to treat psychosis than were in use in Paris because they had found that higher doses could lead to responses in patients with some chronic psychoses. But at doses approaching 500 milligrams of chlorpromazine, in addition to Parkinsonism, they saw a range of other extrapyramidal manifestations of the neuroleptics and these motor problems reminded them of what they had seen twenty years before in Zurich. Steck then proposed that the agents were working on the motor mid-brain in some way and that it was this action which brought about their benefits.

To appreciate this, one needs to know that in addition to the motor problems consequent on encephalitis lethargica, some of the psychiatric patients in the Burghölzli who developed encephalitis lethargica showed improvements in their mental state.[116] In the case of a number of patients the intensity of their delusional beliefs and of their hallucinations diminished markedly as they became Parkinsonian. This was exactly what appeared to be happening with the administration of chlorpromazine to psychotic patients. In both encephalitis lethargica patients and patients given chlorpromazine there was diminished initiative, limited movement, a fixed facial expression, sometimes trembling, and often, with higher doses, abnormal movements. Once pointed out, these commonalities are striking and the idea that the therapeutic benefits and the motor problems with the neuroleptics go hand in hand does not seem far-fetched. But it required a series of accidents and a set of prepared minds to see this.

This idea was accepted by Deniker and Delay in Paris and ultimately led to the famous definition of the new drugs as neuroleptics. When Laborit introduced chlorpromazine into his cocktail, he was trying to produce a ganglioplegic (ganglion-paralyzing) cocktail. The idea was for a combination of drugs with a variety of actions to block all the different ganglions that might mediate the effects of stress. The phenothiazines began life as ganglioplegics. Impressed by the indifference induced by the new drugs, Laborit also introduced the term ataractics (from the Greek ataraxia, a state of being without agitation) to describe it. As it became clearer that chlorpromazine was primarily a neuroplegic (nerve-paralyzing) part of the cocktail, leading to a sedated central nervous system that was less sensitive to the effects of stress, it came to be called a neuroplegic drug.

But the emphasis was still primarily on sedation, as can be seen from the fact that another phenothiazine, levomepromazine (Nozinan), rapidly became the second most used medication for psychosis after chlorpromazine and it was even more sedative than chlorpromazine. Reserpine, although likely to cause turbulence, was also intensely sedative. Not until the discovery by Broussolle of the "disinhibiting" effects of prochlorperazine did it become clear that sedation was not needed. This opened up the possibility that an effect more specific than hitting all nerve junctions was needed.

Deniker and Delay put forward a theory about what that specific effect might be in an article published soon after Broussolle's description of the effects of prochlorperazine.[117] Conceding the importance of Broussolle's discovery, they upstaged Lyon by explaining that the importance lay in the fact that this discovery supported the idea of a neuroleptic, which Delay and Deniker claimed they had introduced at the 1955 conference on chlorpromazine.[118] Acknowledging the contribution of Steck, they argued that the new drugs created a state of psychomotor indifference, which was effective in treating states of excitement and agitation. These drugs produced a gradual reduction in both acute and chronic psychotic problems and by the same mechanisms produced both extrapyramidal and vegetative symptoms. The common action was on the basal ganglia or extrapyramidal system, which showed that the agents were specifically neuroleptic rather than merely generally neuroplegic.

Ideas were evolving differently in the English-, German-, and French-speaking worlds, and so a symposium was convened at the Second World Congress of Psychiatry in 1957 in Zurich to discuss what to call the new drugs. Speaker after speaker came forward with proposals. Delay finally argued that his idea of neuroleptic was more appropriate than names like tranquilizers, ataractics, neuroplegics, ganglioplegics, or anything else. His view carried the day in Europe.[119] But the Americans, separated by an ocean and generally less committed to classical neologisms, clung to the term major tranquilizer, until a later, less cautious generation adopted the term antipsychotic.

HALOPERIDOL: THE ULTIMATE NEUROLEPTIC

In 1953, Paul Janssen, a chemist influenced by a father who was both a physician and a representative for the Gideon Richter Pharmaceutical Company of Hungary, decided with some colleagues to set up a research-based pharmaceutical company.[120] The plan was to develop novel compounds to the point where they had potential therapeutic applications and then to license them to larger companies. The Janssen company went on to

make significant discoveries in the field of analgesic, antidiarrheal, and antifungal agents and across a wide range of therapeutic applications.

After discussing analgesia with Arnold Burgen of London,
Janssen was persuaded that he could improve on pethidine's analgesic effect and speed of action by removing a methyl group from
it to make it more fat soluble (lipophilic).[121] The resulting agent
would, he thought, penetrate the brain more quickly and therefore act faster and more effectively than pethidine. These ideas
about pethidine and about lipophilicity were both wrong, but the
history of psychopharmacology makes it clear that having a theory is scientifically useful primarily because having a theory leads
to action. The skill lies in detecting what actually happened
during tests rather than what the theory suggests must have
happened.

Janssen's new compound, norpethidine, was a more effective
analgesic than pethidine, and efforts were made to improve it further. He and his chemists experimented with the molecule by
adding side chains to it, changing the compound slowly from an
opioid to a butyrophenone. They found that when they did so the
characteristics of the molecule began to change. At the time only
a small number of screening tests were available to identify what
they had created. The new agents they had produced could be
checked to see if they produced effects similar to those produced
by morphine or atropine or amphetamine, or blocked those effects. Both the new compounds and chlorpromazine blocked the
effects of amphetamine. The new compounds also produced
experimental catatonia (catalepsy) in laboratory rats in the way
that chlorpromazine did.

This blocking of the effects of amphetamines was intriguing.
Amphetamines were widely used at the time in Belgium and
France by cyclists and other sportsmen to enhance performance
and increase endurance. Belgian cyclists regularly won the Tour
de France but frequently when crossing the finishing line looked
confused and stereotyped in their responses and in some cases

borderline paranoid. There were certain similarities between these states and milder forms of schizophrenia, but nobody in the West at the time seems to have remarked on these similarities.

It was different in Japan. After World War II a large supply of methamphetamines came onto the Japanese market.[122] They had been used by Japanese troops to enhance vigilance and improve performance. The companies that were producing them as part of the war effort continued to produce them thereafter and the drugs were used widely. By the 1950s, Japanese psychiatrists had recognized that an increasing number of patients admitted to their hospitals had ingested significant amounts of methamphetamines. In 1955, M. Tatetsu theorized that stimulants might trigger acute paranoid disorders and proposed that methamphetamine-induced psychosis could act as a model for chronic forms of both schizophrenia and manic depression.[123] This was ten years ahead of comparable work in the West.

Meanwhile, intrigued by the amphetamine-blocking abilities of his new set of compounds, Janssen sought to maximize these and finally in 1958 produced a molecule, R1625, later to become known as haloperidol. But what would it do clinically? There were suggestions from screening in animals that it had features in common with chlorpromazine. Haloperidol was produced in a clear liquid form and 10 milligrams of it were put in vials. No one knew what the dose should be. At the time chlorpromazine, which initially had been given in doses of 10 or 25 milligrams, was being used in doses of hundreds of milligrams without ill effect. Based on the idea that haloperidol might be of some use in treating psychotic patients, Janssen gave some to the closest large psychiatric hospital in Liège and asked psychiatrists to test it

The vials of haloperidol remained untested on a shelf for some time, until the son of a physician was admitted one night in a state the French call bouffée délirante, an acute and florid psychotic breakdown that may have either a good or a bad outcome. Often these states cleared up with few aftereffects. A susceptible person might have one or two more episodes during his life or might have no further episodes. In these good-outcome cases, the patient essentially experiences a stress-induced transient psychosis. But in some patients a florid episode of acute onset might be the first manifestation of a much longer lasting disorder, such as schizophrenia.[124]

When this young man came to the hospital, the resident, André Pinchard, gave him a 10-milligram injection of haloperidol. The results were dramatic. The patient immediately became quieter, disengaged from his environment, and quite manageable. Janssen was invited the following morning to witness the surprising effects of his new drug. He came and saw a young man who was still composed. Janssen was impressed and so were the young man's father and the senior doctors in the hospital.

It was clear, however, that the patient had been given a higher dose than was needed. Could this be possible with what seemed to be such a small dose? No one could guess what the right dose might be. Since haloperidol came in liquid form, the arrangement was to try administering a 1-milligram dose in the patient's coffee once a day. This dosage appeared to work well and several weeks later he went home. He subsequently went to college, became an architect, got married and had children, all the while continuing to take the medication. But was the drug producing his cure, or had he simply experienced one of the good-outcome episodes that would have been resolved without treatment within weeks?

The treating hospital team, Janssen, the patient, and his father met yearly to review the situation and yearly opted to continue with the 1-milligram treatment. After seven years, they decided to discontinue treatment on the grounds that they were not sure that the patient had ever had schizophrenia. The haloperidol was stopped. Three weeks later, the patient was readmitted in an acutely psychotic state. His subsequent responses to treatment were never as good as the initial response had been.

In the meantime, studies of haloperidol were being conducted in several places in Belgium. One was carried out in Liège by Jean Bobon despite the opposition of his superior, Paul Divry, a professor of psychiatry of the old school who believed that schizo-phrenia was an irreversible dementing condition and that by defi-nition no drug could help it. If a drug appeared to help a patient who had been diagnosed with schizophrenia, then the diagnosis was wrong. Bobon, hoping to succeed Divry, decided to bolster his research record by testing haloperidol on some patients. Bobon found the effects of haloperidol dramatic and powerful, and even though he did not understand how or why it worked, he decided that virtually every patient in the hospital should be given it. He found the new drug beneficial in treating agitated states, whether stemming from mania, schizophrenia, delirium, or dementia, as well as in treating neurological conditions such as Sydenham's chorea.

In psychiatric hospitals and wards in the 1950s and 1960s, there were a significant number of people who were merely be-having oddly rather than exhibiting signs of insanity, and there are such patients even in today's institutions. They may show little evidence of delusions or hallucinations but their behavior is in some way bizarre. For example, today there may be patients with a gross lack of feel for social boundaries, such as those with Asberger's syndrome. In the 1950s, psychiatric hospitals housed some patients who in the course of an otherwise normal conversa-tion might interject curses and expletives for no obvious reason. This odd behavior was at the time generally seen as in some sense mad by the outside world. Several such patients were in a hospital at Rekem in Belgium, where Jean Waelkens worked, and in the hospital in Liège where Bobon worked; Waelkens and Bobon gave haloperidol to all of these patients.

Haloperidol produced some of its most clear-cut benefits in these patients. Their response made it clear that theirs were cases of Tourette's syndrome, which had been described in 1885 by Giles de la Tourette, although its history can be traced back even further.[125] Tourette's descriptions of the condition had not led to wider recognition of the syndrome, and it was infrequently diag-nosed during the first half of the twentieth century. Following the response of patients with this syndrome to haloperidol, however, it was rediscovered. In fact, Waelkens and Bobon had seen and reported positive responses to haloperidol four years before the publication of the paper that is traditionally cited as marking this rediscovery.[126]

Janssen, somewhat skeptical of physicians, had given haloperidol to investigators from several different countries. On Delay's advice, he approached Juan Lopez-Ibor in Madrid, Felix Labhardt in Basel, and investigators from Portugal, Germany, the United States, Denmark, Sweden, Finland, and Turkey. Delay gave haloperidol to Pierre Pichot. In the pecking order in the Department of Psychiatry in Paris, Pichot theoretically was higher in the hierarchy than Deniker, but Deniker's role in the discovery of chlorpromazine had catapulted him to a greater international prominence. Possibly, Delay gave haloperidol to Pichot in part to balance things out. Pichot, however, was less interested in drugs than in psychometrics, so Thérèse Lempérière, working alongside him, was effectively the primary investigator.[127]

At that time, no money was provided for the conduct of clinical studies. In contrast, in the year 2000, between $5,000 and $10,000 usually is spent on every patient involved in the a study of an antipsychotic, but the money does not guarantee that senior clinicians will be involved in assessing whether there is anything truly novel about the compound (see Chapter 7). In the late 1950s, however, the drugs being investigated were so dramatically different from their predecessors that senior clinicians could not resist the opportunity to use them. The answers to important questions might lie in the treatment of the next patient, especially one given a drug as powerful as haloperidol.

On 5 September 1959, Janssen reconvened the investigators at his laboratories, where they all reported essentially the same response to the drug.[128] It was effective in controlling agitated states. It had a profile different from that of chlorpromazine. It was much less sedative. It seemed to work better in the management of hallucinations than chlorpromazine. It was more likely to cause extrapyramidal symptoms than chlorpromazine, but many investigators did not mind this because they had begun to think that if a drug did not cause extrapyramidal problems, it probably could not be a neuroleptic.

One problem with the new drug was finding the right dose; after experimenting the investigators settled on what seemed to be low doses. Haloperidol was clearly much more potent than chlorpromazine. In Namur, André Paquay conducted his study using doses between 1 and 7 milligrams of haloperidol per day, trying to avoid the motor side effects that had appeared in patients previously treated with higher doses. His success rate was the highest of all the studies, some of which had been using up to 15 milligrams per day.

Janssen approached the Searle Company in the United States to see if it was prepared to license haloperidol. Searle had already taken Lomotil, an early Janssen compound, still in use today for the management of diarrhea. The contract for Lomotil gave Searle rights of first refusal on any subsequent Janssen compound. However, the head of the company, Jack Searle, had already tried out two other neuroleptics, Dartal and Mornidine. Dartal was very similar to an already existing compound, perphenazine, marketed very successfully by another company, and so it had little success in the marketplace. Mornidine caused a lot of side effects. Both compounds failed, and Jack Searle lost interest in the "antipsychotic business."

Furthermore, by this time a study conducted in New York had cast doubts on haloperidol's usefulness. This study had been undertaken by Herman Denber, who often visited Europe and frequently took compounds he obtained there back with him to Manhattan State Hospital, hoping to be the first to try them out in the United States. Denber visited Janssen and took samples home with him. He then reportedly gave the new compound to ten patients. It apparently did not work. The results of the study suggested that haloperidol was a peculiar drug that benefited Europeans but not Americans.[129] But Denber was, in fact, not present when the studies were done. A research assistant gave out the drugs and assessed the results.

This one study could have been dismissed, but instead it confirmed Searle's prejudices. He refused to market haloperidol in the United States, although his company did later market haloperidol in the rest of the world as Serenace. There was a further disaster for Janssen. A study conducted by D. Goldstein in Florida also reported that haloperidol was ineffective. Reviewing Goldstein's work, however, Janssen found that he had conducted an earlier study in which up to 4 grams per day of chlorpromazine was apparently no more effective than a placebo. This outcome he found unbelievable. Janssen visited Goldstein and found a man who ran a punchcard operation and never saw patients. He had employed untrained and unskilled people to assess the effects of the drug. The methods used were so insensitive that no differences even in side effects were discovered between chlorpromazine and a placebo.[130]

Finally in 1964, a study conducted in California using low doses of haloperidol demonstrated the drug's effectiveness in American patients. Janssen broke the terms of his agreement with Searle and approached the McNeil Pharmaceutical Company, which undertook to market haloperidol in the United States. It became available in 1965 and was used increasingly, becoming in the 1980s the most commonly used antipsychotic in the country. As a result, the Janssen Company later became part of Johnson & Johnson rather than part of Searle, as it might otherwise have done.

Haloperidol therefore became available in the United States ten years after it had been launched elsewhere. It became the best-selling neuroleptic there as it had elsewhere, but bizarrely, as late as the mid-1970s, French psychiatrists who had been using the drug for fifteen years would be told when they attended lectures in the United States that the benefits of haloperidol had only recently been discovered.[131]

THE NOBEL PRIZE

The discoveries of reserpine, chlorpromazine, and haloperidol naturally led to speculation about whether any of those involved in the work would win a Nobel Prize. Other prizes had, as we have seen, already been awarded. Nathan Kline and Robert Noce had shared in the 1957 Lasker Prize for their work in the discovery of reserpine, even though Leo Hollister's data was more convincing than theirs. In 1964, Kline became the only man to be awarded a second Lasker Prize, for the discovery of the antidepressant properties of iproniazid. He seemed a good candidate for a Nobel Prize, but then the second award of the Lasker prize to Kline was contested by a coworker, Jack Saunders, and the ensuing legal wrangle put paid to any chances of Kline's winning the Nobel Prize.[132]

The other candidates for the Nobel Prize of course were Deniker and Delay, for their work on chlorpromazine. Of course, Jean-Marie Harl's name was on the first reports of their studies, and as the junior doctor on the ward Harl was probably the person most knowledgeable about the patients and most aware of the impact of chlorpromazine on them. He was, however, at the hospital only to be trained; he quickly moved on to private practice and very shortly thereafter was killed in a climbing accident. He had no prospect of being nominated for the prize.

Delay was probably the most senior psychiatrist on the world stage. By the mid-1950s, however, he was seeing very few private patients and appearing on the wards only rarely. Delay's contact with ward patients was probably restricted to the case conferences he chaired, where it was the practice to interrogate the patients. However, Delay appears to have had a shrewd grasp of the general importance of the work on chlorpromazine. Moreover, he certainly made distinctive contributions to emerging ideas about how the neuroleptics worked, and even coined the term neuroleptic to describe both the action and the class of drugs.

Delay always thought that he and Deniker should have received the Nobel Prize. It came to obsess him. Even if they were not the first to use chlorpromazine, they were the first to proclaim its distinctive antipsychotic properties. And after all, the honors often go to those who alert the world to the existence of and importance of a phenomenon rather than to its discoverers. Delay's realization that chlorpromazine was beneficial in treating psychoses gave decisive impetus to developments in the chlorpromazine story at a time when many of his contemporaries doubted its therapeutic potential in treating such conditions.

But events did not favor Delay. In 1957, the Americans had awarded the Lasker Prize to Pierre Deniker and Henri Laborit, along with Heinz Lehmann, for work on chlorpromazine, and to Kline and Noce, and to Rustom Vakil, whose paper on the use of reserpine in the treatment of hypertension had triggered Western interest in the compound. Once one prize committee of stature had decided who the key players were in the discovery of chlorpromazine and had not recognized a specific contribution from Delay, another committee, the Nobel committee, was unlikely to do so. Why not give the Nobel Prize then to Deniker and Laborit? Because Delay sat on the Nobel Prize committee and blocked any efforts to award even part of the prize to Laborit. When no prize was offered for the discovery of chlorpromazine, none could later be offered to Kuhn or Kline for the discovery of an antidepressant, a derivative discovery of lesser importance.

There was tremendous hostility between the Sainte-Anne camp and Laborit. Deniker and others from Sainte-Anne played down Laborit's contribution to the work on chlorpromazine. Throughout the 1950s and 1960s, Delay assiduously staked out claims for his priority. He reacted with anger and hostility to efforts by others to propose classification systems for the new antipsychotics. Pierre Lambert and Louis Revol from Lyon, for instance, proposed a classification system ranging from sedative to incisive types of neuroleptics, with levomepromazine and thioridazine typifying the sedative type and prochlorperazine and later haloperidol typifying the incisive types. When Lambert presented the outlines of this scheme at the first CINP meeting in Rome in 1958, he was attacked by Delay for daring to transgress on his territory. Delay even tried to have Lambert dismissed from his position.

Another candidate for the Nobel Prize was Paul Janssen, who was nominated for the innovative drug development that produced haloperidol and later other drugs. Janssen never got the prize. Some argue that because he made so much money out of his discoveries adding a Nobel Prize would not have been appropriate. In any case, Janssen was the last of the major figures in the story of the development of the new drugs to be considered for the Nobel Prize. Daniel Bovet's Nobel Prize, awarded in 1957, was the closest the prize came to any of the central players in the drama.

The war between Laborit and the Sainte-Anne camp continued into the 1980s. In the late 1960s, an American, Ann Caldwell, came to Paris to write the first history of the discovery of chlorpromazine. She met the participants, sided with Laborit, and produced a book that all but wrote Deniker and Delay out of the script. This was followed in 1974 by Judith Swazey's *Chlorpromazine in Psychiatry*. Swazey's book is a model of historical scholarship that tried to set the record straight. It gave credit to both parties. The Sainte-Anne camp was not satisfied. Deniker said that Swazey had managed to write the chlorpromazine story without reference to the concept of a neuroleptic. Her scrupulous delineation of detail elicited from Deniker the comment that some people had tried to write the history of chlorpromazine in terms of bills of sale of the product.[133] After Swazey's book appeared, Deniker wrote a piece on who had discovered the neuroleptics, to which of course there could be only one answer.[134] In 1992, the fortieth anniversary of Deniker's use of chlorpromazine, Rhône-Poulenc marked the occasion by publishing a volume that noted Laborit's work in the field of anesthesia but credited the clinical breakthroughs to Deniker and Delay.[135]

In 1980 Jean Thuillier wrote an account of the chlorpromazine story at Sainte-Anne that gives full credit to Delay as an important figurehead.[136] But he also outlined the distinctive contributions of Laborit and Deniker and made it clear that without Laborit the chlorpromazine story might never have unfolded. Although a celebration of chlorpromazine, written with the panache of a prize-winning author and at a time when antipsychiatry still threatened at the gates of psychiatry, this account won Thuillier few friends in Paris, even though he suppressed entirely the hidden secret at the heart of the Nobel disputes—the story of what happened to Delay in the student revolutions of 1968. Despite Thuillier's book, Laborit felt cheated, and died bitter.

In 1994, on the two-hundredth anniversary of the foundation of the Val de Grâce, a plaque was placed on the wall of the hospital to honor the discovery of chlorpromazine there in 1952—by Laborit, Hamon, Paraire, and Velluz.

4

Psychiatry outside the Walls

The bitterness of the priority disputes about chlorpromazine has meant that there have been no Nobel Prizes in psychiatry since World War II, despite the impact psychiatry now has on all our lives. This bitterness stems from more than the egos of scientific prima donnas. It is indicative of a fundamental difference in worldviews. On the one hand is Laborit's identification of a behavioral effect caused by chlorpromazine that could be beneficial. This was a discovery with ambiguous implications. It opened up the possibility of social engineering, critics of psychiatry quickly noted. On the other hand is Delay and Deniker's claim that chlorpromazine's effect on the mentally ill was to bring about an unambiguously beneficial restoration of social order.

Psychiatry's critics argue that chlorpromazine was not of great value because mental hospitals were starting to close before its introduction. Just as streptomycin emerged at a time when social measures had done much to reduce the impact of tuberculosis, the most prevalent illness of the nineteenth century, so chlorpromazine, the critics argue, emerged at a time when the management of mental illness was rapidly being transformed by a series of social initiatives. The acceptance of such criticisms means that few mental health professionals know much about the history of psychopharmacology, in contrast to the history of psychoanalysis. But arguably, the main impact of chlorpromazine, like that of psychoanalysis, has been on the culture in which we live, and a failure to appreciate that makes it very difficult to understand the origins of antipsychiatry, or the possible social construction of addiction, or even the fate of Jean Delay.

THE PRE-CHLORPROMAZINE MATRIX

The Impact of War on Psychiatry

The supposed alternative to chlorpromazine is social, or milieu, therapy, which sprang from the work of several practitioners. In the 1920s in Vienna Kurt Lewin worked with patient groups and Juan Moreno experimented with psychodrama. Both of these therapies rejected the exclusive focus of psychoanalysis on the individual. Lewin and Moreno emigrated to the United States, where their work was continued within psychiatric circles by Trigant Burrow, Louis Wender, and Paul Schilder. In the late 1920s also, Harry Stack Sullivan established a six-bed unit at the Sheppard & Enoch Pratt Hospital in Baltimore for young male schizophrenic patients, and treated them by trying to modify their personal and social environments.[1] His emphasis was on growth through the experience of interpersonal relations.

This therapeutic approach sprang from social psychology, a field that developed after Gustav Le Bon published his book on the behavior of crowds in 1896. Le Bon's thesis was that crowd behavior in Europe's revolutions was a manifestation of a group hysteria whose laws could be deduced.[2] World War I and the Russian Revolution led to further studies of crowd behavior by Wilfred Trotter and William McDougall.[3] This theoretical work had an immense impact on the way military commands managed psychological casualties in World War II; the emphasis was on group work of the sort developed by Lewin and Moreno. This treatment of war-ravaged patients firmly established the social psychiatry and interpersonal treatment approaches, which formed the backdrop against which chlorpromazine was introduced.

For battlefield casualties in the World War II, in contrast to deteriorated psychotic patients, it was appropriate to emphasize responsibility and independence and to provide a setting more collegial than that offered by the traditional hospital. Medical and nursing staff on these wartime units rarely wore white coats. Patients and staff called each other by their first names. The social hierarchies of prewar European life were dissolved in this milieu. Visitors to such units in Britain at hospitals like Belmont and Northfield described the experience as "mind-blowing."[4]

The medical staff envisioned a new form of therapy. If appropriate group experiences with enriched interpersonal exchanges were therapeutic for the victims of war, why not for conventional psychiatric patients? Thomas Main coined the term "therapeutic community" in 1946 to characterize this new approach.[5] And Maxwell Jones, David Clark, and others established therapeutic communities in psychiatric hospitals after the war.[6] In addition to kindling enthusiasm for therapeutic communities, the experience of treating war casualties led to a disregard for genetic theories of mental illness; progress through manipulating the environment seemed to be the way to remedy social ills, including mental illness.

The experience of therapists in wartime units coincided with the experiences of a cadre of young military medical officers, men who had no prior interest in becoming psychiatrists and no pre-conceptions about the nature of mental illness. They were faced with a mass of recruits with varied backgrounds slotted willy-nilly into different units. It was a gigantic social experiment. It became clear to some of these medical officers that simple administrative steps might make a profound difference to a soldier's mental health. The feeble-minded, who should not be allowed to fire weapons, could be transferred from the front lines to other duties, as could the shell-shocked, the neurotic, and others. If trying to fit square pegs into round holes caused mental breakdowns in the military, would it not also do so in civilian life? And if breakdowns in soldiers could be helped by social interventions, would the same hold for breakdowns in civilian life?

The war also increased understanding of the importance of morale. Regiments that had high rates of infection of venereal and other diseases were often demoralized units, whose problems needed to be solved by replacing the commanding officer as well as treating the soldiers. Medical officers returning from the war to asylum posts were struck by the demoralization and brutality of life in asylums. Inured by the brutality of war to the brutality of asylum life, many of these individuals, who in other times would have flinched from the dehumanizing effects of the asylums and gone into other branches of medicine, ended up as superintendents and set about changing the conditions in the asylums. Most psychiatrists returning to the United States went into private practice, but the brutality of prewar asylum life was brought to public attention by conscientious objectors who had worked in the asylums.[7] Their exposés focused attention on "records . . . of patient deaths following beatings administered by brutal attendants."[8] "Frequent active assaults," one observer noted, "have resulted in broken bones, lacerations, bruises, and a consequent deterioration of the mind. Favorite weapons have been the buckles of heavy straps, the loaded end of heavy keyrings, metal plated shoes, and wet towels which leave no marks after choking."[9]

Even before the war there was a growing recognition that "normal" people might "break down." In the 1930s and 1940s facilities in many countries had started accepting voluntary admissions, and an increasing number of patients had availed themselves of the opportunity. For these patients the authorities created more pleasant "neurosis" or admission wards, where the staff treated patients with ECT, insulin coma therapy, barbiturates, or stimulants. Moreover, patients in these wards spent less time in the hospital than did patients on traditional wards. Altogether, these developments intensified the pressures for change in asylums. The patients were more likely to be known socially to the staff, and this also put pressure on the old asylum style to change.

Among the patients admitted in greater numbers were alcoholics. In 1950, one of the first of the new psychotropic drugs, disulfiram (Antabuse), became available. Useful though it was for some people, many of the medical superintendents quickly realized that far more useful was a new psychosocial approach, Alcoholics Anonymous. What was this if not a therapeutic community?

The establishment of therapeutic communities was associated with a policy of unlocking wards. In Britain, this happened first in 1948 in Warlingham Park Hospital—long before the advent of chlorpromazine. In addition, in many places occupational therapy, rehabilitation facilities, and work therapies were provided, and some institutions even moved toward granting patients more participation in day-to-day operations. All these efforts were aimed at counteracting the institutional neurosis that old-style authoritarian hospital structures were thought to engender. The hospitals were, therefore, clearly being transformed before the introduction of chlorpromazine.[10] Indeed, this movement had become so firmly entrenched in certain hospitals that Aubrey Lewis said, in a passage that was to become famous, "If we had to choose between abandoning the new psychotropic drugs and abandoning the industrial rehabilitation units and other social facilities available to us, there would be no hesitation about the choice: the drugs would go."[11]

In many respects this was the perfect setting for the emergence of pharmacotherapy, because after patients had been retrieved from chronic psychotic states by drug therapies, many of them needed other kinds of therapy to fully rehabilitate them.[12] Clinicians such as Pierre Lambert in Lyon, Jack Durrell at the NIMH,[13] Vernon Kinross-Wright in Texas, and Leo Hollister in California found that patients were beginning to talk to them for the first time.[14] Some of these patients became able to sustain activities for the first time since entering the hospital, so that it was possible to include them in occupational therapy programs and to inculcate the interactional skills many of them had lost. Far from being competitive with pharmacotherapy, Raymond Battegay, Luc Ciompi, and others in Basel, for example, even intentionally exposed recovering patients to groups, so that the patients could see for themselves that failure to adhere to treatment would quickly lead to relapses.[15]

The programs that sprang up were fueled by the enthusiasm of nurses and other staff members, who had begun professionalizing in the 1950s.[16] In that decade, the magic of the changes that chlorpromazine produced had not yet worn off. The doses used were lower than those used later. The patients were a much more homogenous group than patients admitted after 1960, with many fewer patients who had personality disorders, forensic histories, or neurotic disorders. Problems such as tardive dyskinesia had not yet emerged.

This enthusiasm for chlorpromazine elicited a reaction from socially oriented psychiatrists, who from the late 1950s on pointed to the many beneficial treatments that had been developed before the advent of chlorpromazine. They dismissed chlorpromazine's role in the postwar psychiatric revolution—sometimes using the words of the new psychopharmacologists to brand it as no more than a refined form of lobotomy. Sometimes the evangelism of biological psychiatrists helped evoke such reactions. Sometimes they were ideologically based: some viewed social therapies as ethically superior to biological interventions.[17] And of course it is true that if inappropriately used in a more coercive climate or more restrictive setting, chlorpromazine could be an instrument of oppression rather than of liberation. Between 1955 and 1966, the number of psychiatric beds in Japan quadrupled, and it continued to rise through the 1970s.[18] The inappropriate use of chlorpromazine and other neuroleptics facilitated this rise, as it did similar rises in other countries. These facts lend considerable force to the claims of the social psychiatrists.

The changes produced by social psychiatrists before the advent of chlorpromazine clearly brought about benefits, but there were problems with the milieu approaches. These approaches had been developed for the management of wartime casualties, many of whom were neurotic or psychopathic, and the success of the approaches led to the admission of greater numbers of such patients. The wartime experience had also led to an appreciation of the benefits of breaking down boundaries, and by the end of the 1950s this trend was also increasingly leading to an indiscriminate mixing of psychotic and psychopathic patients. In a situation where diagnostic boundaries were blurred, it was easy for dramatic benefits to be produced in some patients labeled as having schizophrenia. Beneficial effects achieved in such patients were used to justify continuing with the new approaches, even though many psychotic patients almost certainly got worse. This deterioration probably contributed significantly to the ultimate discrediting of milieu approaches.

Despite these divisions of opinion between what were later called social and biological psychiatrists, there were probably very few psychiatrists in the 1950s who would have opted for either drugs or social measures to the exclusion of the other. Characteristic of the intermingling of views in this period is a statement by Jules Masserman: "We all have seen the leveling of the bizarre and rich instinctual features of fantasy life in patients taking antipsychotics, the low lying dysphoric energy leading to creative inertia in patients during the early months of lithium treatment, the talkative impersonality of patients prescribed the tricyclic antidepressants, ... the tightening up and organizing effect of the amphetamines in some loose thinkers, the relative imperviousness to criticism of the erstwhile fearful paralyzed patients who have been treated with tricyclics, ... the trips into new spaces out of old cognitive ruts of the middle-aged hallucinogen user, a shift in marital dominance pattern when the bully has to take reserpine for high blood pressure."[19]

For many psychiatrists, such as Heinz Lehmann, the first to publish on chlorpromazine in North America, drugs made it possible to do therapy.[20] Drugs and "therapy" obviously went together.

Epidemiological Psychiatry

The war gave rise to another form of social psychiatry, now called epidemiological psychiatry. The spectacular triumphs of bacteriology at the turn of the century took center stage in medicine. The identification of specific microorganisms as the cause of one after another of the infectious diseases reinforced the view that disease was a biological process. The previous triumph of sanitary measures to improve hygiene was reinterpreted as having removed the specific causes of disease, which could have been as readily and perhaps more effectively removed by a magic bullet. This bacteriological vision led orthodox medicine to focus on the pathogenesis of diseases, neglecting the social context in which disease became manifest.

But, in fact, epidemiological findings powerfully demonstrated the role of social class and other factors in health and disease. Why otherwise would black ghettos and poor suburbs have a higher rate of infective disorders?[21] By the 1930s, therefore, there was some recognition that the diseases that afflicted men and women were shaped by how and where they lived, with whom they lived, what they worked at, and the resources they commanded. These factors influenced rates of exposure, malnutrition, comorbidity, and morale, all of which nonspecifically increased vulnerability to specific diseases.[22] The decline in tuberculosis long before the advent of the effective antitubercular agents graphically illustrated how even a clearly biological disorder could respond to social interventions.[23]

In the case of psychiatry, George Rosen in the United States and Aubrey Lewis in Europe in the 1940s took a new social approach that involved surveying large numbers of patients to search for factors that cut across all patients with disorders such as hysteria or schizophrenia—age of onset, season of birth, social class, and so on.[24] This is clearly an epidemiological approach, but was not so designated at the time because then epidemiology was a term restricted to the field of infectious diseases. The epidemiological input to the study of heart disease and lung cancer had yet to make an impact; its proponents saw themselves as doing social medicine. The approach of psychiatrists like Rosen and Lewis was essentially preventive. If risk factors could be identified, steps could presumably be taken to minimize degrees of exposure. Work of this kind was as far removed as it was possible to get from psychodynamic approaches, where hypotheses about what was important stemmed from the intense examination of individual cases.

Just as the war fostered new social treatments, so also it promoted the development of social medicine in psychiatry. To avoid charges of liability, national armies were concerned to establish the illnesses of recruits before combat, from tuberculosis to their propensity for nervous breakdowns.[25] In the United States, such efforts inspired the research of Mandel Cohen and Paul Dudley White on combat fatigue and effort syndrome (see Chapter 7). In Britain, the public health approach implicit in this effort laid the basis for the later creation of socialized medicine in the form of the National Health Service, where the population was treated as a unit, in contrast to a system where individuals are consumers in a marketplace.

There were differences between this kind of social psychiatry and the socially active psychiatry that gave rise to therapeutic communities. Both were concerned with poverty, unemployment, old age, workers' compensation issues, social failure, and malingering. But socially active psychiatrists wanted to manage these factors in order to reduce the dependency of patients.[26] Social activists saw little difference between changing society and psychotherapy. The new social epidemiologists, in contrast, were hostile to analysis and skeptical of therapy.[27] They viewed psychiatric disorders as indistinguishable from other medical disorders. Their approach originated in the social psychiatry unit at the Maudsley Hospital in London and the work of "biometricians" in the United States such as Morton Kramer and other practitioners in St. Louis. The epidemiological approach in both Britain and the United States required an interest in diagnostic criteria. Ironically, by delineating psychosyndromes clearly and establishing their prevalence in the community, epidemiological psychiatrists probably did more than anything else to create later markets for psychotropic medicines.[28]

Despite social psychiatrists interest in pure research, two treatment themes emerged from their work. Researchers at the Maudsley Hospital studying patients discharged to families began to recognize the deleterious effects that families could have on schizophrenic patients.[29] Therapeutic approaches aimed at minimizing such effects were created but never had much success. An alternative approach emphasized the need for training in social skills. Drug treatments could ameliorate acute episodes, but psychotic or institutionalized patients needed social psychiatry's help in achieving resocialization.[30] However, while this form of social psychiatry was medically oriented, there was still an inclination to regard drug treatments as appropriate in managing acute exacerbations of schizophrenic illnesses but not as curative in themselves.[31]

The boundaries between social activism and epidemiological psychiatry were often difficult to determine in an era where the transformation of society seemed eminently possible. As John Ryle, who became the first professor of social medicine at Oxford in 1943, noted, unemployment was bad for health. "Many of the social evils, so widely manifest by disease . . . call not for medical action but for drastic social and economic reform. For these the electorate, through their representatives, and not the doctors, must become responsible. But who unearths and exposes the evils? . . . We have reached a time in which 'the physician' . . .

must assume leadership in the struggle for the improvement of conditions."[32] But is it the role of the doctor to work to increase levels of employment rather than to treat the illnesses that result from unemployment? If the majority of psychiatric disorders are found among the unemployed and the poor, surely then psychiatry must be at huge risk of medicalizing distress and blurring the boundaries between the sociopolitical universe and the domain of mental illness.

What, indeed, was the proper domain of social psychiatry? For practitioners to leave the asylum, even if only to deal with the statistics of public life, involved a great extension of the psychiatric reach. As one commentator put it: "In the past decade it has become increasingly fashionable to attach the adjective 'social' to 'psychiatry' and to suggest that practically every field of human activity falls within the province of the social psychiatrist . . . subjects as diverse as drug addiction, criminology, mental disturbance and art, architecture and psychiatry, problems of sleep and dreaming, the biochemistry of the mind, electronics and psychiatry and the theory of sexual perversion."[33] Postwar psychiatry, therefore, occupied an entirely different universe from that of prewar psychiatry, with consequences no one could easily have guessed at.

The Impact of War on Psychoanalysis

The factors that led to the creation of social psychiatry also transformed psychoanalysis. Before the war, analysis was an almost entirely European approach with very little interest in the treatment of schizophrenic psychoses. Freud had rescinded his earlier claims that analytic approaches might benefit patients with schizophrenia and had confined himself to treating neurotic disorders. True, Jung had from 1908 spent time analyzing the content of psychoses and arguing for a possible psychogenesis in some cases, but his work had little impact in the world of psychodynamic therapy. And Eugen and Manfred Bleuler advocated supportive approaches to the management of schizophrenia that involved enduring with patients and keeping alive a recognition of their humanity, but achieved little more.

With the rise of the Nazi Party in Germany, psychoanalysts began to migrate to the United States, and by the end of the war a majority of the world's analysts were based there. These immigrants were joined by the returning military psychiatrists. The situation in the United States was completely different from that in Europe, where the military recruits to psychiatry returned to asylums and socializing medical systems. In the United States, army recruits could return to private practice and psychoanalysis was a passport to an office practice. This situation, combined with an exodus of psychiatrists from public hospitals, meant that by 1955 more than 80 percent of U.S. psychiatrists were in office practice.[34] Foreigners filled their places in the asylums. Uniquely, therefore, power and influence in American psychiatry resided in the community.

The insights and enthusiasm generated by the war that led many Europeans to social psychiatry led American psychiatrists such as Karl and William Menninger to expand psychoanalysis. Karl Menninger, the lead American military psychiatrist, was enthusiastic about the psychoanalysis spawned by the war.[35] There was no clear understanding at the end of the war that group therapy and individual psychoanalysis were quite different therapeutic approaches. Analysts had taken the lead in applying group approaches and group therapists had appealed to the writings of analysts. Nothing in wartime experience suggested that individual therapy would not be able to achieve as least as dramatic benefits as group approaches.

Traditional Freudian analysis viewed everyone as at least latently ill and as being in need of treatment. Nothing about the group approaches in the war did anything to dispel this idea either. The new analysis that emerged in America after the war was to make the idea that everybody needed treatment a public health issue: the way to right the world's wrongs was not just to treat mental illness but to resculpt personalities to promote mental health.[36]

In 1946, William Menninger helped establish the Group for the Advancement of Psychiatry, which among other things saw it as its mission to gain control of American psychiatry. As early as 1948, three quarters of all committee posts in the American Psychiatric Association were held by analysts. By 1962, most psychiatric departments were headed by dynamically oriented psychiatrists, all graduate programs except one in St. Louis were based on analytic principles, and thirteen of the seventeen most recommended texts were psychoanalytically oriented.[37] As a director of the NIMH later put it: "From 1945 to 1955, it was nearly impossible for a non-psychoanalyst to become a chairman of a department or professor of psychiatry."[38]

Although this psychoanalytic psychiatry was largely office based and, accordingly, dealt almost exclusively with neurotic disorders, never penetrating the public hospital system to any great extent, it was nevertheless important for the hegemony of psychoanalysis that it be seen to contribute to the treatment of the psychoses. This, and the perception that the group work going on in therapeutic communities was in some sense psychodynamic, perhaps contributed to the extraordinary influence of what was a relatively small body of work on the psychoanalysis of the psychoses.

One of the milestones in the psychotherapeutic treatment of the psychoses was the work of Frieda Fromm-Reichman at Chestnut Lodge Hospital in Baltimore.[39] This work became the subject of a celebrated popular account, *I Never Promised You a Rose Garden*. She introduced the notion of a schizophrenogenic mother, which captured both the public and the academic imagination. Another influential figure was Madeline Sechehaye, who also claimed that schizophrenia involved aberrant mothering. Given a license to interpret behaviors symbolically, even the most normal mothering could be made to appear dangerous.

Other major figures were Harold Searles of Chestnut Lodge, Elvin Semrad at Massachusetts Mental Hospital,[40] and Silvano

Arieti in New York. As the editor of the 1959 *American Handbook of Psychiatry*, Arieti had extraordinary influence. His sections in this handbook dealt with the psychotherapy of schizophrenia, the difficulties of which he portrayed as yielding to a new scientific approach.[41] Semrad's approach stressed identification of the life impasse that had occasioned decompensation in the patient and efforts to resolve it.[42]

These approaches focused mostly on the defense mechanisms of the patient. An alternative was to intervene directly with the primary processes that were supposed to be disturbed in schizophrenics. This idea led to direct analysis, whose foremost advocate was John Rosen. Direct analysis could involve a barrage of punishment, abuse, and shame as well as rewards and intense group pressure, aimed at countering infantile processes with direct communications of a kind that even infants could understand. Startling results were claimed, and Rosen's work was initially widely hailed as a significant breakthrough. As late as 1968, he remained one of the great heroes of the analytic establishment.[43] In due course, however, a darker picture emerged, and his work has since been comprehensively discredited.[44]

All these approaches had two things in common. One was the challenge to the therapist. Unlike the management of neuroses, management of schizophrenia appeared to require intervention in the underlying primary processes of mental life rather than just the tinkering with the secondary defense mechanisms done in standard office therapy. These supposed primary processes appeared alien and threatening even to the therapist. Dealing with them tested the therapist himself. How well had he conquered his own ghosts? Any therapist worth his salt had to feel that he should, at least once, venture into these rough waters. The work of Jung, who had apparently at one point in his career descended into what has been termed a psychosis, loosely supported the view that a psychosis was in some sense a good thing, a growth experience.[45] Jung had recast the experience as a journey to the ground of his being, where he came in contact with the archetypes of myth making in humanity. The implication was that any therapist who wanted to achieve true grandeur should follow suit.

The other factor common to psychoanalytic approaches was the conviction that they dealt with the real source of mental illness. This idea stemmed from the notion that drugs provided only symptomatic relief. Psychotherapeutic approaches, which were based on a theory of causation, in contrast, were tackling the supposedly basic mechanisms involved with the psychoses. In theory, then, psychotherapeutic approaches were more likely to be effective in the long term and also were more ethical—provided of course that the theories as regards basic causation were right. A new psychotherapeutic language arose from the analytic treatment of schizophrenia, giving rise to a range of ideas that permeated popular culture, such as the notions of double binds and split personalities. Hollywood found these ideas compelling and produced movies such as *The Three Faces of Eve* that generated considerable public support for the efforts of therapists.

One of the features of these developments was that a rootless patois of dynamic terms seeped into popular culture to create a psychobabble. People became familiar with terms such as the ego and the id, transference, defense mechanisms, and libido. Where before authenticity had been conceptualized in terms of holiness or a life lived in accordance with the dictates of conscience, now it became redefined in terms of adjustment and awareness. Another feature was the way the analytic establishment handled both the failures of patients to get well and the refusal of critics to admit they were wrong. These were viewed as further indicators of the psychopathology afflicting patients and critics, respectively.[46]

By 1965, when the catecholamine theory of depression, the first biological theory of a major psychiatric disorder, was published, the article following it in the *American Journal of Psychiatry* focused on the psychoanalytic consequences for the nation of the death of John Kennedy. This was a time when analysts were listened to when they argued that if only statesmen were analyzed there would be no more wars. The reach of both analytic approaches and social activism was imperial, but far from being natural allies, social psychiatrists and psychoanalysts were at loggerheads and could not cooperate in mounting a coherent response to the challenges to psychiatry thrown up by the changing world of the 1960s.

The Fracturing of Psychiatry

While American psychiatry was developing in power and influence, almost undisturbed by the advent of chlorpromazine and imipramine, the back wards, which had seen the failed experiments of psychosurgery and the management of psychoses by drainage of abscesses, were being staffed by nonanalytically oriented Europeans, and they were the first witnesses to the new psychopharmacotherapy. Thus Heinz Lehmann in Montreal and Vernon Kinross-Wright in Texas reported on chlorpromazine and set about establishing milieu therapy settings very similar to those found in Europe. Pharmacotherapy spread like wildfire in these deprived settings. Initially there was very little conflict between analysts and drug therapists because their spheres of influence did not overlap much.

The emergence of tranquilizers such as Miltown and later "antidepressants" such as Marsilid (iproniazid) and Tofranil (imipramine) began to change the picture. Ultimately, it was not so much the new drugs as their availability on a prescription-only basis that made the difference. The implication was that the one thing that differentiated a doctor from other health professionals was the ability to issue a prescription. This combined with the fact that office-based psychoanalysis had brought psychiatry to Main Street created the matrix in which the biological, social, and psychological engines of psychiatry would ultimately begin to pull in opposite directions.

A harbinger of what was to come came in 1964 in a study by Philip May, an English immigrant working in the California public hospital system. May compared the effects on schizophrenics of treatment with psychoanalysis alone, psychoanalysis plus drugs, drugs alone, and ECT or milieu therapy on their own. He had difficulties getting the study funded by the state of California, which suspected him of a psychoanalytic bias because his wife was a psychoanalyst.[47] The study showed that chlorpromazine on its own produced better results than any other treatment, with ECT the next best option. The study was criticized because it was conducted in state hospitals where the staff consisted of student or trainee analysts rather than fully trained psychoanalysts.

This criticism prompted a second study, conducted under the aegis of Jack Ewalt in Boston, who believed that it was important to show that nonpharmacotherapeutic methods worked. A cohort of chronic schizophrenics was transferred from Boston State Hospital to the Massachusetts Mental Health Center, then the mecca of psychoanalytic training in the United States. Selected patients daily got group therapy, rehabilitation therapy, and intensive individual psychotherapy; others were treated only with drugs. Patients getting psychotherapeutic input did not do as well as those getting thioridazine (Mellaril) alone.[48] In retrospect, it seems possible that the patients in the first group were overstimulated. But the continuing failure to demonstrate the benefits of psychotherapy were to have a long-lasting effect.

One of the striking features of the 1950s and 1960s, at least in the United States, was how much the turf wars concerned the treatment of the psychoses. Of course at that time, as I have pointed out, it was possible to produce apparent responses in many patients who had unquestionably been misdiagnosed as having schizophrenia when in reality they had other conditions. Some had drug-induced psychoses; others had manic-depressive disorders; and yet others had borderline and other personality disorders with psychotic features, and many of them would have either experienced spontaneous remissions or shown improvements with psychotherapeutic inputs. Furthermore, the more chronic and intractable patients had been transferred to state hospitals before this decade. This inversion of the standard practice in other branches of medicine, where the university department of psychiatry was usually the place to which the most difficult clinical cases were referred, was rarely commented on.[49] But also the legendary ability of major figures such as Elvin Semrad to elicit responses from truly psychotic patients when others couldn't held out hope that others could learn to copy his methods.[50]

The emergence of office-based psychoanalysis and the availability of the new drugs on prescription in the 1950s began to bring the neuroses, personality disorders, and substance misuse within psychiatry's remit. Conceptually, however, the psychoses were still at the heart of psychiatry, with the anxiety disorders on its periphery. This may explain why the mass treatment of the anxiety disorders with Miltown and later benzodiazepines and anti-depressants passed without as much complaint from psychotherapists as might have been expected. The triumph of physical therapies over analysis in the treatment of severe conditions within hospital settings was to have dramatic implications for the kind of psychiatry being practiced outside the walls of the asylums.

FROM COMMUNITY PSYCHIATRY TO ANTIPSYCHIATRY

Was it the analysts, the social psychiatrists, or the biological psychiatrists who closed the asylums? The surprising answer is that it was primarily a combination of analysts and social psychiatrists. Hospital closure was advocated by many close to the levers of political power. In the United States the key figures were the Menningers, Frances Braceland, and Robert Felix, the first director of the National Institute of Mental Health (NIMH). In Britain, Aubrey Lewis was the key figure. Biological psychiatrists, less concerned about institutionalization and more inclined to value hospital beds, were much less likely to advocate closure.

In the United States, the recognition that neuropsychiatric disorders had been the primary cause of medical discharges from military service and the leading cause of rejection of possible recruits to the military led to passage of the National Mental Health Act in 1946. The plans for this were formulated by Felix, Braceland, and William Menninger.[51] This act set up the NIMH and provided grants to establish outpatient facilities. Legislators were persuaded by psychiatrists' arguments that the early detection of problems in outpatient clinics or private practices would in due course reduce the burden of caring for chronic patients. Some of the larger states followed suit in succeeding years by authorizing funds to support outpatient facilities.

In 1955 the Joint Commission on Mental Illness and Health was established, and in 1961 it issued a report entitled *Action for Mental Health*, which in turn led to the passage in 1963 of the Community Mental Health Centers Act. This law mandated the establishment of community mental health centers as an alternative to hospitals.[52]

Community psychiatry began in France and Britain at roughly the same time.[53] In Britain, hospital doors were opened during the late 1940s and early 1950s. Voluntary admission had become possible in the 1930s. But in these countries, unlike the United States, there were few psychiatrists trying to influence government opinion. In university settings across Europe the leaders of the profession were committed neuropsychiatrists, uninterested in the problems of the asylum and all too willing to believe that schizophrenia was an incurable condition that would require long-term hospitalization. Nevertheless, in France in 1960, spurred by successful treatments with chlorpromazine, the first moves were taken to establish sectorization.[54] Psychiatric teams in future would be charged with looking after the mental health needs of the people in a specific geographic area, only some of whom were patients in asylums. In Britain, from the 1950s on, there was a surge in the establishment of outpatient facilities and day hospitals, and in the placement of new psychiatric beds in district general hospital units rather than in asylums.[55]

Along with legislative reforms to permit voluntary admissions, this drive to the community appeared to remove many of the "problems" of old-style psychiatry. "Community psychiatrists" trumpeted the reduction in the proportion of detained patients to one in ten of the hospital population.[56] The virtual disappearance of catatonics was held up as a triumph of the new psychiatry. Social psychiatrists credited the improved nutritional status and physical health of patients as well as the new hospital routines with preventing the extremes of withdrawal and isolation found in catatonia.[57]

But the psychiatric reforms of the 1960s fed into another dynamic. The decade saw the rise of the civil rights movement, the rise of feminism, and an invigorated labor movement, all of them focused on oppression. All used a rhetoric that was adapted for psychiatry and these movements in turn borrowed from the example of psychiatry. It was a time of concern for the colonization of women's minds by men, black minds by white, the young by the old, the rich by the poor. Psychiatric patients were viewed as yet another oppressed minority, their psyches manipulated by therapists. They symbolized the oppression inflicted on all other minorities.

In this matrix a new movement began to take shape that borrowed heavily from the findings produced by social psychiatry and from the institutional changes produced by social activism. At first, the leading figures in this new movement were relatively indistinguishable from the social activists within mainstream psychiatry, but soon there was a transmutation into something quite different, something that became known as antipsychiatry.[58]

One early contributor to this movement was Ronald David Laing, a Glaswegian who trained at the Tavistock Institute in London.[59] His 1960 book *The Divided Self* became an instant classic.[60] In it Laing juxtaposed the angst of prolonged adolescence with the fragility and sensitivity of a schizophrenic breakdown, suggesting that the two were in many respects indistinguishable. He set up Emil Kraepelin as the prototypical psychiatrist, a figure who alienated rather than healed. Orthodox psychiatry was one large effort on the part of an older generation to control the young, made even more menacing by the new capacities of the old to drug the young. Laing followed this book up with *Self and Others*, *The Politics of Experience*, and other books written with Aaron Esterson and David Cooper.[61]

Then in 1967, David Cooper, who had moved to Britain from South Africa, published *Psychiatry and Antipsychiatry*, which proposed that the major stumbling block to the recovery of schizophrenic patients was orthodox psychiatry with its alienating physicians and debilitating milieu.[62] What better way to learn how to be mad than to be incarcerated on a psychiatric ward? Cooper's vision was social psychiatry taken to its logical extreme. Clark and Main and others had not denied the existence of mental illness, but Cooper, Laing, and their colleagues appeared to be doing just that.

In the United States, Erving Goffman published *Asylums*.[63] In it, he demonstrated how institutions such as asylums and prisons stripped individuals of their dignity and humanity, potentially becoming, in the case of the mental hospital, the problem rather than its solution. Thomas Scheff in 1966 introduced the further sociological notion that it was the act of labeling someone mentally ill that caused the illness.[64] According to Scheff, this simple act led to obvious and clearly harmful consequences, such as institutionalization, and also to a range of other, more subtle problems and covert discrimination, not much less harmful than the obvious consequences and potentially even more problematic because of their insidious nature.

In 1961, Thomas Szasz published *The Myth of Mental Illness*, in which he claimed that the very concept of mental illness was a logical absurdity.[65] Szasz's volume was largely aimed at the psychotherapy industry in the United States, which borrowed the language of medicine, talked about medical models, and sought to treat neurotic disorders that, even by the definitions of the psychotherapists of the day, did not have a biological basis, with treatments which clearly were not physical interventions. This kind of "mental illness" was one that many European psychiatrists could agree was a myth. But psychoanalytic thinking was in the mainstream of North American psychiatric thinking and attacking the staple of office practice in the United States was perceived as an attack on all of psychiatry.

Orthodox psychiatrists missed the drivers that made 1960s antipsychiatry a story of supreme relevance to the rest of society in a way that previous psychiatric reforms had not been. There have always been reformers in psychiatry, but there was nothing remotely like antipsychiatry before 1960. There couldn't have been, for the simple reason that until World War II no "normal" people ended up in psychiatric hospitals. There was no outreach of psychiatry into the wider world and no means of incarcerating people without chains in the midst of their communities. Occasionally unmarried women who got pregnant were hospitalized in order to avoid family shame, but until World War II the vast majority of those who were committed to asylums were clearly psychotic, severely epileptic with behavioral disturbances, or mentally handicapped. Thereafter increasing numbers of neurotic people and people with personality disorders enter the asylums. The community mental health centers did nothing to reduce rates of admission to public hospitals; indeed, these rose dramatically, in some cases tripling[66] and in others rising by even greater amounts.[67] It became more and more conceivable that the people whom the antipsychiatrists Laing, Szasz, and Goffman addressed in the 1960s could themselves end up in the hospital at some point and almost certain that they would have friends or relatives who had been hospitalized.

The psychiatric reach had extended out into the community in many ways. Not only were the formerly psychotic now discharged to the community but the arrival of a range of new tranquilizers and later antidepressants available only by prescription brought quotidian distress within the psychiatric remit. Psychiatrists of the 1960s were faced with the alienation of everyday life in a way that no earlier generation of practitioners had been.

A further factor was the development of existentialist philosophy in Europe. The appalling horrors of the war posed extraordinary challenges to the prevailing social order. The Christian churches had not spoken out against the Holocaust. The structures of the state appeared capable of engineering mass oppression and barbarism, in the case of Germany, or complicity, in the case of France and Italy. Philosophers who assumed that society was stable and there was order in the universe appeared outdated. A generation of Marxist and existentialist philosophers, Jean-Paul Sartre, Albert Camus, and others, echoing the earlier work of Henri Bergson and Friedrich Nietzsche, came to the fore with works that challenged the validity of the social order. Sartre reviewed an early copy of Laing's *Politics of Experience* and agreed that "mental illness is the revolt that the free organism in its total entity invents in order to live in an unbearable situation."[68]

In France, the principles of therapeutic communities had been championed by François Tosquelles, a psychiatrist on the Republican side of the Spanish Civil War, who had set up a therapeutic community at St. Alban's Hospital in the south of France. St. Alban's never had walls. While thousands of patients died in other hospitals during the war, none died there. In the 1950s, St. Alban's captured the public imagination. Many people made pilgrimages there and came away feeling that the struggle of the Popular Front against tyranny and oppression was not yet over but had to be extended into the rest of bourgeois society.[69]

St. Alban's most notable staff member was Frantz Fanon, a black psychiatrist from the French colony of Martinique. Fanon's encounter with racism led to his writing a thesis entitled "Peau noire, masques blancs" ("Black Skin, White Masks") that was rejected by the medical faculty in Lyon. It articulates the effects of colonization on the psyche. Fanon later became a military psychiatrist in the Algerian War. Initially he treated French casualties, but soon he switched to the guerilla side. He became a fierce critic of the French, who accused Islam of inducing fatalism and laziness and viewed North Africans as lobotomized Europeans, totally neglecting the effects of colonization. He removed straitjackets, opened wards, stopped basket-making, and set up a typical North African café in a hospital outside Algiers.[70] On one level this was orthodox social psychiatry, but Fanon's language made it seem that giving a cigarette could be an act of therapy or of oppression. Assimilation had to be resisted and decolonization striven for, for both the colonized and the mad. These ideas resonated at a time when people hoped that the oppressed throughout the world could draw strength from each other as civil rights movements from India to the United States had done. Fanon's final book, *The Wretched of the Earth*, became one of the gospels of the era.[71]

In France, also, Michel Foucault put forward the thesis that there had been an unnoticed confinement of the mad and deviant through the eighteenth century.[72] Some feature of the Enlightenment had led "civilization" to lose its tolerance for madness and deviance. Efforts to move the deviants and the inefficient into asylums suggested that the capitalist order was behind this reorganization of society. If no one knew for sure what was going on, who could say whether anyone was safe? The issue at stake was a new dialectics of power. Scholars have subsequently shown conclusively that the details of Foucault's account were wrong, since what confinement there was occurred in the nineteenth rather than the eighteenth century, but the notion of a dialectics of power resonated with the work of Fanon and social psychiatrists from Belmont Hospital in Britain to the therapeutic communities in the United States. Foucault and Fanon mounted a critique of all of society that went far beyond the idea of simply making conditions in asylums more humane.

These new movements gained an unexpected ally from the ranks of orthodox psychiatrists when in 1983 Edward Hare of the Maudsley Hospital claimed that schizophrenia, the prototypical disorder of modern psychiatry, had appeared only recently.[73]

Reviewing the historical record, he found descriptions of mania and depression all the way back to the ancient Greeks but no mention of schizophrenia. Perhaps schizophrenia, Hare said, had appeared with industrialization and that was what had led to the growth of the asylums. Andrew Scull responded that far from schizophrenia appearing and medicine responding, there had been a progressive extension of the psychiatric enterprise: if you increase the provision of service, you increase the number of people identified as lunatics to fill the beds.[74]

Meanwhile in the United States, from New England through Chicago to California sensitivity groups and encounter groups had sprung up. In these groups, inspired by the work of Lewin and Moreno and therapeutic communities, normal people were being told that they were not realizing their full potential. They were finding everyday life degraded.[75] What was psychiatric illness if not an exaggerated form of this feeling?

There was also, of course, the psychedelic movement, spawned by the discovery of LSD and its seepage into mainstream culture around the mid-1950s. It spread quickly in the early 1960s.[76] Suddenly a previously inhibited generation had the scales removed from its eyes and began to see the world in three-dimensional Technicolor, a world permeated with meaning and spirituality, where conformity, status, and hierarchy appeared oppressive, a world where it appeared that this oppression might stop at nothing to achieve its ends, including driving its victims mad.

The use of psychedelic drugs was endorsed by a formidable critic of the social system, Herbert Marcuse, a cofounder of the Frankfurt School of Social Relations. Influenced by the work of Le Bon, the Frankfurt school had adapted Marxism to the new social psychiatry. A professor of philosophy variously at Columbia, Harvard, and Brandeis, in 1964 Marcuse delivered a powerful message in *One-Dimensional Man:* "the persecuted, the unemployed and the unemployable . . . exist outside the democratic process; their lives illustrate the urgent, inescapable need to put an end to institutions and conditions that are intolerable. Their opposition is revolutionary, even if their consciousness is not."[77] This book sold hundreds of thousands of copies, and it was carried around by students from New York to Rome and Tokyo. Marcuse became the ideological leader of the New Left.

The message was the same as that of John Kenneth Galbraith's *Affluent Society*,[78] that people were increasingly producing and consuming the unnecessary, but Marcuse made it revolutionary by tacking on the thesis that the capitalist system manipulated the mind of the bourgeois to make it desire what the system could produce and to call the license to consume freedom. Analyzing the resulting conflicts on the couch was for Marcuse a means of perpetuating rather than resolving the problem. For Marcuse and others on the left, the new psychedelic drugs, in contrast, offered a possible way to raise consciousness.[79]

The idea that psychiatry might help achieve progress had been fatally weakened. Until the 1960s, psychiatrists and their historians could relatively unselfconsciously talk about Pinel and Freud as psychiatry's heroes. The humane and benevolent impulses that lay behind Pinel's famous liberation of the insane from their chains had previously been seen as symbolic of all that psychiatry aimed at. A new generation saw it as a derisory gesture, likely to have sprung from ulterior motives that boded ill for the patient. Pinel and his disciple Esquirol were after all also the foremost proponents of asylum care, and French antipsychiatrists delighted in cataloguing the apparently barbarous physical interventions inflicted on the patients in asylums.

In the 1950s, a range of new chemicals from pesticides through antibiotics had appeared, and the DuPont Chemical Company coined the slogan "Better living through chemistry." Humanity was seen to be taming nature and the results could only be good. A heroic era. But in 1962, Rachel Carson's *Silent Spring* appeared, the first book to cast doubt on this heroic vision.[80] This book heralded a return to Nature and foreshadowed the birth of a Green movement later in the decade (see Chapter 8).

In the midst of this ferment not only was normal psychiatric practice seen as degraded, but psychosurgery, ECT, and neuroleptic-induced tardive dyskinesia were held up as visible degradations, symbols of all that was wrong in psychiatry. In most countries, from the United States through Europe to Japan, there was a growing clamor opposing the use of ECT. In the public mind it was indistinguishable from psychosurgery. In 1962 Ken Kesey's book *One Flew over the Cuckoo's Nest* analogized society's oppressors with psychiatric ward staff and the means of oppression with physical treatments, especially ECT.[81] Significantly, the book's hero, Randle McMurphy, though his personality was shot through with antisocial elements, could not ever have been diagnosed as psychotic. The message was that if ECT was inflicted on McMurphy it could be inflicted on anyone.

The first psychiatric survivor groups had emerged by this time, often united by their opposition to ECT. In the United States, legislatures in states from Massachusetts and Alabama to California drafted motions to ban the use of ECT.[82] In many states and many countries, it became effectively impossible to use ECT. Books critical of ECT appeared; Thomas Szasz commented on Leonard Roy Frank's *History of Shock Treatment* (1978): "what the rock and the stake were to the inquisition, what the concentration camp and the gas chamber were to national socialism, the mental hospital and electroshock are to institutional psychiatry. *The History of Shock Treatment* is a carefully researched documentation of psychiatry's 'final' solution."[83]

For British and American activists references to a final solution were largely metaphorical. But French and German psychiatrists and their activist opponents knew at first hand what the fate of psychiatric patients had been.[84] Therapeutic community meetings had inspired some large hospitals to hold meetings that often included everyone from the psychiatrist to the gardeners as well as the patients. Many participants in these meetings were against all forms of coercion. If psychiatrists suggested that methods of treatment should be subject to observation and experiment, the responses were likely to be that experimentation was a slippery slope that ended in experiments in the concentration camps.[85]

APOCALYPSE IN THE AIR

The crisis toward which the era was heading took shape in the period from the mid-1960s to the mid-1970s. From the early 1960s, the war in Vietnam and civil rights in the United States were constantly in the news. In 1967, world headlines announced the death of Che Guevara, the start of the Northern Irish Troubles, Israel's Six-Day War, and the bloody war between Nigeria and Biafra.

In early 1968, the Tet offensive in Vietnam was a major reversal for the United States. It became conceivable that America could lose the war. In Eastern Europe, the Soviet army invaded Czechoslovakia to crush the Prague Spring. In the process, however, it became clear that Soviet power was at its limit. The Eastern bloc would remain intact only by force of arms. These twin reversals for the superpowers forced them toward détente. It seemed as though the Algerians, Cubans, and Vietnamese were winning. The air of crisis was heightened by the assassinations of Martin Luther King and Robert Kennedy.

During the late 1960s there was much unrest. There were student revolutions both east and west of the Iron Curtain. In Poland, there were uprisings in 1968. In Paris in May 1968 there were protests, which ultimately led to the retirement of de Gaulle. In Italy, student protests led to $100 million damage to universities. In Mexico, army units combating student and worker protests before the 1970 Olympic Games killed several hundred. Leading intellectuals, from Bertrand Russell in Britain to Jean-Paul Sartre in France, along with Susan Sontag, Norman Mailer, and James Baldwin in the United States, joined campaigns of civil disobedience. Protests at the 1968 Democratic National Convention in Chicago, which in retrospect appear relatively small, were much magnified by the police reaction and the media coverage.

What was happening? At the time, the Western economies had been through their greatest period ever of sustained growth.[86] This success had led throughout the Western world to huge rises in the proportion of the population that were students. At the same time, the rise of feminism and the availability of the contraceptive pill were leading to dramatic changes in gender roles. The 1960s, for instance, was the first decade when the French women's clothing industry produced more pants than skirts. And television spread these political and economic changes throughout the culture.

It was a time when guerilla theater made the sit-in an art form, and Andy Warhol made an art of trash, an innocent time before rock concerts were marketed, before rule-breaking had become institutionalized, before anyone guessed that the key youth leaders would later become figures of the establishment. It was the first time that Western icons from Malcolm X to the Beatles traveled to other cultures in search of values rather than in an attempt to export supposedly superior Western values to others.

By 1972, the establishment had begun to respond. In France, most tellingly, the universities were reorganized and established hierarchies were abolished. Plans to drastically curtail access to university/college education were dropped and France as well as other Western nations moved toward a new, knowledge-based economy. In 1973, the Organization of Petroleum Exporting Countries (OPEC) dramatically increased the price of oil, and the Western world had other things to think about than how to distribute the fruits of affluence. This crisis led to the eclipse of Keynesianism and the rise of monetarism, which had extraordinary consequences for psychiatric research and culture (see Chapter 7). But neither the role of psychiatry in contributing to the crisis nor the effects of the ferment on psychiatry have been catalogued.

The Changing Face of Medicine

Psychiatry was not the only branch of medicine to undergo fundamental change in the period, although no other branches were affected to the same extent. Until 1966, there had been a general perception that the first duty of physicians was to the patient rather than to the community or to the goals of research. Physicians were still likely to cite the maxim of Claude Bernard that a physician should never perform an experiment on anyone that might harm the person in any way, even though the result might be highly advantageous to science and ultimately therefore to the health of others.[87]

This understanding of medicine was challenged for the first time around 1850 with the development of anesthesia. With anesthesia, physicians had to take the risk of killing the patient even before surgery was performed. Could one take such risks? Could one do evil in order to do good? Mainstream medicine accepted the fact that in the long run a greater number of people would benefit from surgery with rather than without anesthesia.[88] An ethical calculus was introduced into medicine concealed by ever more frequent professions of the hallowed maxim to first do no harm.

During World War II, many antidotes and vaccines were tested on retarded or mentally ill patients. Jonas Salk, for example, who was later to win fame for the creation of a vaccine against polio, tried a vaccine for influenza on mentally ill patients. There was a tacit understanding that participation in such studies, even though it was rarely voluntary, was a means by which prisoners, the mentally ill, the mentally handicapped, and others could contribute to the war effort. At the Nuremberg trials, one of the defenses put forward for the medical experimentation undertaken by the Nazis was that experimentation during the war was not confined to Nazi Germany, that at least superficially similar experiments had been performed in the Allied countries also.

Things were changing, however. The war provoked a vast

increase in research efforts related to the national interest. In the United States, the Office for Service Research and Development was established. During the war work was undertaken on antidotes, vaccines, and antibiotics, with the work on penicillin in particular leading to its vastly successful commercial production. Penicillin produced what seemed to be miraculous cures, and its example provided the impetus for continuing planned and coordinated medical research after the war. The United States established the National Institutes of Health (NIH), whose research budget grew rapidly from $700,000 in 1945 to $1.5 billion by 1970.[89] Research centers proliferated and physicians' career paths increasingly led through research.

Research by the Soviets put Sputnik into orbit, and the Americans immediately tried to emulate that technical achievement. The space race hogged the headlines, but there was a race to develop technologies in all areas and in particular in the health field. It was at this time that the hitherto small pharmaceutical divisions of chemical companies began the rapid growth that was to transform these companies into the most profitable multinational corporations on the planet.[90]

Despite the explosion of research, as of 1966 there were no institutional review boards in hospitals and no formal procedures for informing patients of the risks of a study or obtaining their consent to participate in research. It was assumed that the relationship between researchers and patients was the same as that between doctors and patients, where the interests of the patients were supposed to be paramount. In 1966, Henry Beecher shattered that assumption when he published an article detailing twenty-two cases of research studies in the United States where the subjects either clearly had not been or were unlikely to have been informed that they were participating in a research project rather than receiving routine medical care.[91]

The impact of Beecher's article was immense. The NIH and the FDA were forced to design consent forms and institute ethical review boards. A series of Senate hearings on these and related issues demonstrated that the medical attitude was that doctors should decide what patients were told. Beecher's work showed that such positions were no longer tenable. Rather he made it clear that an increasing number of clinicians were putting research ahead of clinical care. There seemed to be an unavoidable conflict of interest between patients and researchers and/or the corporations they liased with.

At this point philosophers came out of the ivory towers of linguistic philosophy and began to get involved in the emerging field of bioethics. This new set of dilemmas intersected with the emerging civil rights movements, as well as feminism and antipsychiatry. Doctors and investigators, who had previously seen themselves as heroic, were increasingly recast in the role of oppressors. Like all authority figures—teachers, husbands, parents, prison wardens, the police, and social workers—physicians were considered potential agents of the state.

Where before physicians had been permitted a certain amount of discretion, which it was assumed would work to the benefit of the patient, now there was concern that they might be chiefly motivated by self-interest. Where differences in individual practice had previously been seen as a manifestation of local conditions and interests, variations between practitioners began to be held up to scrutiny and even to be castigated.[92]

The encounter between doctor and patient was becoming less personal. Admissions to the hospital were briefer than they had been and increasingly for the purpose of undergoing a battery of tests rather than for being healed. Conversation between doctor and patient might occur during this process, but it was no longer intrinsic to it. Several books chronicled the changing nature of medical care. One of the most striking was Elisabeth Kubler-Ross's *On Death and Dying*, published in 1969, which noted that people were dying in intensive care units more profoundly alone and isolated than ever before in human history. Something was very wrong.[93]

Other problems were also cropping up. The invention of dialysis machines in 1960 was a breakthrough but one that introduced rationing. Who would decide who should live and who die?[94] The first kidney transplant in 1963 raised even larger ethical issues. Clearly a doctor acting for the patient who needed the transplant was trying to do the best for his patient, but what would the same doctor say to the person about to lose a kidney? It is often said that there is nothing new under the sun. But physicians had never faced anything quite like these ethical issues before.

The situation became even more acute with the first heart transplant in December 1967. What was a triumph to some was an agony for others, who still saw the heart as the seat of the soul. Can I still claim to be the same person with someone else's heart beating in my chest? For many, this was no simple rhetorical question. Surgeons and physicians were usurping the role of God, to such an extent that a new definition of death was required. Previously, death had been considered to occur when the heart stopped beating, but now hearts could be kept beating if it was vital that they remained in good working order until they were transplanted. In such cases how could one define death? In 1968 the Harvard Brain Death Committee was established to grapple with just this question.[95]

Medicine had the power, it seemed, not only to decide who should live and who should die, but to redefine death. A series of right-to-die cases, of which the most famous involved Karen Ann Quinlan, painted a new picture of physicians as technicians dealing with human material rather than doctors enduring with their patients. Medicine was changing from a healing ministry to an engineering profession. The desacralization of life had proceeded to the extent that the imminent end of a tax year might influence decisions as to the best date on which to turn off a respirator. Render to Caesar that which is Caesar's took on a whole new meaning.

Community efforts to have some say about the appropriate uses of the new technologies were resisted by physicians, who saw such responses as attempts to circumvent medical discretion and circumscribe medical power. Part of the problem was that physicians did not perceive that the new technologies would be produced by corporations answerable to shareholders rather than to the community at large. They also did not perceive that a process had begun whereby medical research would follow the money, potentially benefiting a favored few rather than the community at large.

In 1976, Ivan Illich articulated a new perception of medicine that turned social medicine inside out.[96] According to Illich, health technologies were developing in a manner that would ultimately threaten human well-being. In the New Medical Theocracy, a lack of belief in the importance of health would be the supreme virtue, but it would be in practice unattainable owing to the power of industrial propaganda. Illich was not alone. Discontent increasingly emerged in the mid-1970s as the medical establishment was transformed from an exclusive club into a medico-pharmaceutical complex.[97] The development of cosmetic surgery showed just how difficult it was to confine new technical developments to the traditional spheres of medicine.[98] Everything was becoming plastic and throwaway, it seemed—even people.

In the realm of psychiatry, lawyers and others fought to ensure the rights of patients to refuse treatment and to avoid detention. They campaigned to save patients from the clutches of psychiatry.[99] Clearly, therefore, the changes in psychiatry in the decade from 1965 to 1975 mirrored changes in the rest of medicine. There were major differences though. Some of those posing the greatest problems in medicine, such as the heart surgeon Christian Barnard, were public heroes. Psychiatry, in contrast, was apparently breeding monsters such as Walter Freeman, a zealous advocate of psychosurgery, and Ewan Cameron, who was responsible for psychic driving, an explicit attempt to depattern behavior by administering massive doses of ECT—work that was funded by the CIA.

Other branches of medicine had treatments that became increasingly newsworthy, but only psychiatry had treatments that were made illegal. Only psychiatry had treatments that it was thought might have political consequences, just as today only psychiatry has disorders which warrant interventions in the affairs of other countries. Given this situation, it is astonishing that the role of psychiatry has been written out of the history of the period.

The fate of LSD exemplifies this scotoma. LSD crept into clinical use in the 1950s, a twin to chlorpromazine (see Chapter 5). It was both a therapeutic agent and a research tool, which, allied with chlorpromazine, many thought might make a science of psychiatry. As part of a study to determine whether the changes it produced in any way mimicked schizophrenia, for example, Leo Hollister gave it to Ken Kesey.[100] But its spread outside the therapeutic arena in the 1960s occasioned increasing concern on the part of the establishment. An incident in Holland typified the reaction to LSD. The Dutch crown princess was engaged to marry a former German soldier. An anarchist group, Provo, campaigned against the marriage and in February 1966 threatened to spike the drinking water of the police horses controlling the crowds at the wedding with LSD. The media made much of this episode, warning that the public was "vulnerable" to such attacks. Within a month the Dutch parliament had made LSD and other hallucinogens illegal.[101] Few knew that most Western countries had detailed military plans to use hallucinogens as weapons.

In 1965, New York passed a law imposing penalties for the possession, sale, or exchange of LSD. Reports of violence, suicide, and other disturbances attributed to LSD became circulated widely. Few if any were ever substantiated. In 1968, the *New York Times* ran a story about LSD takers who under the influence of the drug had stared at the sun a long time and become blind; a few days later this story was revealed as a hoax.[102] Previously drug abuse had been seen as a working-class problem, but 1960-style substance misuse had become a political issue that put governments at odds with large sections of their political base, the middle class. These developments led, on 27 October 1970, to the replacement of the Harrison Act with the Comprehensive Drug Abuse Prevention and Control Act and the start of a war on drugs.[103]

The Social Nature of Substance Abuse

The new act classified drugs into five different schedules. Schedule 1 included drugs with a high potential for abuse and no accepted medical use. Both cannabis and LSD were placed in schedule 1, even though cannabis had been a staple of psychiatric pharmacotherapy in the nineteenth century and had a growing list of medical uses, and even though at the time LSD still held promise as both a therapy and a research tool. That a drug might cause physical dependence was an important element in the decision to place drugs in one or other of the new schedules, with the opiates, supposedly the most dependence-producing agents, also placed in schedule 1, but the example of LSD makes it clear that this was not the only consideration.

A quarter of a century later, Patricia Gilbert and her colleagues published an article on the effects of discontinuing antipsychotic medication.[104] After examining data from over a hundred trials, they were able to show that although many people could discontinue antipsychotics without adverse consequences, others could not do so. The *Archives of General Psychiatry* invited a distinguished set of experts to comment. All agreed that this was a new area deserving of close scrutiny. Far from being new, however, this was an old corpse rising to the surface, bearing on it clues to events that had occurred around 1968.

There is a considerable mystery as to why surprise and disbelief should have rippled through the psychopharmacological community in the mid-1990s following the publication of Gilbert's article. The antipsychotics were known to induce the involuntary movement disorder called tardive dyskinesia, which was first described in the 1960s. It was very visible proof that psychiatric treatment might be worse than the disease it was meant to cure. It brought the production of new antipsychotics to a halt in the 1970s. But even though tardive dyskinesia first came to attention in patients discontinuing antipsychotics and therefore is a symptom of withdrawal, somehow tardive dyskinesia got disconnected from the question of dependence. And this happened even though in the 1970s and 1980s there were good grounds to think that many patients taking an antipsychotic who developed tardive dyskinesia might never be able to stop taking the drug regardless of how hard they tried. This dependence was an order of magnitude worse than the problems faced by the takers of any other drugs—the opiates included.

How could tardive dyskinesia have got disconnected from the story of drug dependence and vanished, when as early as 1957 Leo Hollister had clearly demonstrated withdrawal problems with chlorpromazine? In the 1950s, despite the advent of streptomycin and isoniazid, every new drug that showed evidence of tuberculostatic activity in a test tube was still being tested to see if it could cure tuberculosis.[105] Still working at the time as an internist, Hollister had tested chlorpromazine on tuberculosis patients in a randomized controlled trial. It had no effects on tuberculosis but when treatment was halted after six months, six of the seventeen taking chlorpromazine had clear discontinuation problems while none taking a placebo had. Hollister made nothing of the data at the time, much to his surprise later.[106] Why not?

Trying to answer this question makes it clear how socially sensitive definitions of addiction are. The introduction of morphine in the 1820s was not associated with concerns about dependence, despite a recognition that opium could lead to addiction. Morphine was a pure compound, whose isolation from the poppy was a triumph of science. No longer were people subject to the vagaries of dosage that they got with poppies, which sometimes produced effective pain relief and sometimes did not. It was only with the introduction of the hypodermic syringe in 1856 that the first hints of problems appeared.[107] Clear recognition of a new reality came in 1878, with Edward Levinstein's book *Morphiumsucht—Morbid Craving for Morphine.*[108] Despite this, one of the first things heroin was used for was to alleviate morphine dependence.[109] At the same time, in the 1880s, Sigmund Freud was famously using cocaine to treat nervous problems, including dependence on morphine. There was no recognition that cocaine might cause cravings and dependence.[110]

By 1900, though, addiction had become increasingly recognized as a social problem, leading to the passage of Harrison Act in 1914, which made the opiates and cocaine available on prescription only.[111] The rationale behind making these drugs available only by prescription was the hope that coopting physicians as a legal source of supply would undercut the black market. Medical input might also wean addicts from their drugs. But physicians for the most part refused to participate in the new arrangements.

The modern eye can easily miss the perceptions at work here. The problem was not seen as one caused by a drug. Addiction was associated with low-life elements, with illegal trafficking in drugs, and with opium dens. Even though some famous medical practitioners did become addicts, the predominant view until the 1950s was that addiction was a matter of personality. Only sociopaths or people with personality disorders became addicts. It is easy to see how such perceptions formed. Addicts hooked on opiates and cocaine almost certainly became manipulative and engaged in crime to finance their habits, and their behavior was then interpreted by senior figures in the field such as William Martin of the Addiction Research Center in Lexington, Kentucky, as evidence of a personality disorder. Psychopathy was the real problem; addiction was just one more symptom.

That thinking changed only after World War II, when Martin's colleagues Abe Wikler and Harris Isbell put forward the notion that specific withdrawal syndromes might maintain addictions by deterring addicts from stopping. Alcohol had been known to cause delirium tremens for many years, but before

Wikler it was not clear that alcohol caused a specific physical dependence.[112] Wikler's work suggested that the addict might in fact be chemically trapped. Withdrawal syndromes were established also for the barbiturates and the opiates.

The opiates, barbiturates, and alcohol also produce tolerance. As people grow accustomed to these drugs they may have to take ever increasing doses to produce the effects they initially obtained. In addition, these drugs generally induce pleasure. Against this background Hollister's findings did not register. Chlorpromazine was not a euphoriant. When addicts were asked about it, they typically replied that it would have no street value.[113] Nor did chlorpromazine cause tolerance. Hollister's trial provided evidence of physical dependence, but this finding ran against the emerging clinical expectation that people with schizophrenia might have to take chlorpromazine throughout their lives. No one was very surprised when patients became unwell after discontinuing treatment.

Hollister also investigated Librium for the Hoffman La Roche pharmaceutical company. In 1960, he gave it in doses of up to 120 milligrams to patients with schizophrenia and then discontinued it abruptly. Within a few days many of the patients developed withdrawal syndromes, and this led Hollister to predict that there would be dependence problems with the benzodiazepines.[114] But although there was significant public debate about the benzodiazepines during the 1960s and 1970s, it did not arise from concern about their addictive potential. There were concerns that the mass tranquilization of misery might lead people to drift rather than engage in fruitful lives, and there were concerns that Roche was overpricing the benzodiazepines.[115] The failure to recognize benzodiazepine dependence is linked closely to the eclipse of LSD and the failure to recognize comparable problems with the antipsychotics.

In the 1980s, the scene changed rapidly. Peter Tyrer, Heather Ashton, and Malcolm Lader in Britain all described dependence on benzodiazepines. It began to dawn on clinicians that part of the reason why consumers continued taking these drugs was that some of them had become dependent on them. Symptoms of withdrawal, including convulsions, were described. The association between these difficulties and the pills became increasingly clear as shorter-acting benzodiazepines were introduced. The advent of Mead-Johnson's buspirone, an anxiolytic that acts on the serotonin system, raised the stakes. Mead-Johnson had an incentive to publicize the evidence of the problems caused by benzodiazepines. Lectures and symposia on these problems were sponsored and they spawned journal articles and supplements which were widely disseminated.[116]

Although traditionally addicts had been the focus of social opprobrium, in the case of benzodiazepines the hostility transferred from the supposed addicts to the medical practitioners and pharmaceutical companies that had between them, it was claimed, engineered the situation. In an antipsychiatry view of the addictions, these new addicts were seen as the unwitting victims of a medico-pharmaceutical complex.[117]

The benzodiazepine story offered a brew of politics, morality, and medicine that became one of the media events of the decade, helping in the process to place health in the forefront of media interest. Where before health had rarely featured on the front page of newspapers and had rarely received much television or radio coverage, newspapers during the 1980s developed a health page and often ran health stories on their front pages. Health became news for investigative journalists.

The professional response was one of surprise. The APA set up a committee to investigate dependence problems. This group drew attention to the fact that benzodiazepine use was not associated with tolerance and that for the most part it was only used medically. Addicts were not interested in these drugs. Escalating doses were not a feature of their use, and although the benzodiazepines were pleasant to take, they were not euphoriants. The APA accordingly drew distinctions between addiction and dependence.[118]

This action inescapably returns us to the 1960s. By the mid-1960s, even Wikler's emphasis on the role of withdrawal symptoms in maintaining addictions could not account for the emerging picture. Neither cocaine nor the amphetamines were associated with dependence syndromes, at least of the type associated with the opiates or alcohol. In addition, although there was a growing problem with LSD and other psychedelic drugs, these did not appear to produce any dependence. Users took them episodically rather than regularly.

Research efforts intensified, leading to a major discovery in behavioral pharmacology. The key early discovery had come about by accident in 1953, when James Olds found that when electrodes were placed in certain locations in the brains of rats, the animals would self-stimulate.[119] Indeed, their urge to do so could override natural appetites for food or sex, so that an animal might stimulate itself to death. In the mid-1960s, Jim Weekes, Maurice Sievers, and Robert Shuster in Michigan and Leonard Cook at SK&F found that laboratory animals could learn to self-administer drugs. In general, drugs that caused addiction in humans were preferentially self-administered by animals.[120] A way to screen for abuse liability had been discovered as well as the fact that some drugs cause cravings. Cocaine and amphetamine, which did not cause opiate-type withdrawal symptoms, turned out to be drugs that animals appeared to crave.

The concept of drug dependence emerged. Within a year of being minted the new concepts of abuse liability and drug dependence were framed in the legislation of the Comprehensive Drug Abuse Prevention Act (1970). What was written out of this script was the fact that self-administration of these drugs by animals clearly was connected with the degradation of their environment.[121]

Using the ease with which an animal can be induced to crave a drug as a yardstick, researchers found the abuse liability of the benzodiazepines was low to nonexistent.[122] Consequently, in the 1980s it made perfect sense for an addiction specialist to state that physical dependence on the benzodiazepines was possible but that they caused neither addiction nor drug dependence. This was a semantic step too far not just for the public but for most of the medical profession. In the laboratory the benzodiazepines might not be seen to be drugs of addiction, but saying that they were not drugs of addiction did not solve what had become a pressing public problem.

If the benzodiazepine problem was not an addiction problem, what was it? There was no comparable problem with benzodi-azepine use in Japan, where the market for benzodiazepines remains strong and anxiolytics are still considered useful. The strength of the Japanese anxiolytic market, furthermore, is inversely corre-lated with the small size of the antidepressant market. As of 2000, no SSRIs were available in Japan for the treatment of depression. In contrast, in the West the terms anxiolysis and tranquilizer had fallen out of use almost completely. The failure of buspirone to succeed as a nondependence-producing anxiolytic led to a switch from developing anxiolytics to developing SSRIs as antidepres-sants. If the addiction card had not been played, Prozac would probably not have been the phenomenon it was in the West and the 1990s would not have been the Age of Depression.[123]

When SSRI withdrawal was shown to exist in the late 1990s,[124] the medical establishment denied that SSRIs could be addictive. Critics responded that the SSRIs were proving to be simply an-other group of drugs in a sequence that now included the opiates, the bromides, the barbiturates, and the benzodiazepines. In all cases there had been early categoric assurances that these drugs did not lead to dependence. But some years later, when millions were taking the drugs, users faced the prospect of inadvertently becoming hooked. Depending on the slant of the commentator, the critique might include the gullibility of the medical practi-tioners, their subversion by corporate sponsorship, or the failure of regulators to insist on adequate research.

A further aspect to the developing controversy was Eli Lilly's promotion of Prozac as less likely to cause dependence than other

SSRIs.[125] This echoed Mead-Johnson's support for efforts to draw attention to the dependence produced by benzodiazepines,[126] which was in turn a replay of the tactics Roche had used to undermine the barbiturates.[127]

The establishment of SSRI dependence may finally force the psychiatric profession to face up to its demons. This will involve pinpointing the factors that for twenty years inhibited the recognition of benzodiazepine dependence. It should be remembered that, in contrast to dependence on benzodiazepines, dependence on antipsychotics had been clearly recognized in the mid-1960s but that this recognition was then lost. A series of studies in the mid-1960s demonstrated conclusively that when patients stopped even low doses of antipsychotics (such as 1 milligram of haloperidol) taken for brief periods of time (six months), significant withdrawal problems could ensue.[128] Indeed, some patients were unable to discontinue using their drug. Findings such as this led to discussions in the mid-1960s, especially at the CINP meeting in Washington in 1966, in which the concept of dependence of a nonaddictive type was accepted.[129]

But this concept of dependence of a nonaddictive type vanished almost as quickly as it appeared. It was incompatible with every theory about addiction and drug dependence that emerged from the late 1960s onward. Most theories of science stress that such an incompatibility should be the stuff of scientific breakthroughs. But the science was enmeshed with a political requirement—to dissociate therapeutic from recreational drug use. The psychopharmacological mind-set could barely begin to guess at the dimensions of the issues at stake. Antipsychotic dependence was written out of the picture so comprehensively that when the review by Gilbert and her colleagues hinted at it in 1995, the most senior experts in the field hailed the points made as entirely novel.

Dependence on the antipsychotics and SSRIs points to profound problems with theories of addiction. Current theories of addiction remain almost exclusively focused on the point when the "addict" discontinues treatment. But in the case of the antipsychotics, one of the classic withdrawal problems, tardive dyskinesia, appears commonly in the course of treatment. Tardive dyskinesia is better thought of as a stress syndrome, a term coined by Ross Baldessarini.[130] What other problems could emerge during antipsychotic treatment?[131]

When Raymond Battegay discontinued antipsychotic treatment in 1964 in a group of patients with various psychoses, only a quarter of those who experienced withdrawal symptoms had neurological problems such as tardive dyskinesia. The other three quarters exhibited increased sensitivity to heat or stress, abdominal problems, rapid alterations in mood, and a range of other symptoms. Clearly, these manifestations were not a reemergence of the original illness. First, they appeared almost instantly on withdrawal, whereas an illness relapse would have been expected only weeks or months later. Second reinstituting treatment with a low dose of the antipsychotic drug very quickly fixed the problem, whereas treating a new illness episode usually requires hefty drug doses and can take weeks or months to become effective.

If this condition can be easily managed by reinstituting treatment, where is the problem? The serious but manageable problem is that people having these types of difficulties who want to discontinue treatment may be unable to do so without experiencing lengthy and significant discomfort. The potentially unmanageable problem is that it becomes impossible once patients have taken antipsychotics for some time to know where the treatment ends and the disease begins. It is conceivable that part of the neurotic and dysthymic features that are considered negative features of schizophrenia today are treatment-induced phenomena rather than manifestations of the illness (see Chapter 7). There has been since 1968 a substantial body of evidence indicating that just this may in fact be the case.[132] Similar problems may beset the SSRIs.

This is a prospect that the pharmacotherapy establishment cannot view with equanimity. But what of the alternative, which essentially comes down to recognizing that while dependence is a pharmacological issue, addiction is a social one with political implications? The concepts of drug dependence that first took shape in the late 1960s set the stage for disease models of addiction, which came to dominate in the 1990s. The historical evidence that therapeutic communities might do more for a larger number of addicts than drug treatments was nowhere to be heard when in the late 1990s two new agents, naloxone and acamprosate, hit the market (see Chapter 8).

Tackling these issues would mean revisiting the late 1960s and trying to figure out exactly what happened—trying to establish the social factors that could in the 1990s make methylphenidate (Ritalin) a drug widely prescribed for children, and used with few if any qualms by millions of parents, even though it differs little in its pharmacological profile from cocaine. By the 1990s, the perception of physicians was that Valium is more addictive than heroin.[133] This perception, which has no basis in pharmacology, makes it entirely possible that a combination of events and forces similar to that which led to the demonization of the benzodiazepines could remove Prozac from the therapeutic arsenal. The examples of Ritalin and Valium suggest that addiction and theories of addiction are context dependent, and these examples also point to a link between the role of disease concepts in psychiatry and social order.

SIGNS OF THE TIMES

In the late 1960s, psychiatry was faced with the enemy at the gate. Given that of all the branches of medicine in 1968 psychiatry had the most flourishing counter-culture, the most vigorous ethical debates, and the most doubtful legitimacy, one of the astonishing features of what happened in the 1970s and 1980s was that psychiatry ended up being the medical discipline least affected by the emergence of bioethics. Far from leading medicine to a new value system or a new engagement with social realities, psychiatry retreated from the social domain and hewed to a strict biomedical model, as exemplified by the development of the dopamine hypothesis of schizophrenia, a story outlined in Chapter 5.

Just the year before Gilbert's article appeared, DSM-IV, the manual in which psychiatric disorders are now classified, stated: "A diagnosis of substance dependence should be considered only when, in addition to having prolonged physiological dependence, the individual using the substance shows evidence of a range of problems (e.g., an individual who has developed drug seeking behavior to the extent that important activities are given up or reduced to obtain the substance)."[134] A committee of the great and the good had decided that antipsychotic, antidepressant, or benzodiazepine dependence could not occur.

But as will become clear in Chapter 6, the way the antipsychotic story evolved cannot be understood without reference to the peculiar neuroleptic withdrawal syndrome tardive dyskinesia. Efforts to get to grips with this led in the 1990s to the replacement of neuroleptics with antipsychotics. The story also cannot be understood without the realization that psychiatry's legitimacy was sharply challenged from 1965 to 1975. The scientific methods used in response to this crisis, a recourse to operationalization and measurement, I will argue in Chapters 7 and 8, far from solving the problem, have in fact led to a deepening of the crisis.

In the short term the slippery slope facing psychiatry in the late 1960s led not to anarchy but to DSM-III. Ironically, in *The Divided Self*, a poetic volume, Laing drew attention to Emil Kraepelin, and thereby did as much as anyone to resurrect the reputation of the man whose apparent delineation of discrete mental illnesses became the defining feature of a neo-Kraepelinian movement in the United States. This resurrection, ultimately through the institution of DSM-III, was to reimpose an order on world psychiatry. Ironically, however, when the psychiatric establishment fought to overthrow antipsychiatry and reinstitute an order that would make the world safe again, it did so for a generation of psychiatrists many of whom came into psychiatry because of the appeal of the works of Laing, Szasz, and Foucault, as well as of the encounter groups that had sprung from the work of Lewin and had given rise to humanistic psychotherapies.

Those moving into psychiatry in the 1980s entered a corporate psychiatry, quite unlike anything that had existed before. These newcomers knew the patient movements well and played a part in turning groups like the National Association for the Mentally Ill (NAMI) and others away from the radical end of psychiatry. NAMI provided the model for the formation of patient groups such as groups of OCD sufferers, of those with social phobias, of depressive patients, and others, most of which by the 1990s were extensively penetrated by the pharmaceutical industry, which had recognized that patients were often the best lobbyists for new treatments. Meanwhile the insights of Lewin that had influenced military psychiatry and led to deinstitutionalization played less and less of a part in clinical psychiatry from the 1970s on and an ever greater part in the evolution of the science of corporate management.

But all this lay in the future. While they waited in times of trouble for a messiah, psychiatrists and their patients witnessed many dramatic scenes that were signs of the time. One was a debate in the Stephen Leacock auditorium at McGill University in Montreal in 1971 on the validity of psychiatry. The protagonists were Herbert Marcuse and Heinz Lehmann, chlorpromazine's first advocate in North America. Marcuse's invitation had come from Frederick Qunes, who was the seconder on his side of the debate. During the debate, while Lehmann was speaking, Qunes flung a cream cake in his face. Lehmann, apparently unperturbed, kept on speaking.

This gesture achieved mythic status in the annals of biological psychiatrists as an example of the vilification the early proponents of chlorpromazine had to endure at the hands of the psychoanalytic establishment.[135] This was ironic because Marcuse's thesis was that the psychologization of social distress was the key problem. As one who believed that drugs like chlorpromazine acted to open patients up to psychodynamic approaches, Lehmann had volunteered to debate Marcuse when none of Montreal's psycho-analysts would. Even more ironically, none of the participants in the debate referred to or appeared to be aware that they were de-bating within miles of the Allan Memorial Hospital, where Ewan Cameron had engaged in "brainwashing" research, funded in part by the CIA.[136] This involved an alarming physical degradation of patients undertaken by a man who had been one of the Allied psy-chiatrists at the Nuremberg trials.[137]

Other signs could be found in Japan. In 1969, following visits to the country by Szasz, Laing, and other antipsychiatrists, Japan-ese students revolted and occupied the department of psychiatry at Tokyo University.[138] This was a revolt against biological psy-chiatry, against the dominance of Tokyo in the Japanese hierarchy, and against authority in general. Hiroshi Utena, the professor of psychiatry at the university, was forced from office by student dis-approval of biological research he had done in the 1950s. The university department was to remain occupied by students for ten years, bringing all research to a halt.[139]

But the most potent sign of the times must surely be the ran-sacking of the office of Jean Delay in the department of psychiatry at the University of Paris by French students in 1968. Not only was Delay, by virtue of his position, a symbol of the hierarchical order the students hoped to destroy, but he was intensely commit-ted personally to that hierarchy. He relished its trappings and honors and celebrated its capacity to bring about progress.[140] Chlorpromazine for him was a symbol of the capacity of psychia-try to restore order to the world. But an older world order based on hierarchy and deference was giving way to a new world, which had no sympathy for him, a world that chlorpromazine had done much to create, in ways he could never have understood. The stu-dents, guided by Laborit's view that chlorpromazine caused indif-ference, proclaimed it a means of buttressing a madness-inducing social order. Where chlorpromazine had been hailed as liberating the mad from their chains sixteen years earlier, it was now seen as the dreaded camisole chimique (or chemical straitjacket) and its self-professed creator was a target for the revolutionaries. Where psychiatrists had acclaimed the new silence that reigned in psychiatric hospitals, the students took up the cry of the antipsychiatrists that this was the silence of the cemetery. Delay's office was invaded and ransacked. When the university proposed a reorganization in the face of student demands, Delay resigned.[141]

5

Twisted Thoughts
and Twisted Molecules

In 1938, Albert Hofmann and his colleagues in the laboratories of Sandoz Pharmaceutical Company synthesized a series of ergot derivatives, to see whether they could produce synthetic derivatives that would be more effective than the naturally occurring alkaloids of ergot. Ergotamine, which had first been isolated in 1918, was used extensively by midwives in managing labor because it caused the uterus to contract. It was also known to cause blood vessels to constrict and to stop hemorrhages.[1] Synthetic forms therefore had considerable medical potential.

Ergot has been known from antiquity. It is found in a fungus growing on rye and other grains, which was long known to cause a variety of conditions such as St. Vitus's Dance and St. Anthony's Fire. These conditions got their names from the disturbances of blood flow to limbs, which led to gangrene, or from the behavioral frenzy that ergot produces. The visions and mass hysteria that it causes may conceivably have played a part in what were considered for centuries to be religious or transcendental manifestations.[2] Some of the midwives using ergot almost certainly were perceived as witches.[3] A strong case can be made that the events leading to the Salem witch trials in 1692 and the grande peur that preceded the French Revolution in 1789 were related to outbreaks of ergotism.[4]

Hofmann devised a method of adding a methyl group to ergotamine to produce methergine. This was more effective than ergotamine for the management of labor, testifying to human abilities to improve on natural products. Lysergic acid is the core molecule within ergotamine, and Hofmann produced a series of lysergic acid derivatives, the twenty-fifth of which was lysergic acid diethylamide, which accordingly was named LSD-25.[5] There were hopes that these other derivatives might produce quite different effects than did methergine. Some of the molecules in the series resembled nikethimide, a stimulant used in anesthesia at the time. Ernst Rothlin, the head of the laboratories, gave the new series to animals and found some cardiorespiratory stimulation as well as some oddities of behavior, but these were not further explored at the time.

In 1943, Hofmann returned to the LSD series and in a tale of mythic simplicity accidentally discovered a new world. While working in the laboratories, he felt unwell, went home, and found that his world had been transformed. His perceptions were unstable and fantastic. He seemed to be seeing sounds. This disorienting experience lasted several hours. Wondering afterward what had happened, he concluded that he must have inhaled some dust of LSD-25 by accident. If this was the origin of his extraordinary experiences, the changes in behavior had been brought about by an improbably minuscule amount of the compound.

Several days later he repeated the experiment under supervision, preparing for himself a dose of 0.25 milligrams of LSD, which he considered the lowest conceivably active dose. His hunch proved correct. LSD-25 had caused his first bizarre experience. He was overwhelmed again with strange experiences of even greater intensity and duration than previously. His second hunch was wrong. A 0.2-milligram dose was higher than the lowest active dose.

One of the reasons why LSD did so much to shape thinking in

the 1950s is the lowness of the dose that causes effects. The fact that a vanishingly small amount of drug had to dissolve in and disperse through the body before affecting behavior, and that an even smaller dose penetrated the brain, suggested strongly that there must be a receptor or specific site of action on which LSD was acting like a key that would unlock the changes it brought about. Mescaline, in contrast, had to be given in doses of hundreds of milligrams to produce similar effects. At dose levels this high, it was easy to see mescaline as a poison that overwhelmed brain functioning, but this was not the case with LSD.

Doses of mescaline large enough to cause hallucinations were large enough to be detected in the body at postmortem, and the argument against the relevance of exogenous toxins such as mescaline to mental illness lay in the failure to detect postmortem traces of any possible toxin in the brains of psychotic patients. LSD, which produced comparable "psychotic" effects without leaving visible traces, revived the possibility that the body produces an endogenous psychotogen, reactivating a line of thinking that had lain dormant for a hundred years. In 1845 Jean-Joseph Moreau de Tours had written a famous book, *Hashish and Mental Alienation*, in which he described the results of the experiments of the Club De Haschischins in Paris.[6] Members of this club included the poet Charles Baudelaire and others who took hashish with results that were very like those found in Thomas De Quincey's celebrated *Confessions of an Opium-Eater*. Moreau de Tours went on to speculate about correspondences between experiences induced by hashish and the forms of mental illness then being seen in the recently created French asylums. Moreau de Tours's extraordinarily imaginative leap was even more perceptive than it might first seem, since the exemplar of insanity in 1845 was still the delirious state and for this state hashish-induced disturbances still are an excellent model.

The next foray into this new field came in the 1890s when Arthur Heffter isolated mescaline from the peyotl cactus. It was known that the Indians of New Mexico and Mexico had been using this cactus for religious purposes and that it was a hallucinogen of some sort. The hallucinogenetic use of mescaline, which was named after the mescal buttons the cactus produced, brought new players into the story. One of the most famous neurologists of the day, Silas Weir-Mitchell, took mescaline and described the effects. Mescaline-induced experiences formed an important part of William James's book *The Varieties of Religious Experience*, in which he argued that these drug-induced alterations of consciousness held lessons for students of religious experience.[7]

Notwithstanding these famous experiments, the dominant view within psychiatry was that drug-induced alterations of consciousness and experience had little clinical relevance. The leading philosopher of psychiatry, Karl Jaspers, argued that drugs producing such effects were poisons which overwhelmed normal brain functioning, and that the disturbances induced by these exogenous triggers were actually quite different from the endogenous disturbances of classic mental illness.[8] All this changed with LSD and demonstrations that chlorpromazine could block or reverse LSD-induced psychoses.

Initially Sandoz kept quiet about its problem child. But word began to leak out. In 1950 there was an outbreak of ergot poisoning in France in the town of Pontorson. Jean Delay was asked to investigate and gave Jean Thuillier the task.[9] Thuillier approached Sandoz because he was aware of its work on ergot derivatives. Rothlin gave him LSD to take back to Paris. In a famous series of experiments Thuillier and others gave LSD to a variety of animals to see its effects, for example what impact there was on the way spiders wove their webs. The hope was that if they could produce an animal model of madness they might be able to screen for new therapeutic agents.[10]

Coincident with the emergence of chlorpromazine, investigators began giving LSD, mescaline, and other psychotomimetic compounds to both patients and volunteers, including their colleagues, with a number of aims. One was to explore resemblances between these model psychoses and the naturally occurring psychoses. On the assumption that there was overlap, some clinicians wanted to have such compounds to gain some insight on the world of the insane. But in addition, chlorpromazine, and later haloperidol, when given beforehand, blocked the effects of LSD and mescaline and when given afterward helped resolve the conditions they induced. Psychiatry, it seemed, had overnight become scientific. Madness could be induced and resolved within hours. If this was the case, it could surely be studied systematically and would quickly yield up its secrets.[11] The model psychoses flourished hectically but they were to die out almost as quickly and comprehensively as they had first appeared when LSD was banned in the late 1960s.

LSD intersected with psychiatry in many other ways. It was used as a treatment for neuroses, personality problems, and alcohol dependence.[12] But of central importance was its contribution to two ideas. One was the notion of the receptor, the specific target mechanism, on which LSD appeared to act so sensitively. The other was the transmethylation hypotheses of the cause of schizophrenia, which became the dominant biological theories for twenty years, but which have since disappeared almost completely from both popular and scientific consciousness.

THE TRANSMETHYLATION HYPOTHESES

In 1951, John Smythies, a registrar at St. George's Hospital in London, and a medical student, Julian Redmill, noticed, as others had, that mescaline was chemically related to epinephrine. In 1932, for example, Henk de Jong, in a paper on experimental catatonia, pointed to the same structural similarity and suggested that a disturbance of epinephrine metabolism might result in the production of a mescaline-like compound in the body that would cause catatonia.[13] Since catatonia was one of the primary forms of schizophrenia, the implications for schizophrenia in general were clear.

Smythies' observations themselves, then, involved no great discovery, but what he did next led to important developments. He wrote for further information to a psychologist, Robert Thouless of Cambridge, whom he had met at the Society for Psychical Research. Thouless introduced him to John Harley-Mason, an organic chemist, who had done work on epinephrine metabolism. Harley-Mason worked at the Cambridge Department of Physiology, where the first steps had been taken to identify the metabolic pathways through which norepinephrine and epinephrine were broken down. Derek Richter and Herman Blaschko had discovered the enzyme monoamine oxidase there in 1938, and it later became famous as a site on which some antidepressants acted.[14] Richter had also found a breakdown product of epinephrine, which he called adrenochrome, because it was pink.

Smythies's question for Harley-Mason when they met in his room after dinner was whether there were breakdown products of adrenergic metabolism that could produce altered mental states. Harley-Mason's response introduced a theme that was to resonate through the following two decades. He pointed out that the addition or subtraction of methyl groups was one of the main synthetic or degradative steps in the body for amines like epinephrine. He outlined a number of metabolic pathways that might produce compounds, some of which could conceivably be psychotomimetic. In the ordinary course of events, dopamine is a precursor of norepinephrine; norepinephrine, in turn, is O-methylated to epinephrine. One possibility was that rather than norepinephrine being O-methylated to epinephrine, dopamine might be inappropriately N-methylated to di-methyl-phenylethylamine (DMPA). And since phenylethylamine and amphetamine are structurally similar, there seemed a real possibility that DMPA could be an endogenous psychotogen. Harley-Mason called the process that led to inappropriate methylation transmethylation.

There were a number of distinguished psychiatrists at St. George's at the time, but none was interested in this new hypothesis. The only person to show any interest was Humphrey

Osmond, a senior resident, who thought the transmethylation hypothesis was worth testing clinically.[15] Several months later, Osmond moved from London to Saskatchewan, to take up a position as the assistant director at the main mental hospital in Weyburn. The director was an ex-patient and former drug addict whose chauffeur appeared at times to be running the hospital. Osmond took over and invited Smythies to join him.

The recently appointed provincial director of research was Abram Hoffer. Hoffer and Osmond hit it off and in conjunction with Smythies they wrote a paper on endogenous psychotogens. But rather than Harley-Mason's DMPA, they plumped for adrenochrome as the likely candidate.[16] An asthmatic patient had provided a lead. During attacks he injected himself with an epinephrine solution. If this solution was left lying around for a while it developed a slightly pink color—it oxidized. When the patient injected himself with this pink solution he developed psychotic symptoms. Osmond and Hoffer prepared doses of adrenochrome, took them, and reported that the agent produced a psychotomimetic response.

At a time when chlorpromazine had not yet been produced, this discovery offered attractive treatment possibilities. Hoffer and Osmond were quick to come up with one. The B3 vitamin, nicotinic acid, is methylated in the body to nicotinamide. Conceivably, then, giving large doses of nicotinic acid would mop up all the methyl donors in the body that could be used to convert norepinephrine to epinephrine, and if epinephrine were produced in smaller amounts, its potentially toxic by-product, adrenochrome, would also be produced in smaller amounts.

At this stage there was no evidence that epinephrine or adrenochrome occurred in the brain, but there was nevertheless a real plausibility to these hypotheses. In 1915 Walter Cannon had been the first to implicate sympathin, as he called the extracts from the adrenal gland, in mediating stress responses. In the 1950s, the stress theories of Hans Selye were influential, and it was firmly established that norepinephrine, epinephrine, and cortisone, the hormones of the adrenal gland, mediated stress responses. The synthesis and commercial production of cortisone led to demonstrations of its beneficial effects in treating a variety of conditions, from respiratory disorders to rheumatoid arthritis. It made sense that abnormalities or derailments of the stress response could lead to mental disorders. Claims that this was so led to some of the earliest controlled trials in psychiatry, using cortisone. These failed to find any beneficial effects of cortisone.[17]

Hoffer and Osmond's work serendipitously appeared at just the same time as the discovery of norepinephrine in the brain by Marthe Vogt,[18] along with the discovery of 5HT (serotonin) in the brain by Irvine Page and Maurice Rapoport in the United States[19] and by Tom Crawford and Jack Gaddum in Britain.[20] The possibility that an endogenous psychotogen might actually exist in the brain was opening up. This, allied with the emerging awareness of the psychotomimetic effects of LSD, put Hoffer and Osmond's work at the forefront of biological speculation.

Hoffer and Osmond gave nicotinic acid in large doses to three schizophrenic patients and obtained apparently good responses. They applied to the Canadian Association for Mental Health for funds to do further research and were told they needed to undertake a placebo-controlled trial. This they did, publishing the first results in 1954, which showed that nicotinic acid did enhance recovery among schizophrenics. In subsequent studies, they included chlorpromazine and claimed that the combination of nicotinic acid and chlorpromazine produced responses that were superior to those produced by chlorpromazine alone.[21] These were among the earliest randomized clinical trials (RCTs) in psychiatry. Hoffer has since decried RCTs, saying that it would have been more appropriate to study further the populations who apparently did and did not respond to nicotinic acid before proceeding to clinical trials. Interestingly, just as the transmethylation hypothesis has been written out of history, Hoffer and Osmond's RCT is seldom cited when the history of such trials is written.

The work of Hoffer, Osmond, and Smythies was important

for three reasons. They had produced a coherent theory of schizophrenogenesis, along with a treatment that appeared to produce some benefits and certainly provoked considerable interest. In addition, their ideas tapped straight into an increasing public awareness of the hallucinogens, which as a group were referred to as the psychedelic drugs, a term coined by Osmond. The heady buzz that resulted made Saskatchewan in the 1950s one of the focal points of the psychiatric universe. Famous figures such as Aldous Huxley made the pilgrimage to meet Osmond and Hoffer to learn more about the science of the psychedelics.[22] Huxley's *Brave New World* put the notion of the psychopharmacology of behavioral control on the map.[23] His *Heaven and Hell* and *The Gates of Perception* and other works put the psychedelics on the literary and cultural maps as well as the scientific map.[24]

In addition, a flurry of confirmatory reports of the benefits of nicotinic acid came from researchers around the world.[25] Smythies drummed up support from Heinrich Kluver in Chicago, one of the most distinguished neuroscientists of the day. From Chicago Smythies traveled to Canberra to visit the laboratory of John Eccles, a neurophysiologist and Nobel laureate. With this kind of backing, the scientific world took notice. After all, in addition to treatment implications, there were testable consequences of the hypothesis. If some process in the body was functioning abnormally and producing psychotogens, then these metabolic products should be detectable in blood or urine. This idea was fed into the mainstream of neurochemical science in the 1950s, when much effort was expended to elucidate metabolic pathways and discover the enzymes responsible for converting one biochemical molecule into another more or less active product or breakdown metabolite. Urine, blood, and other bodily fluids were being screened for just the kind of product that the transmethylation hypotheses predicted.

One of the key players in this emerging field was Seymour Kety, the chief of the neuroscience laboratories at the National Institute for Mental Health in the United States. Kety was possibly the most distinguished neuroscientist of his generation. He gave the Osmond, Hoffer, and Smythies papers to Julius Axelrod, suggesting that Axelrod try sorting out the metabolic pathways for epinephrine. Axelrod did and discovered the enzyme catechol-O-methyl-transferase (COMT), an enzyme whose existence was predicted by the hypotheses of Harley-Mason and Smythies. COMT, along with monoamine oxidase (MAO), were steps on the breakdown pathway for epinephrine and nor-epinephrine. The combination of MAO and COMT enzymes, however, did not account for the termination of the actions of norepinephrine, and efforts to find other mechanisms led Axelrod to the discovery of monoamine reuptake mechanisms, for which he won a Nobel Prize.[26]

This search for metabolites drove research in biological psychiatry for over two decades. Laboratories throughout the world engaged in the hunt not just for adrenochrome but for metabolic products of various sorts. One of the major triumphs of the period was the discovery of the cause of phenylketonuria. This devastating and common mental handicap turned out to be due to a simple inborn error of metabolism. Infants after birth could be tested and screened for the disorder, and if phenylalanine was removed from their diet mental handicap did not result. In this period were discovered such compounds as vanillylmandelic acid (VMA), a breakdown product of epinephrine found in the urine, 5-hydroxy-indole-acetic acid (5HIAA), a breakdown product of 5HT, and homovanillic acid (HVA), a breakdown product of dopamine.[27] In the mid to late 1950s, some of these metabolites were found to be elevated in carcinoid syndrome (5HIAA) and pheochromocytoma (VMA) to levels that have made them useful ever since as diagnostic markers of these conditions.[28] Such discoveries opened up the prospect that, even if an endogenous psychotogen could not be found, a diagnostic marker for schizophrenia or other psychoses might be.

Along with the triumphs of insulin replacement strategies for diabetes, thyroid hormone replacement strategies for thyroid disorders, and vitamin replacement strategies for diseases such as pellagra, which sometimes had cerebral manifestations, the decade between 1957 and 1967 saw the flourishing of metabolic psychiatry. Psychiatric disorders, according to the new breed of biological psychiatrists, were clearly physiological or biochemical disorders that had functional or behavioral manifestations. There was a belief that if everything being taken in by the body and being put out by the body could be measured, answers to pressing questions would surely appear. Rolf Gjessing was an early exponent of the approach, conducting experiments in the 1930s that appeared to show a metabolic abnormality in patients with periodic catatonia (Chapter 2).[29]

Given the role of phenylalanine in the production of phenylketonuria, one of the obvious things to do was to administer other amino acids in loading doses to see whether any of them caused people prone to mental illness to decompensate. Loading with L-tyrosine, the precursor for norepinephrine, or with L-tryptophan, the precursor for 5HT, might produce problems. Neither did. Loading with L-methionine, however, did produce problems. This has been one of the most widely replicated findings in clinical psychiatry. Subjects with major mental illness given methionine become more perplexed, confused, disoriented, and unwell.[30] This was exactly what might have been predicted by Hoffer and Osmond's theories. Methionine is a methyl donor.

Then in 1962 came what seemed like an almost inevitable breakthrough. Arnold Friedhoff reported that he had discovered a pink spot in the urine of patients with schizophrenia.[31] That pink spot appeared to be Harley-Mason's di-methyl-phenylethylamine (DMPA). Up to fifty groups attempted to replicate the finding. Many confirmed Friedhoff's finding, but others could not find the pink spot or suggested that it was a metabolite of chlorpromazine, or raised the possibility of a dietary component.[32] The biggest study, of eight hundred patients, was undertaken by Raymond Bourdillon and Cyril Clarke in Liverpool.[33] Controlling for clinical types of the disease, they found that certain forms of schizophrenia were associated with the production of pink spots in up to 90 percent of cases, whereas other forms showed little or no evidence of pink spot activity. When DMPA was injected into experimental animals, it produced experimental catatonia. And since catatonia was then still thought of as a schizophrenic disorder, this finding seemed further strong confirmatory evidence that some form of the transmethylation hypothesis was correct.

Further discoveries were made. Steven Szara, working on the serotonin pathway, postulated that transmethylation might lead to the production of di-methyl-tryptamine (DMT), another known hallucinogen.[34] DMT was never found in the urine of patients with schizophrenia, but bufotenine, another potentially hallucinogenic breakdown product of 5HT, was.[35] Adrenochrome was also confirmed as a hallucinogen.[36] Daniel Efron, who had moved from Yale to be head of research at the NIMH, reported that there were reductions in methylated metabolites of histamine in people with schizophrenia.[37] It was also noted that transmethylation could interrupt the production of melatonin, which had already been recognized as a by-product of serotonin that played a role in biological rhythms. It also appeared that transmethylation might cause the production of metabolites in the sweat of patients with schizophrenia, which would in turn produce unusual odors—and in fact a regular feature of clinical descriptions of schizophrenia over the previous century was that patients exuded unusual odors.[38]

The great volume of work being done meant that any doubts about transmethylation were easily shrugged off. Pink spots had been identified through the use of paper chromatography. Metabolites of chlorpromazine and of tea as well as DMPA clustered in the same spot when this technique was used. It was impossible to control for all three at the same time. Later, when more sophisticated techniques such as spectroscopy became available, it became clear that whatever was happening had, in most cases, nothing to do with DMPA.[39] But even this finding had little effect on the transmethylation story.

Another major figure was the Nobel Prize–winner Linus Pauling, who suggested that schizophrenia might involve a deficiency of the enzyme nicotine adenine deaminase (NAD). A deficiency of NAD could lead to a cerebral form of pellagra, which might be treatable with large amounts of niacin or nicotinic acid. This approach fitted well with Hoffer's ideas. The philosophy behind these theories was ultimately to give rise to a new branch of therapeutics called orthomolecular psychiatry. This has at its core a therapeutic approach to psychiatric disorders that involves giving patients vitamins, metals involved in biological processes, or other naturally occurring elements and sometimes administering very high doses of these substances to absorb toxic by-products—megavitamin therapy.

If variations on the pink spot story remained at center stage, neither Hoffer nor Osmond did. Eager to push the hypothesis further, Hoffer bought chromatography equipment and used it in his research; in 1958 he published an article the *American Journal of Psychiatry* claiming that he had found adrenochrome in blood.[40] This claim ran counter to the findings in studies conducted by the NIMH, and the NIMH sent an investigator to check Hoffer's procedures. The unpublished NIMH view was that Hoffer had detected ascorbic acid rather than adrenochrome. Hoffer refused to back down. This created a difficult situation. The organizers of meetings could not ask him to present data that were generally thought to be false. Although he was a participant in all the early psychopharmacology meetings, Hoffer slipped off the stage after 1958.

Meanwhile, the findings of potentially hallucinogenic metabolites lent weight to a reformulation of the transmethylation hypothesis by Seymour Kety. Kety suggested investigating a general disposition to transmethylation. The new focus should be on instabilities of the methylation process rather than on any toxic by-products, which might vary according to individual constitutional types and accordingly would not be detected in a general population of schizophrenics. One schizophrenic might have a quite different toxic metabolite than did another. This new hypothesis, if true, would explain why the clinical presentations of schizophrenia were so diverse.[41] Smythies formulated another version of the same idea called the one-carbon-cycle hypothesis.[42]

These variations on the original hypothesis helped explain why a loading dose of methionine, particularly when given in combination with a monoamine oxidase inhibitor, led to a decompensation in patients with schizophrenia. They also suggested that S-adenosyl methionine (SAMe) should be of benefit in the management of some nervous conditions. A series of studies reported favorable results, suggesting that SAMe had restorative properties of some sort, almost more antidepressant or tonic in nature than specifically antipsychotic. SAMe went on to achieve considerable sales in southern Europe as a liver tonic and in a range of other countries as an over-the-counter health adjuvant.[43] Studies by Ross Baldessarini and his colleagues, reported in 1979, showed, however, that methionine loading increased SAMe but did not increase transmethlyation.[44]

The Eclipse of Transmethylation

By the time of Baldessarini's 1979 finding, the transmethylation hypotheses had already been eclipsed. In 1963, Arvid Carlsson sowed the seed of what was later to become the dopamine hypothesis of schizophrenia, an entirely different type of hypothesis. The transmethylation hypotheses proposed a pathological mechanism as the source of the clinical features of psychosis. From that kind of theory, logical therapeutic strategies can be derived. The dopamine hypothesis of schizophrenia, in contrast, argued backward from the efficacy of the treatment to what might be the cause of the disorder. That made little more sense than arguing that because aspirin was useful in treating rheumatoid arthritis there must be some kind of aspirin deficiency implicated in rheumatoid arthritis. Yet, despite its weakness, the dopamine hypothesis of schizophrenia was successfully used by the pharmaceutical industry to sell drugs.

Many clinical trials to investigate the utility of nicotinic acid were set up by the Canadian Association of Mental Health, and these were unable to confirm the original reports of Hoffer and his colleagues.[45] By the time this series of studies were fully reported, however, transmethylation and nicotinic acid were all but dead. Hoffer's reaction was that he and his colleagues were being foiled by the powerful pharmaceutical industry and by the NIMH. No one could take out patents on nicotinic acid or on any of the agents he and Osmond had proposed. Hoffer continued to insist on the benefits of the orthomolecular approach. But while transmethylation had once been at the heart of biological psychiatry and had been railed at by the critics of biological psychiatry, it now was the alternative biological psychiatry, attracting criticism from the pharmaceutical industry and mainstream biological psychiatry.

It remains completely unexplained to this day why methionine loading causes decompensations in psychotic patients, and the transmethylation hypotheses continue to have considerable face validity. It turned out that there was comparatively little epinephrine in the brain, compared with the amount of norepinephrine or dopamine found there, and therefore comparatively little opportunity for adrenochrome to occur in the brain and cause symptoms. But norepinephrine and dopamine are metabolized to noradrenochrome and dopaminochrome, and oxidative stress can give rise to a variety of semiquinones in the brain that are highly toxic. These may well turn out to be involved in the pathogenesis of a range of disorders from Parkinson's disease to some psychoses.[46] Nevertheless, current neuroscientists and biological psychiatrists have completely forgotten about the transmethylation hypotheses that dominated the field for over two decades and were espoused by Nobel Prize–winners, Nobel candidates, and other senior figures in the field.

The Eclipse of LSD

The transmethylation story became an almost classic 1960s story, and therein may lie one explanation for the demise of these hypotheses. In part they had depended on the LSD model of psychosis to underpin them. By the mid-1960s, the validity of LSD as a model for schizophrenia had been investigated extensively. One of the primary investigators was Leo Hollister, who gave LSD to volunteers and patients, and by comparing their experiences with that of psychotic patients demonstrated that there were profound differences between the two groups.

LSD had also been used to treat alcoholism, as well as other substance misuse and neurotic conditions. In many places, such as the Allan Memorial Institute in Montreal, LSD or other hallucinogens were given to break down the defenses of neurotic patients.[47] One of the unusual features of these therapies was that many patients exposed to LSD reported childhood abuse of varied sorts (see Chapter 7). The standard response from psychiatrists was not to take these reports as evidence of the actual occurrence of abuse. Most psychiatrists thought that such reports of abuse had been shown by Freud to be elements of the fantasy life of patients. This notion was what gave rise to the idea that LSD could cut deep into the fantasy life of patients, potentially breaking down their defenses.[48] But as the claims made for these approaches began to be tested systematically, little evidence emerged of benefits produced by LSD.[49]

Furthering the eclipse of the LSD and endogenous hallucinogen hypothesis was the societal reaction to LSD in the 1960s. LSD was perceived as an agent of the counter-culture, and this alarmed the political establishment. Sandoz stopped production of LSD, and its use was increasingly proscribed even though it was not habit forming.[50]

Before the 1960s substance abuse, except for alcohol abuse, was not considered in the purview of psychiatry, for the very good reason that the asylums were not where drug users wanted to go.

But the mental health system was transformed by the antipsychotics, and in the 1960s offered treatment at outpatient clinics and community mental centers. For in-patients, the fabric of the hospitals had improved dramatically. Because of these developments, a rising tide of LSD users and abusers of other drugs became psychiatric patients. Mixed in with a growing number of patients with personality disorders, this new patient group increasingly led mainstream psychiatrists to take a jaundiced view of LSD and the hypotheses that went with it.

A final element in the eclipse of LSD is the use of LSD and other hallucinogens by the military. From the start it was clear that LSD could be used as a weapon of war, to disorient populations.[51] LSD and other agents were also used as a means of breaking down individuals. The CIA had a secret research program to investigate just such uses of LSD.[52] The possible military uses of LSD made people suspicious of experiments involving volunteers, patients, or others taking psychotropic drugs. These suspicions were fueled by the establishment of institutional review boards in response to increasing bioethical concerns throughout medicine. None of them was likely to support such experiments without strict oversight. By 1970 studies on volunteers also had to be insured, and the high cost of the insurance put the conduct of such experiments beyond the resources of many university departments.[53]

The LSD story has a backdrop of considerable historical resonance. It seemed that under the influence of LSD mainstream cultures were inhibited, that a dose of LSD would lead to a humanizing of society and a democratizing of values. A similar story had played out two hundred years earlier with the development of mesmerism (hypnosis). Mesmerism led to a perception among "therapists" that the entire social order could have resulted from suggestion. Many viewed mesmerism not just as a means of correcting the problems of an individual but as a means of changing society. Quite a few of the men who signed the early documents triggering the French Revolution were also members of Franz

Mesmer's Society of Harmony.[54] One of the responses of the establishment was to proscribe mesmerism, and later hypnosis. Mesmerism remained officially banned for almost a hundred years; it took the influence of the most famous clinician of his day, Jean-Martin Charcot, to bring it back into the scientific domain.

But work by Charcot and Janet on hypnotism created further problems. It began to seem that many religious phenomena, including the stigmata of saints were hypnoid phenomena, and this perception led to the suggestion that saints exhibiting such effects in fact were hysterics. Hypnosis fell under a further cloud when its use by Freud was associated with his claims that hysteria was linked to sexual abuse during childhood (Chapter 7). There was widespread disquiet. The Catholic Church, for example, proscribed hypnosis in the 1880s, and the ban was not lifted until 1955.[55]

LSD caused a similar ferment in the political and religious domains. The LSD users of the 1960s became the revolutionaries of 1968. This revolution, like the French Revolution before it, did lead to dramatic changes from authoritarian, hierarchical societies to looser, more democratic ones, symbolized eloquently by the student protests in Paris and in particular by the ransacking of the office of Jean Delay. The establishment mobilized against it in a manner that bore marked resemblances to the backlash against hypnosis. In the process transmethylation was swept away.

TWISTED THOUGHTS AND TWISTED GENES

In addition to his work on transmethylation and his role in fostering a laboratory in which many of the key neuroscientific discoveries were made, in the 1960s Seymour Kety got involved in genetic research. Genetic research in psychiatry had been neglected since World War II. The 1960s were the decade when nurture had seemingly finally triumphed over nature. It had triumphed to the extent that children born with ambiguous genitals might be brought up as girls even though chromosomal testing revealed they were male, in the confident expectation that it was rearing that would determine gender and personality.[56] To attempt to rescue genetics was the equivalent of Charcot's efforts to rescue hypnosis in the 1860s. But if anyone in the 1960s was equivalent in stature to Charcot, it was Seymour Kety.

Kety linked up with David Rosenthal and Paul Wender, researchers at the NIMH. He had become aware of an opportunity to investigate the genetics of schizophrenia. Most Scandinavian countries had stable ethnic mixes and kept national registers of illnesses and adoptions. Denmark's records were particularly good. They gave Kety and his colleagues several possibilities. They could study the incidence of schizophrenia in the adopted-away children of schizophrenic mothers. This incidence could be compared with the incidence of schizophrenia in adopted children set against the incidence of schizophrenia in both their adoptive and biological parents. Finally they could look at what happened to children born to normal parents who grew up in a house where one of the adoptive parents later developed schizophrenia. They opted to research all three questions.[57]

At the end of June 1967, when the studies were nearing completion, but before anyone knew the outcome, Kety convened a meeting at Dorado Beach in Puerto Rico. He invited all points of view. The clinical grandees of the schizophrenia universe, such as Manfred Bleuler, were there. Also present were proponents of schizophrenogenic mother hypotheses, such as Theodore Lidz and Yrjo Alanen, and of deviant family communication patterns, such as Lyman Wynne and Elliott Mishler. Sociologists such as John Clausen and Lloyd Rogler were present, along with social psychiatrists such as Leon Eisenberg. Also attending were the few psychiatrists prepared to acknowledge themselves as geneticists—Eliot Slater, Einar Kringlen, Jon Carlsson, Irving Gottesman, and Leonard Heston. There was no effort made to avoid confrontation.[58] Lyman Wynne collapsed and had to be flown out.[59]

The meeting put genetics back into psychiatry. The fact that one of the senior geneticists in psychiatry, Eliot Slater, from the Maudsley Hospital, was the editor of the *British Journal of Psychiatry* and that Kety of the NIMH was the editor of the *Journal of Psychiatric Research* helped. But there was nothing like having Kety actually fighting on the front line. One of the reasons for Kety's importance was that he was American. As Eliot Slater said, "if American psychiatric opinion can be moved to the point of admitting that human genetics has a contribution to make to the behavioral sciences, we can hope that many gaps will be bridged between psychiatry, medicine and biology, and between Europe and America . . . [there could be] fantastic changes taking place over a very wide front, including psychology, sociology, and educational theory."[60]

Even as he said this, Slater and his contributions were being sidelined by the new findings of Kety and Rosenthal, which pointed to a polygenic input to the schizophrenic disorders and substantial interactions between the environment and genes. An older generation of geneticists such as Franz Kallmann and Slater had studied the genetics of schizophrenia in the postwar years, but their methods were faulty. They made a number of errors, all in the direction of overestimating the genetic contribution. Their work was done on twins at a time when schizophrenia was overdiagnosed and the ability to establish the zygosity of twins was poor. They failed to correct for the age at onset of the disorder, and in particular there was a lack of established twin registers, which might have minimized any biases.[61]

There was a gulf between the new and the old genetic visions. One of the issues, as Rosenthal put it, was that "the great promise of psychiatric genetics was that it led to specificity, specific genes for specific disorders." This idea resurrected the specter of hereditary taint. Psychobiology for twenty years after the discovery of LSD and the first uses of chlorpromazine had been a force for liberation. The new genetics of Kety and Rosenthal led to concordance rates and heritability estimates for schizophrenia that were not unlike those for tuberculosis. In the case of tuberculosis such figures led no one to claim that the disease was not environmentally caused or could not be tackled by environmental manipulations. This hardly qualified as genetic determinism.[62] Besides, Kety and Rosenthal's schizophrenia was a loose concept and in their model some schizophrenic factor other than dementia praecox was being inherited.

The problem was the reemergence of genetic research at a time when theories about schizophrenogenesis were about to be handed over to drug companies. As attention switched from transmethylation to the dopamine system, the genetic evidence became one more justification for a hard-line medical model in which a single defect in a brain system underpinned all forms of schizophrenia. The problem was that for whatever reason belief in genetic models was rising almost in inverse proportion to incoming evidence from ever more carefully designed studies that led to a scaling back of estimates of genetic input.[63] The zeitgeist was changing.

THE EMERGENCE OF THE RECEPTOR

When the neuroleptics were first introduced, nothing was known about brain neurotransmission. The idea that there were neurotransmitters was an alien one that was resisted for a variety of reasons, one of which was almost certainly a residual vitalism. Until 1950, the dominant theories of how the brain worked were electrophysiological. These views were promoted by physiologists, whose concern was with the functioning of organs within the body at a molar rather than a molecular level. Compared with the electrical view, where the soul was generally viewed in traditional ways, the chemical views emerging in the 1960s broke the soul up into bits. An older chemical tradition had postulated that chemical reactions gave rise to a variety of vital vapors, but this new vision was quite different and profoundly materialistic.[64]

In contrast to the physiologists, the pharmacologists, working on nerve endings, guts, and hearts, had for many years been toying with the notion that hormones and other transmitter substances acted by binding to receptors. Pharmacologically this approach seemed necessary to explain drug actions. One key aspect of drug actions pushed thinking in this direction. Many drugs or naturally occurring compounds, especially the most famous anticholinergic compound, atropine, came in stereo-isomer forms, meaning that their molecules can have two different, mirror-image forms. These mirror-image forms of the same molecule are called the left isomer and the right isomer, the l-form of the molecule or the d-form.[65] Usually only one of the two isomers is active, but if both are active, they may have exhibit different profiles of activity.[66]

The only thing that can easily explain this phenomenon is that in order to act, the molecule of the drug must be binding to some receptive molecule, and in order to bind to this molecule, to fit keylike into the lock, some part of the drug's molecule must itself have a very precise shape. Notions of a receptive substance of this sort were first outlined by John Langley in 1878.[67] These ideas were picked up by Alexander Crum-Browne and Thomas Frazer in Edinburgh, who drew attention to the differences between l- and d-hyoscine, the isomers of atropine. The contribution that seized the imagination though originated in Paul Ehrlich's use of a variety of dyes to stain different bacteria and tissues. Out of this work came the notion that agents related to the dyes might chemically bind selectively and specifically, leading Ehrlich to the notion of the magic bullet. This was to become the dominant therapeutic metaphor of the second half of the twentieth century, and it gave early currency to the idea of a receptor. The term receptor appears to have been first used in 1910 by Henry Dale and George Barger, ironically in an article attacking the concept.[68]

A contemporary of Ehrlich's, Emil Fischer, created the metaphor of the lock and the key. It had become clear by the end of the nineteenth century that enzymes catalyzed chemical reactions within the body and that these enzymes were very selective in the chemical reactions they could catalyze. This realization led Fischer to the notion that the fit between biological substances and enzymes resembled that between a key and a lock.[69] Work with enzymes, however, remained beneath physiologists until World War II.[70]

The physiological alternative to bullets and receptors saw the response to drugs as a matter of the individual sensitivity of an organ or organism. Just as we recognize individual variations in perceptual sensitivity or sensitivity to music or art without invoking receptors, physiologists explained drug effects as a result of variations in innate sensitivities.

Nothing changed until the 1930s and the work of A. J. Clark, who had succeeded to the chair of pharmacology at the University of Edinburgh in 1926. Edinburgh was possibly the premier pharmacology center in the English-speaking world in the 1930s, when there were few pharmacology departments anywhere. Pharmacological studies, if undertaken, were conducted within departments of physiology. Convinced of the existence of receptors, Clark spent years working on mathematical models that would correlate drug concentrations with therapeutic effects, and published his major works in 1933 and 1937.[71]

Clark did his work with acetylcholine (ACh), which had been synthesized in 1865 by Adolf Baeyer. It gained a special place in neuroscience in 1921, when Otto Loewi had a dream that led him to perform an experiment. He removed a frog's heart, which he kept beating in an artificial medium. To this he applied the juice from the vagus nerve. This "vagusstoff" caused the heart to slow its beating, and stimulation of the vagus nerve had no effect on the heart if the vagusstoff was blocked from getting to the heart. Loewi had established the existence of chemical neurotransmission. The vagusstoff was isolated and identified as acetylcholine, a discovery almost as astounding as the demonstration by Frederick Wöhler that urea, an organic molecule, could be synthesized in the laboratory (Chapter 2).

For the pharmacologists who accepted that ACh was a neurotransmitter, there was a further indicator that receptors were involved in its action. It had been known for some time that this neurotransmitter could have two different actions: an action mimicked by nicotine and an action mimicked by muscarine. Atropine blocked the muscarinic effects but not the nicotinic effects of ACh. This fact suggested the presence of two different receptors. Clark was committed to this new pharmacological model and to the idea that the action of drugs obeyed the laws of physical chemistry rather than stemming from some vitalist principle, which would attribute to living matter properties unknown to physical chemistry. His final equations accounting for drug effects were similar to ones that accounted for the adsorption of gases onto metal.

This new quantitative work was alien to the physiology of the day and led to delays in the recognition of Clark's work, even though his models had a passable concordance with experimental observations and predicted the action of many known drugs.[72] Clark's theoretical success was the foundation of modern pharmacology, although that was not recognized at the time. It was to remain a minority viewpoint for almost forty years. Following a routine operation, Clark died prematurely in 1941 from surgical shock of just the type that led Henri Laborit nine years later to experiment with chlorpromazine. The torch passed to his successors.

Although epinephrine and norepinephrine were not as clearly established as neurotransmitters in the body, they were accepted as putative neurotransmitters by many pharmacologists and biochemists. In 1948, on the basis of differences in the effects of norepinephrine and epinephrine on different organs of the body, Gordon Ahlquist suggested that there were alpha and beta receptors within the adrenergic system.[73] This idea, which laid the basis for the development in the following two decades of some of the more important drugs of the twentieth century, provided further grist for the pharmacological mill but was ignored outside pharmacological circles.[74]

Pharmacologists who believed in receptors continued to elicit disdain from the electrophysiologists. They had to talk about "putative" receptors and were commonly met with the rebuff that it was bad science to multiply hypotheses or constructs unnecessarily. Receptors were dismissed as hypothetical entities.[75] The fact of the matter was that from the 1940s to the 1960s receptors could not be seen, touched, or in any other way proven to exist. That they were required according to certain views of drug action was not enough to persuade the scientific establishment that they must exist. One of the key factors was that there were very few effective drugs. Theories of how drugs worked could, therefore, be left vague.

While pharmacologists could not see how there could be resistance to the fact that stereo-isomerism required the existence of receptors, physiologists and others were almost viscerally aware that accepting the role of receptors in drug action involved embracing a materialistic view of human beings. In the 1950s and 1960s, this view went against the grain of how the majority of people wanted to see themselves. Some found the chemical vision abhorrent. At least as many were put off as were attracted by the challenge from Ralph Gerard that behind every twisted thought lay a twisted molecule and that the mission for psychiatrists was to pinpoint "the osmoreceptors of hallucinations and the chemoreceptors of dreams."[76] How could responsibility, free will, and humanity coexist with such a materialistic vision? There was (is) a real spiritual crisis behind this scientific question.[77] It is probably no coincidence that biological thinking crept into psychiatry on the back of a group of drugs like the psychedelics, which gave rise to "spiritual" thinking.

For some time, the discussions of receptors focused on the physiology of peripheral systems. No neurotransmitters had been shown to exist in the brain and in the absence of neurotransmitters receptors were irrelevant. Then, in an elegant series of experiments in 1949, John Eccles, who had been one of the staunchest advocates of the electrophysiological viewpoint, demonstrated that acetylcholine was important in central nervous system functioning.[78] A few years later in Eccles's laboratory, now staffed with proponents of the chemical viewpoint, David Curtis and Jeff Watkins demonstrated that glutamate was a neurotransmitter.[79] And indeed glutamate is now recognized as the leading excitatory neurotransmitter in the human brain; and abnormalities in this system and its receptors, one of which is the NMDA receptor, are thought by many to underpin schizophrenia. But in the late 1950s Curtis and Watkins were still inhibited by prevailing attitudes and, notwithstanding their own data, found it impossible to claim neurotransmitter status for glutamate. It was to be almost two decades before this was finally accepted.[80]

Before the 1950s, the Edinburgh Department of Pharmacology had again become the site of developments. Clark was succeeded in 1942 by John Henry Gaddum. Like Clark, Gaddum was a mathematician as well as a physician. During World War II he had worked on methods to antagonize nerve gas poisonings. This work was compatible with notions introduced by Clark of competitive and noncompetitive antagonism. Against this background and sitting in Clark's seat, Gaddum found it difficult to avoid the topic of receptors. As a mathematician, Gaddum was also sympathetic to the idea of moving science forward by quantification. He instituted a series of experiments aimed at refining Clark's formulations, and they seemed to confirm Clark's theories, at least to Gaddum's satisfaction.[81]

But mathematical theory was about to take a backseat because in 1952, Marthe Vogt, working in Gaddum's department, demonstrated the existence of norepinephrine in the brain. The idea that acetylcholine could act as a neurotransmitter in the central nervous system stood for a few years as a symbol of a possibility rather than an actuality that would dramatically change perceptions of how the brain functioned. The demonstration of norepinephrine in the brain converted a crack in the dam into a clear breach and a small trickle into a noticeable flow that was about to become a flood.[82]

In 1933 in Italy, Vittorio Erpsamer had isolated another compound from the gut, which promoted contractions of the gut wall. Since it was derived from the gut, Erpsamer called it enteramine.[83] What later turned out to be the same compound was also isolated from blood platelets in 1947 by Page and Rapoport, who, finding that it caused blood vessels to contract, called it serotonin.[84] The chemical structure of this compound was established as 5-hydroxytryptamine (5HT), and in 1953 Betty Twarog and Irvine Page demonstrated that 5HT could be found in the brain.[85] In 1953 also, Crawford and Gaddum in Edinburgh, looking for the neurohumor Substance P in the brain, found 5HT instead.[86]

There was little reaction to these discoveries initially. It was thought possible that the 5HT in the brain was simply a residue of blood flow through the brain.[87] The discovery of LSD, however, suggested that there was more to brain 5HT than simply a residue from blood flow. Once the structure of serotonin was worked out, it became clear that there was a striking similarity between LSD and 5HT, leading to suggestions that a 5HT molecule was locked inside LSD. As was fashionable at the time among pharmacologists, Gaddum took LSD himself. On Good Friday 1953, he took some 30 micrograms, hoping to be able to counteract its effects with methidrine. The following day he took more, which produced such severe effects that Marthe Vogt worried that he might go mad. On 9 May at home, observed by his wife and daughter, he took an even larger dose and found as Hoffman had done before him that his world was transformed. This experience prompted him to claim that serotonin in the brain may play a role in preserving sanity.[88] This view was echoed independently by Edward Woolley and David Shaw in the United States and Thuillier in

Paris, raising the profile of brain 5HT and its possible role in nervous disorders.[89]

But of even greater interest was that Gaddum hoped to counteract the effects of LSD with methidrine. This effort to antagonize the effect of very minute quantities of LSD owed much to a belief in receptors. Using LSD to block the actions of 5HT in the guinea pig ileum, Gaddum and Zuleika Piccarelli went on to distinguish between two different serotonin receptors: the M receptor, which was morphine sensitive, and the D receptor, which was diphenhydramine sensitive.[90]

This work was still a far cry from work on the brain, however. Even Gaddum, in whose laboratory two neurotransmitters had been discovered, who had described two different kinds of receptor, and who had shown that a drug which produced major changes in behavior acted on one of these, found it at the time all but impossible to agree that at least some brain operations depended on neurotransmitters. The relevance of work on animal organs to behavior or to the brain itself was at best uncertain.

At a series of meetings held in the United Kingdom from 1955[91] to 1960[92] to debate the significance of the emerging discoveries, Gaddum, Vogt, and their colleagues found it difficult to make the conceptual breakthrough. Outsiders such as Joel Elkes and Arvid Carlsson, who crucially had no background in physiology, argued for a new vision of brain functioning in which neurotransmitters played a central role. They were met with reactions ranging from indulgent admonishments—they might be correct but the brain was far to complicated to study even if they were—to frank disdain.[93]

A key event took place in 1955, in the laboratory of Steve Brodie at the National Institutes of Health in Bethesda, Maryland. Robert Bowman in Brodie's laboratory had developed a new machine, a spectrophotofluorimeter, which allowed much more precise measurement of neurohumors such as 5HT. This breakthrough permitted Brodie, Park Shore, and Alfred Pletscher to demonstrate that when rabbits were given reserpine they became sedated or apathetic and that there was a dramatic lowering of their brain 5HT content, which was restored to normal levels when they recovered.[94] No one could argue with Brodie. No one had the technology to argue.

This experiment, briefly reported in the pages of *Science*, became the most celebrated piece of work in early biochemical psychopharmacology. It signaled that it was now possible for the first time to work on the brain pharmacologically and begin to correlate aspects of brain functioning with aspects of behavior. British, Germans, French, Spanish, Japanese, and other pharmacologists spent time in Brodie's laboratory to learn the new techniques.[95] Young researchers entering the field preferred Brodie's demonstration that new technology could lead to exciting discoveries to the comforting certainties of old-style neurophysiology.[96]

In this new world, the identification of the two isomers of atropine opened up the exhilarating possibility of creating drugs that would be very precise in their actions. It is now clear that this attractive idea is fraught with difficulty, since although a drug may bind with great selectivity to one receptor, it may also have other binding sites, which act on quite different receptors. In fact to achieve the precision binding that is the goal of modern pharmacotherapy, a hugely complex molecule such as a protein is often required in order to produce a molecule that has only one function. The much smaller molecules, such as those of serotonin, norepinephrine, dopamine, along with those of compounds structurally related to them such as LSD, mescaline, and cocaine bind to an astonishing number of different receptors. But this fact did not become apparent until the late 1980s.

THE DOPAMINE RECEPTOR HYPOTHESIS
OF SCHIZOPHRENIA

Traditional accounts of the development of biological psychiatry give center stage to the development of the dopamine hypothesis of schizophrenia. A paper by Arvid Carlsson and Margit Lindqvist in 1963 is cited as the first paper outlining the hypothesis.[97] A second paper in 1966, by Jac van Rossum, is cited as outlining a dopamine receptor hypothesis.[98] The implication of these dates is that almost from the start scientists had raced to find out what exactly the neuroleptics do. In fact, the dopamine hypothesis had little impact in the 1960s. Carlsson and Lindqvist's 1963 paper does not mention dopamine, even though Carlsson was the discoverer of brain dopamine. Receptors were still rather theoretical ideas in the mid-1960s, and van Rossum was an obscure figure who played little further role in the development of the story. But when the dopamine hypothesis did take root, it flourished to such an extent that it overwhelmed all other growth round it. What produced the fertility of the furrow this seed landed in?

First of course was the discovery of dopamine. Dopamine was known to be one of the building blocks of norepinephrine even before norepinephrine was accepted as a neurotransmitter. Once the presence of norepinephrine in the brain was established, provided it was not there as a residue, it was necessary that dopamine also must be present in the brain, if only briefly. It was also known to be present in the periphery but no one thought of it as being a transmitter. It was thought of as simply a precursor to norepinephrine and epinephrine.

Carlsson was one of the first outsiders to arrive in Brodie's laboratory in 1955, the year in which the first reserpine experiments took place.[99] After returning to Sweden, Carlsson and Nils Åge Hillarp set up experiments on rabbits to replicate Brodie's work with reserpine and to take the next logical step. It had become clear that reserpine depleted both norepinephrine and serotonin in the brain. But replacing the serotonin did not reverse the sedation produced by reserpine, and this fact suggested that Brodie might be wrong and that it might be norepinephrine that was the key neurotransmitter system. Replacing norepinephrine, however, did not restore the rabbits to normal either. What was going on?

When Carlsson and his colleagues gave the rabbits L-dopa, a precursor of both dopamine and norepinephrine, they found that it did solve the problem. There were only two ways to explain what was happening. One was that L-dopa was working as a neurotransmitter and the other was that the intermediate between L-dopa and norepinephrine—dopamine—was a neurotransmitter and was responsible for mediating the effects of reserpine. The latter turned out to be the case. Noting the ability of reserpine to cause Parkinsonian states, Carlsson speculated that dopamine might play a role in Parkinson's disease.[100]

Two years later Oleh Hornykiewicz and Walter Birkmaier in Vienna reported reductions in brain dopamine levels in people with Parkinson's disease.[101] Some idea of how these developments were initially viewed can be glimpsed from the experience of Gerald Curzon at the Institute of Neurology in London. Curzon had been hired to do post-doctoral research on the neurochemistry of the brain. At a case conference involving Parkinson's disease in 1960, he mentioned that Hornykiewicz had recently shown that dopamine was lowered in the brains of patients with the disorder. The response from the distinguished chairman of the meeting was that if Dr. Curzon had seen the brain of a patient with Parkinson's disease at a postmortem examination, he would know that this was not a chemical disorder.[102]

Not until several years later did George Cotzias devise a replacement strategy using L-dopa that reversed many of the clinical features of Parkinson's disease.[103] This achievement settled the argument, and it was also a powerful piece of evidence in favor of the neurotransmitter view of central nervous functioning. The second step that led to the acceptance of the importance of neurotransmitters stemmed from work done by Carlsson, Kjell Fuxe, and Hillarp in which they stained the monoamine tracts of animal brains with a fluorescent-labeling substance. On subsequent ultraviolet microscopy, animal brains demonstrated a branching distribution of noradrenergic, serotonergic, and dopaminergic neurones. The orderly pattern of these distributions clearly indicated a set of systems that could influence all areas of the brain, even though the number of neurones was comparatively small. This was powerful evidence for the functional importance of these systems.[104]

This work prepared the ground for the catecholamine theory of depression, which more than any other hypothesis crystallized the new possibilities and formulated them in a way that was ultimately to gain popular acceptance.[105] According to the catecholamine hypothesis, depression involved a lowering of brain norepinephrine. The hypothesis was based on the idea that drugs which lowered norepinephrine, most notably reserpine, were likely to cause depression and even lead to suicide,[106] and that drugs which increased norepinephrine levels or function were antidepressant. The norepinephrine version of the hypothesis held sway during the 1970s and early 1980s. A subsequent version of the hypothesis substituting serotonin for norepinephrine became the dominant biological hypothesis in popular consciousness from the mid-1980s to the turn of the millennium. This dominance stemmed almost entirely from the marketing of Prozac and a range of other selective serotonin reuptake inhibitors (SSRIs).[107]

Early efforts to find out how the antipsychotics work met with a puzzle. Reserpine emptied the presynaptic neurone of its monoamines but chlorpromazine and haloperidol had no effects on the presynaptic neurone. Carlsson and Lindqvist's 1963 paper demonstrated that chlorpromazine and haloperidol reduced activity through catecholamine systems but that they acted on the post-synaptic neurone.[108] In 1966 van Rossum tied the post-synaptic receptor blockage specifically to dopamine, and a dopamine hypothesis of neuroleptic action was born.[109] But the world took no notice. The dopamine hypothesis did not prevail until the

1970s, following the success of Solomon Snyder in radiolabeling the first central nervous system receptors.

Snyder had trained with Julius Axelrod at the NIMH and in 1965 moved from there to set up his own laboratory at Johns Hopkins University, initially with few plans to hunt for receptors—the task seemed beyond the techniques available at the time. In 1970 the first receptor, an acetylcholine receptor, was isolated from the body of an electric eel by Jean Pierre Changeux and his colleagues. At a pharmacology conference in England, Changeux dramatically pulled from his breast pocket a tiny glass tube with a single narrow blue band across its middle, and announced that a receptor had been isolated. Far from bringing the world of receptors within reach, however, this demonstration acted as much to deter as it did to encourage research in the field. Changeux and his colleagues had used cobra venom to isolate the receptor from the electric organ of the electric eel. This organ had the densest concentration of acetylcholine receptors in any organ in any animal—amounting to 20 percent of the protein of the organ. Cobra venom contained a large polypetide, alphabungarotoxin, that bound irreversibly to the acetylcholine receptors in this organ. Radio-labeling this made it possible to isolate the receptor and confirm its existence. But even this huge target had been difficult to hit. Finding neurotransmitter receptors in the human brain appeared to be all but impossible.

In the Department of Pharmacology at Johns Hopkins, Snyder was next door to Pedro Cuatrecasas, who had been trying to find the insulin receptor. In the course of this work Cuatrecasas had developed a vacuum filtration machine. This solved a major problem with radio-labeling receptors, which is that radio-labeled chemicals bind indiscriminately to any piece of tissue. This nonspecific binding makes it difficult to detect the signal coming from specific binding to a particular receptor. This background noise had defeated many research teams. Cuatrecasas solved the problem by washing the preparations he was using and removing the radioactive rich washings rapidly by vacuum filtration. This technique helped him to identify the insulin receptor, a large protein receptor. His new technique, allied with the development of radio-labeling, was about to bring central nervous system (CNS) receptors within reach.[110]

After the invention of the cyclotron at Berkeley, California, during World War II, scientists realized that radioactive isotopes could be produced relatively easily. Some of these could be used to trace biological processes.[111] The production of such isotopes and encouragement to use them became part of the Atoms for Peace program during the Eisenhower presidency. Carbon-14 was one of the isotopes produced, and its use to work out the process of photosynthesis in plants was a major breakthrough. This program later gave rise to SPECT (single photon emission computed tomography) and PET (positron emission tomography) scans. One of the developers of the PET scan was Louis Sokoloff, who worked at the NIMH with Seymour Kety.

Producing radioactive isotopes was expensive and research using them was costly. One of the few places with the resources to do such work was the NIH. Already involved in supporting the development of PET scans, Kety could easily see other research possibilities for radio-labeling. Working on transmethylation, he used radio-labeled norepinephrine to test some aspects of this hypothesis. Julius Axelrod borrowed the radio-labeled norepinephrine to demonstrate the existence of a reuptake mechanism. This discovery, for which he was later awarded a Nobel Prize, encouraged a range of other researchers to use radio-labeled compounds to investigate central nervous system processes.

At this point, in the early 1970s, the federal war on drug abuse was beginning in earnest. The federal government committed large amounts of funds for research to the control of a drug Czar, Jerry Jaffe. Jaffe knew Snyder and asked him to do research on opiates. Snyder was interested and found out about the work of Avram Goldstein on opiate receptors. Goldstein was sure they existed in the human brain and that stereo-specific binding to them should be demonstrable, but he could not distinguish specific from nonspecific binding. He did not have a manifold filter machine.

Snyder had a new Ph.D. student working in his laboratory, Candace Pert. He suggested to her that they should radio-label some opiates and see whether they could demonstrate specific binding. Their first step was to radio-label dihydromorphine, but they found nothing. It later turned out that dihydromorphine was light sensitive and it degraded in laboratory conditions. Snyder and Pert mistakenly concluded that because dihydromorphine was an agonist, an antagonist might be needed to demonstrate binding. This reasoning led them to test radio-labeled naloxone. This showed active binding to the opiate receptor. A range of experiments followed. They localized opiate receptors in different parts of the brain and explained why morphine acting in particular brain areas had an analgesic action whereas in other brain areas it caused nausea and in yet other areas pupillary constriction. The answers to many questions about the pharmacology of opiates were within their grasp.[112]

Not everybody immediately appreciated the significance of their findings. They submitted a paper to *Nature*, whose editors' response was that there had already been a paper on the opiate receptors and that the subject did not call for a further paper. Snyder persuaded the editors to change their minds. Initially, many other laboratories could not replicate the work and there were suggestions that this binding was simply an artifact. But once other laboratories began to get the technical aspects of binding sorted out, a new world opened up. Psychopharmacology meetings, where receptors had not been mentioned before 1972, rapidly became dominated by reports of the labeling of new receptors or of changes in receptor density in various disorders or of changes following treatment.

The discovery of the opiate receptors had another benefit. ACh and insulin receptors were clearly produced within the body to provide a site of action for naturally occurring substances. But did alien drugs, such as the opiates or neuroleptics, act through similar receptors? It did not follow that they did. In fact it was hard to believe that they would. But Pert and Snyder's discovery occurred almost within weeks of the discovery by John Hughes and Hans Kosterlitz of the existence of enkephalin in the brain.[113] At one stroke, this discovery explained why the opiates worked: there were naturally occurring opioids in the human body. The lay public very quickly became enthusiastic about these, and people talked about releasing natural opioids while running or exercising and how these could produce a "high." New understandings of the body were opening up.

In addition, the discovery provided a rationale for treatment with synthetic drugs. The opiates contained a large number of artificial compounds, many of which had already been synthesized in laboratories, and these acted with greater efficacy or safety than naturally occurring salts such as morphine. Many effective drugs bore little resemblance to the naturally occurring enkephalins and endorphins. People concluded that anything that produced a functional change to the body, even though it appeared to be quite an alien substance, must be acting through some naturally existing receptor. This realization overcame Karl Jaspers's original criticism that nothing could be learned from scientific studies involving giving "poisons" to volunteers.

Rather than spend the rest of his career isolating and purifying the opiate receptors, Snyder moved rapidly on to apply the new techniques to other receptors. His next target was the dopamine receptor. Snyder and his group took haloperidol and radio-labeled both it and dopamine. They discovered that there were two different dopamine receptors.[114] This work was confirmed by the independent studies of Philip Seeman in Toronto. Of compelling interest was the fact that D-1 receptors radio-labeled by dopamine did not seem to be implicated in the action of antipsychotic drugs. This was in stark contrast to the picture at the D-2 receptor, where the amount of drug taken to block the binding of a radio-labeled antagonist precisely paralleled the amount of drug needed to produce a clinical effect. These binding studies on the

D-2 receptor brooked no argument. Even now they remain among the most clear-cut findings in psychopharmacology.

The answer to the riddle of schizophrenia appeared to be within reach. All known antipsychotic drugs bound to the D-2 receptor. This explained why all produced Parkinsonian features and predicted the dose at which such features were likely to develop. Surely the abnormality in schizophrenia was in some part of the dopamine system leading into this receptor. Snyder, Seeman, and Herbert Meltzer were all quick to articulate such an explanation. They were beaten to the draw by Daniel Tarsy and Ross Baldessarini, who in 1973 put forward a dopamine receptor hypothesis of tardive dyskinesia, but no one wanted to accept a hypothesis about a problem.[115] Instead, following Snyder and Meltzer, researchers thought they could explain just why amphetamine produced the psychoses it did, and why certain drugs were antipsychotic and others not; and indeed they thought they could predict from a binding assay whether a new drug would be antipsychotic.[116] By this time, it was possible to draw attention to the early work of Arvid Carlsson and others. The binding studies rapidly led laboratories around the world to undertake postmortem brain work in an attempt to measure D-2 receptor numbers in the brains of people who had had schizophrenia. Early reports appeared to confirm an excess of dopamine receptors in people with schizophrenia.

The dopamine hypothesis did more than displace the fading transmethylation hypotheses. It wrote them out of history. And it did so even though Snyder in an article in the *Lancet* in 1982 and others had pointed out the potential errors of logic involved: just because all antipsychotic drugs acted on D-2 receptors did not mean there was an abnormality in the D-2 receptor.[117] A few years after Snyder's article Arvid Carlsson also criticized the dopamine hypothesis.[118] It quickly became clear that the elevations of D-2 receptor numbers in postmortem brains of patients with psychoses were an artifact of prior drug treatment. When this was controlled for, there appeared to be no increase in D-2 receptor numbers in people with schizophrenia.[119]

The story replayed itself in the later 1980s, when the development of PET scans made it possible to look at D-2 receptor density in living brains. In 1983, Henry Wagner and Michael Kuhar and their colleagues demonstrated changes in dopamine receptor numbers in living Parkinson's disease patients that were in line with postmortem findings.[120] The same group then reported elevations of dopamine receptor numbers in living schizophrenic patients.[121] But subsequent studies that controlled for medication intake failed to support their claims.[122]

Nevertheless, the dopamine hypothesis of schizophrenia held sway and indeed established an ever firmer and more comprehensive grip on the minds of practitioners. Why? Several powerful factors can be pointed to. In the late 1960s and early 1970s, psychiatry was battered by the forces of antipsychiatry. Psychologists had demonstrated that psychiatric diagnosis was unreliable to the extent that perfectly normal people might be diagnosed as having schizophrenia.[123] Physical treatments were targeted and ECT was being marginalized or even proscribed in a number of countries and states in the United States. Psychiatric associations worldwide were on the defensive. Presidents of national associations felt obliged to issue statements about the legitimacy of diagnosis and the reality of mental illness.[124] When the dopamine hypothesis entered the fray, the latest technologies appeared to stunningly confirm the reality of mental illness, and they did so in a hypothesis that broke free from the entanglements of the transmethylation hypotheses with the counter-culture. Moreover without access to radio-labels and vacuum manifolds, critics could not even enter the debate.

Receptor binding techniques also produced a common language for psychiatry and the pharmaceutical industry, allowing the advertising power of the industry to support mainstream psychiatry. The dopamine receptor hypothesis and a 1976 beta adrenoreceptor hypothesis of depression,[125] provided a new modus operandi for pharmaceutical companies. Previously, the only way to test whether a drug was an antidepressant or an antipsychotic was in a series of animal models. This procedure was time consuming and involved killing large numbers of animals. At the most a handful of new compounds could be screened per week. Receptor binding assay systems could be set up in which huge numbers of drugs could be screened for their receptor binding profiles in one day, yielding candidate drugs that were much more likely to have effects in animal screening tests than unknown compounds. The pace at which candidate compounds were identified increased exponentially. Soon chemists and pharmacologists found that up to a thousand drugs could be screened in one day. This achievement, allied with developments in robotics, led to the development of combinatorial chemistry, whose use allowed up to 10,000 compounds to be screened per day, sometimes in completely automated laboratories.

In one sense, drug development became a lot more "rational," although the progress that had been made increased the risk that companies would simply produce slight variations of already existing compounds. But more to the point, when company representatives met with physicians they could illustrate their sales talk with graphs of D-2 receptor binding with confidence that their interests in the graphs coincided with those of the clinicians they were selling to. Lecturers at international meetings could pepper their talks to mixed audiences of clinicians and company scientists with similar figures and graphs and be confident that both groups were focused on the receptor as the site of the action. Hitting the D-2 receptor selectively and specifically would make the psychosocial aspects of disorders treated with dopamine as irrelevant as psychosocial aspects were to physicians treating bacterial infections. Internists practicing general medicine had already relegated the need for a good bedside manner or a consideration of the patient's psychosocial situation to the footnotes of history, and now the stage was set for psychiatrists to become "real" doctors and follow suit.

For clinicians, the great amount of money that was available to pursue and in the process endorse this new molecular vision provided a massive boost in self-confidence. Furthermore, in the course of the 1980s and 1990s, patient groups that had been fearsome bastions of antipsychiatry were transformed. They too were seduced by the "science" and by pharmaceutical company funds. Industry had realized that these groups could be the most effective lobbyists for new compounds. In the process, patient groups also learned to deploy a vocabulary of receptor jargon to explain why the latest compounds needed to be made available to all.

This coincidence of interests, however, did exact a price. The cycle whereby scientific ideas rise and fall became linked to the business cycle. The marketing efforts of companies that bolstered certain ideas within the scientific domain inhibited the development of others (see Chapter 6). From the 1990s on, scientific ideas would achieve wider acceptability only if they had commercial value, to some extent regardless of their intrinsic merits. They would rise and fall not so much because of the careers of forceful personalities and good arguments within the field of psychiatry, but because of the laws governing patent duration. Clinicians increasingly had to spend time trying to persuade companies that there was a coincidence of interests between their work and a company's market goals. It is difficult to see how things could be otherwise when the research budgets of pharmaceutical companies dwarfed those of research funding bodies such as the medical research council in the United Kingdom or INSERM in France.[126]

The dopamine hypothesis led to a focus on selectivity and specificity. It became clear that the original antipsychotics acted on a range of adrenergic, cholinergic, histaminergic, serotonergic, and other receptors. The binding to these receptors did not parallel the clinical efficacy of the drugs. The next logical step seemed clear: —produce drugs that bind selectively and solely to the D-2 receptor. If the dopamine receptor hypothesis was right, these should be more effective and should also produce fewer side effects. This idea led to a generation of new drugs such as remoxipride and amisulpiride, whose stories are told in Chapter 6.

There were a number of other consequences of the dopamine hypothesis. One of the most notable was that it rendered invisible the physical dependence on and withdrawal from antipsychotics outlined in Chapter 4. Receptor theory demanded that dopamine antagonists, like the antipsychotics, cause dopamine receptor supersensitivity, which should lead to an acute onset of problems when treatment was stopped. With any other receptor system, receptor supersensitivity is taken as the basis of withdrawal effects, but since dopamine supersensitivity was the supposed basis of schizophrenia, these withdrawal effects were transmuted into strong evidence in support of the dopamine hypothesis of schizophrenia.[127]

Under the influence of the dopamine hypothesis, there was a blurring of the boundaries between the negativity that can characterize a schizophrenic syndrome and drug-induced demotivation and passivity (see Chapter 6). Given such drug-induced passivity and the failure to recognize dependence on antipsychotics, there was an increasing confusion between the illness and the effects of the treatments given for it. Many patients preferred an unmedicated although ill state to drug-induced "normality." Such patients became increasingly alienated from a psychiatric establishment that was likely to interpret their refusal to take the magic bullets of modern psychiatry as a lack of insight and grounds for compulsory treatment.

There was a further significant difference between the dopamine hypothesis and the transmethylation hypotheses. While the transmethylation hypotheses held sway, there was a disjunction between treatment and the theories of what underlay the illness. With the dopamine hypothesis, treatment became theory driven. For scientists, this is a desired state of affairs supposedly, but it opens the door to abuse as well as to benefits. Psycho-surgery, for example, is now portrayed as an empirical, ad hoc approach to treatment, which would not have become abusive if it had been properly informed by science. But in fact this is a rewritten history; as Jack Pressman has illustrated, psychosurgery became the problem it did precisely because it was science driven and was endorsed by scientists from Yale, Harvard, and the Institute of Psychiatry in London.[128]

BEYOND DOPAMINE

In 1980, Solomon Snyder and Stephen Peroutka distinguished between 5HT-1 and 5HT-2 receptors through the use of radiolabeling, confirming the original work of Gaddum that there were two 5HT receptors.[129] This research was conducted at just the time that drugs active on the serotonin system, like Prozac, began to become available. The new receptor techniques permitted pharmaceutical companies to distinguish between drugs active on the 5HT-1, 5HT-2, 5HT-3, and other 5HT receptors. Moreover, the behavioral consequences of binding to these receptors was elucidated. It became clear that 5HT-2A receptors were involved with sleep, while 5HT-2C receptors played a role in appetite and hedonic tone. A particular kind of anxiolysis seemed to be mediated through the 5HT-1A receptor while a different kind seemed to be mediated through the 5HT-2A receptor. Orgasm could be speeded up or delayed by actions on the 5HT-1 or 5HT-2 receptors.

In 1988, clozapine, an antipsychotic that had been withdrawn from the market in many countries, was licensed for use in the United States. It quickly became clear that this drug offered something that previous neuroleptics had not. Clinicians, chemists, and pharmacologists struggled to work out what it was about its pharmacology that made it distinctive. It was not a potent D-2 receptor blocker. This finding posed no immediate threat to the dopamine hypothesis, because the years from 1989 to 1993 saw the identification of D-3 and D-4 receptors. Proponents of the dopamine hypothesis simply switched the locus of interest to these other receptors.[130] Claims of D-4 receptor alterations in schizophrenia produced a race among companies to test D-4 antagonists, but these later turned out to have no effect on schizophrenia.[131]

Clozapine provided an incentive though to look beyond the dopamine system. It blocked 5HT-2 receptors. Could it be that the ratio of D-2 to 5HT-2 blockage was important? This hypothesis, put forward by Meltzer and others,[132] gave rise to a generation of drugs that were marketed as SDA antipsychotics (serotonin/dopamine antagonists). Others suggested that it was clozapine's actions on norepinephrine receptors that made it different. These 5HT-2/D-2 models were old-style models, similar to the dopamine hypothesis, but making some effort to accommodate inconvenient data.

Clozapine, however, also acted on cholinergic and histaminergic receptors. Perhaps its lack of selectivity underpinned its efficacy. Arvid Carlsson, one of the earliest proponents of the selective dopamine hypothesis, now championed a retreat from selectivity and specificity.[133] Carlsson accepted that it was not possible to alter one part of the central nervous system without affecting others. Acting on two interacting parts at the same time might in fact produce completely different effects from acting on one of the systems on its own. His new hypothesis came complete with experimental data, showing that it applied in the real world; the only question was how it applied to schizophrenia. Efforts to test this hypothesis called attention to the fact that schizophrenia consists of more than one disorder. This, however, was not a fact the pharmaceutical industry wanted to deal with. Whereas trainee psychiatrists had been quick to hear about the dopamine hypothesis, few if any heard about the new hypothesis because no company had any incentive to market it.

Should this development have come as a surprise? In the late 1950s, Hannah Steinberg found that a combination of dexamphetamine (a stimulant) and barbiturates (sedatives), which might have been expected to have a neutral effect on activity levels overall, in fact activated experimental animals more than amphetamine alone did.[134] Steinberg and her colleagues had been investigating why this combination was such a marketing success for SK&F (see Chapter 2). Her data, however, were reported came at a time when the FDA regulations had changed, making it all but impossible to register a combination compound. The premium the 1962 amendments put on specificity made polypharmacy one of the cardinal clinical sins of the new era.

Steinberg and her colleagues continued their work through the 1970s and 1980s, for the best of scientific reasons—they had demonstrated a new phenomenon that could not easily be explained. In the process they showed that certain combinations of antidepressants and tranquilizers could produce effects not normally seen naturally—such as backward walking in mice. They quantified these effects.[135] But this work was rarely mentioned at meetings. There was no company to market these drug combinations. But this work did jibe exactly with the models later produced by Carlsson.

It also fit in well with the scientific perceptions of the 1960s. At a CINP meeting in 1964, M. Taeschler from Sandoz had put the issue as follows: "observable drug-induced mood lifting can best be explained in terms of a polyvalent action pattern rather than of a single pharmacological effect . . . Such a concept is indeed valid for other drug-induced psychic changes. Closely related drugs may well prove to elicit qualitatively different effects depending on the quantitative distribution of their various pharmacological properties."[136] Translated, Taeschler's vision was that brain systems might interact the way the different primary color rods in the eye do to produce color vision. Working on one rod only was a mistake. Carlsson's work in the 1990s returned the field to a place it had been before, but nobody recognized this.

In the 1960s and 1970s, polypharmacy had been increasingly discouraged as irrational. With the advent of Carlsson's model, polypharmacy once again became the height of rationality, except that no pharmaceutical company could endorse or foster it. By the 1990s, it had become clear that all psychotropic drugs that acted on monoamine systems were almost of necessity cocktail compounds. Any drug that acted on one of the receptors of any of the classic neurotransmitter systems would inevitably act on two or three of them.[137] Specificity was an almost illusory goal, notwithstanding the regulations of the FDA.

Consequently, although the image of the receptor underpinned concepts of specificity during much of the postwar period, ultimately it was the regulatory framework that put the premium on specificity. Where the history of psychopharmacology is concerned, the all but antibacterial model enshrined in current regulations harked back to the almost metabolic psychiatry that seemed possible in the 1960s. But this regulatory framework seems much less suited to a world in which psychotropic drugs act as network management tools, as cocktail compounds, a judicious combination of which produces benefits in treating a range of nervous states. Such treatment can in some important senses never be the subject of randomized controlled trials and can possibly never in principle be condoned by a regulator.

While these developments unfolded, Snyder had gone on to demonstrate that a range of other brain contents, such as D-serine, that no pharmacologist would ever have imagined could be neurotransmitters were in fact neurotransmitters. Among these were two gases: nitrous oxide and carbon monoxide.[138] The vital vapors of the eighteenth century's Paracelsians and iatrochemists had astonishingly reappeared. The brain had once again begun to seem mysterious. If receptors were the final nail in the coffin of vitalism, the end of a story that began with Wöhler and urea, some of these new transmitters were weirdly like the vapors that arose from chemical reactions that the earliest chemical doctors thought might be able to reconcile the science of chemistry with life.

At the end of the century another focus of interest was Substance P. This neurotransmitter had been out of the frame for so long that no one remembered that it was so called because it had been isolated by Gaddum and Crawford from urine (pee) in the early 1950s. While hunting for it they had discovered the existence of 5HT in the brain and sent history down one road. The Substance P road remained blocked off. From the 1950s on, pharmacology departments and industrial laboratories had tried to produce drugs that would act on the Substance P system. In the absence of tools to manipulate it, knowledge about the Substance P system grew slowly. It became clear that it was associated with sensory systems especially the pain system. An increasingly good case was being made that Substance P antagonists had some utility in treating anxiety disorders, affective disorders, and psychoses—as large a range of actions as chlorpromazine once had. Decades of work got nowhere until in the 1990s researchers at the Pfizer Pharmaceutical Company discovered that a modification of a compound produced by Edward Warawa in 1963 and left on a laboratory shelf at the Aldrich Pharmaceutical Company, blocked Substance P receptors.[139] The mistake had been in trying to mimic nature too closely.[140]

The Substance P story yields two lessons. There are two contrasting views of science that interact throughout this story. One is that science evolves by progressively more adequate theorizing, with theories checked by critical experiments. The other view is that it evolves when there are new technical developments. These reveal new phenomena, which theorists, post hoc, scramble to accommodate. According to the latter view, technology drives both history and science. Any consideration of the neuroscience story makes it clear that this latter view of science has to be at least partly right.

But if this is the case, then we have reached a position where it takes the resources of a pharmaceutical company to produce a compound such as a Substance P antagonist and establish exactly how it works. University departments simply cannot do this.

There is a real sense, then, in which a great deal of the future of neuroscience and with it the future of our understanding of ourselves depends on companies.

Companies, however, are governed by a business ethic. They are happy if their compounds reveal something further about human nature, but if those compounds do not sell, these answers to ancient secrets will be buried in the vaults as thoroughly as the mummies in an ancient Egyptian tomb. To make money out of a compound, companies first have to satisfy the 1962 amendments to the U.S. Food and Drugs Act (see Chapters 7 and 8). In an effort to restrict the ability of companies to hawk worthless medicines and to make drug taking as safe as possible, the government has fettered companies with these amendments, which put a premium on producing specific treatments for specific diseases. These same amendments, however, may conceivably lead to a scenario where a Substance P antagonist that might have considerable utility for treating nervous disorders would never reach the market because it could never be shown to work well enough for one specific disorder that occurs with sufficient frequency in the community to warrant its production. It would definitely not be developed if it were a tool that could potentially tell us more about ourselves and our aspirations but had only marginal clinical utility or an unfavorable political profile—the LSD story can never repeat itself.

6

Positive and Negative

SK&F reportedly made up to $75 million from chlorpromazine in the first year it was sold.[1] The drug was so profitable because it was given to almost all patients in all mental hospitals in the United States. Moreover, the patients treated with chlorpromazine, unlike those who could be treated briefly with antibiotics, might have to be treated for many years. Many drug companies strove to get a piece of the market, and a flood of compounds poured into hospitals. But none of these treatments cured more than a proportion of patients, and there was scope for further innovation and more drugs. Then all of sudden, around 1970, the flow of new drugs for schizophrenia effectively stopped. When new agents began to emerge once again in the 1990s, psychiatrists were concerned about their differential effects on positive and negative schizophrenia—concepts that neither Kraepelin nor Eugen Bleuler would have recognized. The new compounds, moreover, would be antipsychotics rather than neuroleptics.

WHAT'S IN A NAME?

The neuroleptics were initially viewed in many quarters as simply sedatives, drugs that, if they affected a psychosis, controlled behavior until a crisis passed. But it became clear from work in Paris and Lyon that this simple view could not be right. In Paris, from early on it was recognized that some patients sunk in profoundly disturbed states could with time "wake up" from their psychoses. This response was inconsistent with a response to a sedative.[2] Similar responses were seen in Basel by Labhardt, Staehelin, and their colleagues, leading them to use higher doses over longer periods to treat chronic psychoses.[3] In the United States Donald Klein and many others saw patients wake up,[4] and Heinz Lehmann suggested that these drugs might for some patients be antipsychotic rather than simply sedative.[5] Some of Leo Hollister's colleagues did not know what to do with all the patients who were now talking to them for the first time—this response was a long way from chemical straitjacketing of manic behavior until a crisis passed.[6]

Similar observations in Lyon led to the notion that these new neuroplegic agents came in two kinds—sedative agents and incisive agents.[7] And thus was born the first bipolar classification of the neuroleptics, splitting them into those that were containing and those that were stimulating. Paris did not agree with Lyon. The Parisian view was that the bipolarity lay in the patients rather than the drugs. The same drug, chlorpromazine, could be both sedative and incisive. It could act as a camisole chimique or it could awaken schizophrenic patients just as effectively as L-dopa was later arouse patients with encephalitis lethargica.

Some years later, in 1964, the Psychopharmacology Research Center branch of the NIMH ran, in nine hospitals, one of the first multicenter, double-blind studies of chlorpromazine as a treatment for schizophrenia. This influential study showed that chlorpromazine was unequivocally superior to a placebo, and that it was particularly effective in treating the negative features of the illness.[8] This huge study, reporting before the words positive and negative became as loaded as they were later to become, acts as a backdrop for the antipsychotic story in the last decades of the century.

The Tricyclic Antipsychotics

From the mid-1950s on, many pharmaceutical companies looked for ways to circumvent the patents on chlorpromazine and make their own version of it or a similar drug. Geigy, for instance, hung the side chain of chlorpromazine onto a nucleus similar to the phenothiazine nucleus, the imminodibenzyl nucleus (derived from the dye summer blue), and produced the drug imipramine.[9] But even when the dose was increased to 1,500 milligrams per day, imipramine had no beneficial or neuroleptic effects. The fact that it was not a neuroleptic killed it in terms of further development as an antipsychotic at that time.

Geigy, unaware that it had a distinctive compound, continued to search for its own version of chlorpromazine. In 1958, for example, Geigy's scientists noted that chlorination, a recognized way to make a compound more potent and more toxic, had transformed the relatively weak promazine into chlorpromazine. Might it do the same for imipramine? They tried it and synthesized chlorimipramine, a distinctive compound that later gave rise to the SSRIs. In 1958 it went into clinical trials aimed at testing its efficacy in schizophrenia.[10] But chlorimipramine was not a new chlorpromazine. Nor was dichlorimipramine, which Geigy then synthesized. At that point, Geigy lost interest in these compounds, which appeared to be only antidepressants—for which there was then a much smaller and less interesting market.

Owing to Geigy's failure in the schizophrenic arena with what are now thought of as tricyclic compounds, there is today a widespread clinical impression that compounds with a tricyclic nucleus must be antidepressant, whereas compounds with a phenothiazine nucleus are antipsychotic. But this clear division is based in great part on historical accident. There is no pharmacological reason why one group should be antipsychotic and one antidepressant. The concepts of an antipsychotic and an antidepressant are neither chemical nor pharmacological. They are social constructs, and there are in fact a large number of compounds that straddle the boundaries between the two, compounds whose significance is blurred by efforts to force them into a market development straitjacket. In contrast to Geigy, for example, the Japanese company Yoshitomi in 1962 synthesized a series of tricyclic compounds, one of which, carpipramide, had many features that would now place it in the atypical antipsychotic group.[11]

Another interesting compound was trimipramine. This sedative tricyclic agent was made by combining the nucleus of imipramine with the side chain found in levomepromazine and promethazine. When it was first tested by Lambert and Guyotat in Lyon, they suggested that in addition to being an antidepressant it had antipsychotic effects.[12] Its use as an antidepressant flourished during the 1960s and the 1970s, when sedative antidepressants were in vogue, but declined thereafter. It was supplanted in Europe by mianserin, a nontricyclic antidepressant with a pharmacological profile similar to that of trimipramine (and almost identical to that of mirtazapine).

Then, in 1989, the D-3 receptor was discovered.[13] By this time, the dopamine hypothesis was under threat. For the defenders of this hypothesis, believing that the abnormality associated with schizophrenia lay in the dopamine system, there was a hope that a D-3 blocking drug might be worth developing. It was then discovered that trimipramine was just such a drug. Its atypical antipsychotic effects were rediscovered and it was launched on a new career as a drug for treating atypical psychoses.[14] The failure of trimipramine to cure the cases of schizophrenia other antipsychotics could not reach and the discovery of a D-4 receptor then led to a search for D-4 receptor antagonists.[15]

Mianserin had an equally unusual metamorphosis. In the

1980s it was the best-selling antidepressant in many European countries. It was attacked by the ecology groups that sprang up in Europe following the student revolutions of the late 1960s; they claimed that it led to a potentially fatal lowering of white cell counts in some patients. Owing to a quirk of history, this drug never made it to the United States, but a closely related drug, mirtazapine, did. In the meantime in Japan, where mianserin was used widely in the 1980s, it was discovered that it could compete with haloperidol as a treatment for delirium, which had of course once been considered the original form of insanity.[16]

To complicate the issue further there is also a considerable body of evidence that imipramine and other antidepressants can be useful in treating some psychoses. Jean Guyotat in Lyon, who discovered the responsiveness of OCD to imipramine in 1960, went on to describe imipramine's beneficial effects in treating a range of chronic delusional states.[17] In response to such findings, it can be argued that there are antidepressant responsive and nonantidepressant responsive psychoses and that the antidepressant responsive psychoses somehow involve an underlying mood disorder. Alternatively findings such as this stand as indicators that psychiatrists and pharmaceutical companies know much less about what they are doing than either clinicians or pharmaceutical market developers usually admit and that the designation of tricyclic drugs as antipsychotics or antidepressants owes more to business logic than anything else.

Imipramine was not the only "antidepressant" to be in some way antipsychotic. Nathan Kline, Jack Saunders, and Harry Loomer discovered the antidepressant effects of iproniazid in 1957. The discovery led to the award of a second Lasker Prize to Kline and a priority dispute with Saunders that dragged through the courts for sixteen years. Kline claimed that the antidepressant effects of iproniazid were discovered when he gave it to some of his private patients who were depressed. Loomer and Saunders, Kline's coworkers, in contrast, had witnessed its effects on "patients [who] were withdrawn and deteriorated, with a heavy weighting of hebephrenics."[18] As Kline noted afterward these beneficial effects of iproniazid on psychoses remained unexplained.[19]

They remained unexplained because the triumph of haloperidol and the neuroleptic idea mandated a rigid form of development of antipsychotic drugs from 1959 on. The first French classification systems that distinguished between sedative, neuroleptic, and disinhibiting agents gave way to a view that these properties of the drugs were just side effects. According to this view the core effect of the drugs could be expressed in terms of chlorpromazine dose equivalents. This became the standard North American view. It fit with the emerging dopamine hypothesis of schizophrenia, which saw the effects mediated through the dopamine system as the key to the benefits of antipsychotics and all other effects as side effects. The dominance of this view underpinned haloperidol's rise to become the most widely prescribed neuroleptic.

An amphetamine antagonism model had driven the production of haloperidol. Amphetamine and another dopamine agonist, apomorphine, produced a range of extrapyramidal syndromes in animals, such as stereotypies. Haloperidol and chlorpromazine reversed these and produced syndromes of their own. For instance, they made rats cataleptic—they induced experimental catatonia. The blockage of the effects of amphetamine and apomorphine, and the production of catalepsy, quickly became the signs that development teams looked for when screening for new compounds. This process produced a series of increasingly potent neuroleptics. These could be given in such low doses that it became possible to contemplate producing them in long-acting, injectable forms now known as depot neuroleptics. Yet one set of tricyclic compounds that did not fit the behavioral profile of the neuroleptics had been overlooked. It is to the twin developments of depot neuroleptics and the most famous tricyclic antipsychotic, clozapine, that our story now turns.

The Depot Neuroleptics

With the development of haloperidol, potency became king. As opinion settled on the idea that chlorpromazine worked because it was a neuroleptic, it became easier to optimize new drugs for neuroleptic properties. The goal was to produce a drug that antagonized amphetamine and apomorphine at lower doses than chlorpromazine without having the sedative, hypotensive, and other "side" effects chlorpromazine had. Clinically the drug should produce extrapyramidal effects at low doses. A simple modification of prochlorperazine produced trifluoperazine for SK&F, its very own neuroleptic. Another modification produced perphenazine for the Sterling Pharmaceutical Company. These home-grown neuroleptics competed with Thorazine and the even more sedative thioridazine (Mellaril) for the American market in the decade before haloperidol's arrival. In Europe, Janssen's pimozide and Lundbeck's piflutixol and tiflutixol were developed; all three could be given in 1-milligram doses that would produce visible effects several days later.[20] This development trajectory was amplified in the 1970s with the emergence of capacities to radio-label D-2 receptors. These new techniques gave companies the capacity to move beyond optimization by amphetamine antagonism.

In the 1960s, having produced perphenazine, Sterling moved on to produce a fluorinated version of perphenazine, fluphenazine. Perphenazine was at the time rapidly becoming the standard alternative to chlorpromazine and was in the view of many U.S. clinicians superior to chlorpromazine. It was much less likely to cause sedation. At the doses used clinically, it was more likely to cause extrapyramidal problems but given the emerging views of how neuroleptics worked that outcome was almost reassuring. A long-acting injectable preparation of perphenazine appeared to have a real chance of displacing Thorazine, which was not available in a long-acting form.

Sterling, however, became the object of a hostile takeover bid from Charles Revlon, the owner of a cosmetics empire. In order to protect itself, Sterling offloaded stock to make it seem as though its pipeline of drugs was poor and that predators would not get much for their money. Fluphenazine was fostered out to White Pharmaceuticals, a small company that specialized in vitamin supplements and pediatric formulations of different drugs.[21]

At the same time, E. R. Squibb & Company had developed methods of producing long-acting forms of many compounds. Not all compounds could be produced in long-acting injectable forms, but neuroleptics, with their fluorine moiety, were particularly likely to combine with the mixture of lipids that would permit slow release. Hunting for potential compounds suited to the new technology, Squibb became aware that White Pharmaceuticals had fluphenazine, which it had hoped to develop for children. Squibb prevailed on White to give it access to fluphenazine.

When Revlon's takeover bid for Sterling failed, Sterling wanted fluphenazine back. It got it back. White hung on to a pediatric formulation and Squibb was given the rights for the depot formulations of fluphenazine. The first depot, produced in 1963, was Moditen, fluphenazine enanthate, which gave steady blood levels of the drug lasting up to two weeks. A further manipulation produced Modecate, fluphenazine decanoate, in 1965. This lasted up to four weeks.

Depot neuroleptics offer obvious conveniences. They look particularly attractive to physicians, caretakers, and state organizations that view neuroleptics as significantly improving the schizophrenic state or at least controlling troublesome behaviors. They may look much less appealing to patients, who may have adverse responses to neuroleptics, such as akathisia, demotivation, diminution of their sex life, and a variety of other problems, that are not noticed by the medical staff administering the drug. With individual oral treatments, there is the option to take drug holidays or manipulate the doses. With depot treatments, no such options exist. But the times were such that all patients were typically informed of the treatments they would be given rather than consulted about them. Psychiatry in this respect was no different from the rest of medical practice.

Psychiatrists were enthusiastic about depot medications. In the United States, civil libertarian concerns meant that only three depot medications were ever licensed there—Modecate, Moditen, and Haldol. In Europe and the rest of the world, in contrast, these three and a further four were licensed: Rhône-Poulenc's Piportil, Lundbeck's Depixol and Clopixol, and Redeptin.

When Moditen and Modecate came to France, they were given to the CLRTP group in Lyon to test. They found that both were acceptably antipsychotic, that the depot form gave the same results as the oral form, and that the effects of Modecate lasted for three to four weeks.[22] They worked out the appropriate dose levels. They became very enthusiastic about depot drugs. Clearly, this form of treatment could facilitate care in the community. If patients who had previously not taken their medication could be persuaded to take the medication in a depot form or otherwise compelled to do so, many could be released from the hospital and could live in the community more readily than before. Their caretakers and others were assured that the patients were taking their medication.

But there were hazards associated with these drugs. Richard de Alarcon and Michael Carney in Britain reported on a series of suicides committed by patients taking depot neuroleptics.[23] In Lyon, clinicians also observed that some patients, apparently living satisfactorily at home, committed suicide, without warning. It became necessary to alert the community psychiatric nurses visiting these patients to pay closer attention to the patients. Was a patient sitting in front of a television set actively watching TV? Did he know, for instance, what was happening on the program? Or was he sitting there because he was lethargic and demotivated to do anything else? Or, alternatively, was he sitting there, seemingly watching the TV, but actually contemplating suicide?

The next series of depot neuroleptics came from Danish

pharmaceutical company H. S. Lundbeck, which specialized in a different series of drugs, the thioxanthenes. Chlorprothixene, the first of these, combined characteristics of chlorpromazine and the "antidepressant" amitriptyline. In retrospect, chlorprothixene looks as if it had many of the features of what are now called atypical antipsychotics. Lundbeck then, following the lead of the rest of the pharmaceutical industry, proceeded to produce more potent forms of the core molecule, ending up in 1965 with flupenthixol.[24] This, it became clear, could be manufactured in a depot form. Zuclopenthixol followed, which could also be made in a depot form. But none of these drugs reached the United States, even though many European clinicians found that they offered significantly better benefits than did Modecate or Haldol. Lundbeck was essentially only a European company, and the drug market was at the time far from being the globalized business it was later to become.

Later, in 1988, Lundbeck was to add another innovation to the arsenal of long-acting preparations. The company was approached by Rasmus Fog, a clinician from the Saint Hans Hospital in Roskilde, Denmark.[25] One of the times of greatest need for an injectable longer-acting medication, he said, was during the first week of hospitalization. At that time injections were often necessary, but giving repeated injections was unpleasant for both staff and patients. Once the initial crisis had passed, there might not be a further need for injections. This argument led Lundbeck to formulate an injectable form of clopenthixol. The result was a drug, Clopixol Acuphase, that stayed in the system for three to four days. It rapidly became popular throughout Europe.

Megadose Therapy

The student revolutions of 1968 had criticized neuroleptic treatment, calling it simply a replacement for conventional straitjackets. But their protests did not lead to more sensitive treatment regimes; average doses of antipsychotics were on the increase in

1968 and were to rise tenfold over the following two decades. Two engines drove this rise: the availability of depot medications and the dopamine hypothesis of schizophrenia.

In 1968, depot neuroleptics were just emerging. Their use, while of great benefit to some, "trapped" others in a treatment there was no getting away from. Furthermore, these injected drugs are several times more potent than oral preparations, since much less gets broken down by first-pass metabolism in the gut or by the liver. In addition, there was an inevitable tendency on the part of prescribers, mental health staff, and the patients' relatives to think that if the patients were not visibly taking medication by mouth, they were not taking medication at all. As a result, many patients were given cocktails of both depot and oral neuroleptics. And furthermore, because many clinicians believed that different neuroleptics had somewhat different properties, patients might be given two different oral neuroleptics in addition to a depot preparation.

A theory of what the core abnormality in schizophrenia was that did not implicate dopamine might have put a brake on this dose escalation; the emergence of the dopamine hypothesis of schizophrenia did the opposite. If the dopamine system was the site of the lesion in schizophrenia, and the drugs acted on the dopamine system and the patient did not get better, the clinical logic seemed clear: give more of the drug. It was regularly pointed out that there was considerable variation between individuals in rates of metabolism of drugs. Maybe those who were not responding to treatment simply were not getting enough drug into their brains.

Besides, the approach could be justified because there were some patients who did get better when given higher doses of these potent compounds than when they had been given older compounds. They were less sedated and less troubled by blood pressure problems. With relatively low doses extrapyramidal side effects appeared; these, however, could be managed with anticholinergic antidotes, and it became common practice to prescribe an anticholinergic antidote at the beginning of treatment, so that patients ended up taking yet another drug. And oddly the extra-pyramidal effects that appeared with doses of 4–5 milligrams of haloperidol or other neuroleptics, and got worse as doses were increased to 40–50 milligrams, vanished when the dose rose above 60 milligrams per day. An explanation for this effect was worked out in Japan in 1980: at doses above 60 milligrams an action of haloperidol and other neuroleptics on the norepinephrine system kicks in.[26] But like most Japanese discoveries, this finding was not picked up in the West.

The fact that some patients were still able to function when ingesting massive doses was taken by some to indicate a fundamental difference between psychotic and normal people. What normal person could tolerate these doses without being horribly affected? So long as the dopamine hypothesis held sway, there was an apparent scientific basis for this perception. The alternative didn't bear contemplating: that the toxicity that normal people experienced when taking low doses of neuroleptics was being inflicted on psychotic patients in a highly intensified form. A small number of voices drew attention to the fact that some patients got dramatically worse when taking even very low doses of the drugs. But nobody wanted to hear that: not drug companies and not clinicians.

The trends toward ever larger doses culminated with the explicit formulation of megadose therapy approaches. Patients were to be rapidly neurolepticized as soon as they were hospitalized, and doses were increased to the equivalent of 5,000 milligrams of chlorpromazine per day. Haloperidol narcosis became popular. This involved giving 10 milligrams of intravenous haloperidol hourly—potentially equivalent to giving 25,000 milligrams of chlorpromazine by mouth per day. The result was a striking testimony to haloperidol's lack of lethal toxicity. But there was a rising tide of deaths in patients taking high doses of neuroleptics caused by a new and sinister condition called neuroleptic malignant syndrome, as well by dystonias that led to asphyxiation and cardiovascular collapse; in several countries such deaths were investigated by professional groups.[27]

Many of these high-dose regimes were inflicted on young women, a group less likely to have dementia praecox than young men and far more likely to be displaying pseudo-psychotic dissociative symptoms as a consequence of sexual or physical abuse (see Chapter 7). Vagn Pedersen of Lundbeck, for example, had an inquiry from clinicians in Norway asking whether Lundbeck knew of any problems they were likely to encounter if they increased the level of flupenthixol for an eighteen-year-old girl from 1,000 to 2,000 milligrams per day (roughly comparable to an increase from 20,000 to 40,000 milligrams of chlorpromazine per day).[28] Such high doses were also administered to patients with personality disorders, who were becoming increasingly common within mental health services. Drug advertising to physicians in the 1970s and early 1980s regularly focused on young men's antisocial and violent behavior and recommended the use of neuroleptics to bring about behavioral control in patients with personality disorders.

Then in 1988, the megadose approach attracted great criticism. The January issue of the *Archives of General Psychiatry* carried two articles. The first was by Ross Baldessarini and his colleagues, who had studied the clinical trial evidence on the relationship between doses of antipsychotics and optimal clinical responses. They could find no evidence that doses higher than 600 milligrams of chlorpromazine or 30 milligrams of haloperidol per day were likely to produce extra benefits.[29] Maybe, some speculated, this was so because the more severely ill patients were getting the higher doses. But data from randomized dosing studies failed to show this was the case.

On its own, this article would probably have not made many ripples, but the same issue of the *Archives* carried an article on research using the latest in high-tech science that came to essentially the same conclusion. Lars Farde and colleagues at the Karolinska Institute in Sweden had radio-labeled drugs to bind to D-2 receptors and then scanned for D-2 receptor numbers in schizophrenic and normal brains, as well as determining D-2 receptor occupancy with different doses of antipsychotics.[30] There were two surprises. First, the numbers of D-2 receptors in schizophrenic and normal brains overlapped. Second, this and subsequent studies suggested that what until then would have seemed extraordinarily low doses of antipsychotics produced the optimal balance between D-2 receptor occupancy, clinical response, and a lack of extrapyramidal side effects.

In short order, other groups demonstrated that in fact those who were doing least well on neuroleptics were likely to have the most, not the least, amount of drug in the brain.[31] In other words, at least some of those doing poorly were being poisoned. Other randomized trials quickly followed, showing that patients got out of hospital as quickly when dosed with 5 milligrams of haloperidol as when dosed with 20 or more milligrams.[32] But none of this work might have had any impact had it not been for the fact that the antipsychotic landscape had changed. A new drug had come on the market that challenged the idea of a neuroleptic.

THE FALL AND RISE OF CLOZAPINE

By far the most significant of the tricyclic "antipsychotics" was clozapine. In 1958, Fritz Hünziker, with J. Schmutz and E. Eichenberger of the chemistry department in the Wander Pharmaceutical Company, synthesized a series of dibenzepine compounds that had a tricyclic ring structure. Some of them looked like imipramine, but antidepressants were of no great interest to a pharmaceutical company at that time so they were not pursued.[33] Some of the others looked different and these were investigated to see if they had antipsychotic effects, because such drugs were in demand.[34]

The pharmacologist at Wander, Günther Stille, put clozapine through a series of screening tests.[35] At the time, following

Janssen's success in developing haloperidol, the blockage of the effects of amphetamine and apomorphine was becoming the key screening test in antipsychotic drug development. Apomorphine differs from amphetamine, and is even useful in treating acute psychotic disturbances.[36] At high doses it causes vomiting and can be used to test for the anti-emetic effects of phenothiazines. At lower doses in animals, it can induce a range of behaviors, causing a mouse for instance to climb as well as a rat to gnaw and bite in a stereotyped way. At the time it was not clear that what later were to become the classic antipsychotics would block all these effects.

Stille tested the new series of compounds on animals with apomorphine-induced climbing and found that three of his compounds, perlapine, clozapine, and fluperlapine, blocked the effect. They did not block apomorphine-induced gnawing and biting or stereotypy in rats, nor did they induce catalepsy in the animals. Schmutz and Eichenberger later conceded that if the testing of these compounds had taken place later, when the blockage of apomorphine-induced gnawing and biting as well as stereotypy were accepted screening tests for antipsychotics, the failure of their compounds to block these effects would probably have led to their being shelved.[37]

The first compound that was tested in a clinic, perlapine, turned out to be a potent sedative, without clear antipsychotic effects. It was shelved, and was succeeded by clozapine in 1961. Clozapine was first given for clinical testing to Hanns Heimann in Bern, who found that it appeared to aggravate some psychoses, possibly because it can produce anxiety-inducing effects on the heart, respiratory, and other systems. It also caused marked hypersalivation in most patients, and other problems in many patients. He was against further development.[38] The pharmaceutical company gave clozapine to two other groups to investigate. One was Pierre Deniker's group at the Sainte-Anne. Deniker and Pierre Simon gave clozapine to nineteen patients. There were four fatalities, one from an irreversible agranulocytosis and another from malignant hyperthermia.[39] Until then, virtually all investigators had regarded the neuroleptics as extraordinarily safe drugs. In Paris, psychiatrists had never seen anything like the lethality associated with this new drug. The trial was terminated early, and Deniker reported to the company that in his opinion the drug was unsafe for further development. Another study by Gross and Langner in Vienna was more successful, the investigators reporting antipsychotic effects and no serious problems.[40]

The potential of the new drug came to the attention of a group of Swiss and German investigators who had established a network for the systematic investigation of new agents.[41] A large clinical trial involving ten centers in Germany, Switzerland, and Austria was conducted, and it demonstrated that clozapine was efficacious.[42] The drug was released in Switzerland, Austria, Germany, and Italy under the trade name Leponex. Further clinical trials were done, which in general showed that the compound was good but not dramatically more effective in treating standard psychotic conditions than other agents such as chlorpromazine and haloperidol.[43]

Among the German investigators was Hanns Hippius, who along with others realized that clozapine posed a significant challenge to current theories of neuroleptic action, in particular the notion that these drugs had to produce extrapyramidal side effects in order to be effective antipsychotics.[44] Although clozapine might produce akathisia and neuroleptic malignant syndrome, it did not produce the classic neuroleptic extrapyramidal effects. Some other drugs such as thioridazine (Mellaril) and levomepromazine (Nozinan) also had a very low propensity for extrapyramidal side effects, but these too could in some cases cause dyskinesias and dystonias, especially when given in high doses. Clozapine seemed different, and not just because epileptic convulsions inhibited its use in high doses.

Although in treating ordinary psychotic cases it might not be strikingly more effective than other antipsychotics, in treating cases that were refractory to other antipsychotics, it sometimes produced significantly better effects than any other treatment.

But there was a further benefit to clozapine. If patients with gross tardive dyskinesia were medicated with clozapine, over time this problem cleared up in many cases.[45] This effect of clozapine on tardive dyskinesia led Nathan Kline to obtain, from Jules Angst in Zurich, supplies of the drug and bring them back to the United States to treat a number of patients, thereby introducing clozapine to the United States. Finally, there was another advantage to clozapine. Patients who could not be stabilized on any other drug but who could be stabilized on clozapine showed a gross deterioration in their mental state if clozapine was discontinued. The possibility that this reaction might be a specific withdrawal syndrome was not considered at the time. The paramount clinical view was that this drug was needed.

All these arguments were to be needed when clozapine ran into problems in Finland. In 1975, a number of patients put on clozapine there developed unrecognized agranulocytosis. Twenty died, and that outcome led to the withdrawal of the drug from Finland and a suspension of all applications to have it licensed in other countries, including the United States. The investigation of the Finnish problems produced no clear answer.[46] There had already been a recognition that agranulocytosis occurred after the administration of neuroleptic and tricyclic compounds and that northern Europeans seemed to be more susceptible to it than southern Europeans.[47] That there is some ethnic component to the problem is shown by the fact that studies of clozapine in Japan produced no cases of agranulocytosis. Clozapine did not achieve a widespread use there, however, because it seemed more likely than traditional neuroleptics to cause a neuroleptic malignant syndrome. Differing ethnic susceptibilities to side effects has, therefore, been the traditional explanation for what happened in Finland.[48] Modern developments in pharmacogenetics might now rescue a compound that caused a problem related to ethnicity, but in the 1970s such a problem doomed the drug.

The chemists at Wander went back to the series of compounds from which perlapine and clozapine had come and selected other compounds. One was NT201252. This seemed a good antipsychotic. It did not appear to cause extrapyramidal effects. But it was prone to cause another of clozapine's problems, convulsions. It was withdrawn. The group moved on to another compound, fluperlapine. This was put into clinical trials and proved an effective antipsychotic. It did not cause extrapyramidal problems and did not appear to cause agranulocytosis.[49] But it did cause liver problems and for that reason it was withdrawn.[50]

By this time Wander had been taken over by Sandoz, which decided to do more work on clozapine. The company had to for a number of reasons. First the drug was still on the market as Leponex.[51] Was it safe to keep selling it? The initial decision within the company was to remove it from all markets because the legal liabilities were too great. This decision elicited furious opposition from clinicians such as Angst, Hippius, and Battegay who argued that clozapine was a singular compound.[52] It needed to be kept on the market both for the sake of those patients who benefited uniquely from it and for the negative implications its withdrawal would have for the development of antipsychotic drugs. Initially it looked as though Sandoz would not be persuaded, even in the face of legal action from some of the clinicians. Finally the drug won a champion within the company, Hanns Bühlmann, who was the head of the Sandoz branch in Germany. Bühlmann was persuaded by Hippius and others that the compound was too valuable to drop and that every effort should be made to preserve its place in the market. His voice carried weight within the company and clozapine survived.[53]

Once Sandoz decided to keep selling clozapine, the company had to decide whether to try to get it onto other markets. Fortunately, another developmental possibility opened up. Clozapine was in clinical trials in the United States when the agranulocytosis problems emerged. The original plan to apply for a license was dropped, but the drug was still used to treat psychosis associated with severe tardive dyskinesia by a small number of investigators, notably Nathan Kline, George Simpson, and Jonathan Cole.[54]

Sandoz's Gil Honigfeld then undertook a study that showed that when given to patients with tardive dyskinesia, clozapine both controlled their psychoses and effected significant improvements in their tardive dyskinesia.[55] This finding was not sufficient to persuade the FDA to license clozapine for the treatment of tardive dyskinesia, but it did lead to a recognition that this compound deserved further investigation.[56] Meetings in the company and discussions with international investigators and in particular with regulators from the FDA persuaded Sandoz to push ahead.

The result was Study 30. This study was designed and coordinated by John Kane and Herbert Meltzer. It enrolled patients who were apparently resistant to other antipsychotics. To enter the study patients had to have had lengthy courses of at least three different antipsychotics, and had to undergo treatment with haloperidol in doses of up to 60 milligrams a day without showing any response to the treatment. If these conditions were fulfilled they could then participate in a trial where they received clozapine or chlorpromazine in a dose of up to 1,800 milligrams a day.

The results of the study were dramatic. These patients, some whom were among the most severely ill patients in any psychiatric hospital, showed little or no benefits when receiving haloperidol or chlorpromazine, but when receiving clozapine many showed improvements, with some making dramatically good recoveries, while others at least became less agitated. The results were clear cut. The investigators did not need sophisticated statistical analysis to demonstrate changes that might be of dubious clinical significance. These were findings of a kind investigators were not accustomed to seeing since the early testing of chlorpromazine and other antipsychotics in neuroleptic-naive patients.[57]

On the basis of this study the FDA licensed clozapine for use in dealing with treatment-resistant schizophrenia. In theory, the number of such patients should be small. Accordingly, Sandoz set a high price for a year's supply of the drug, $9,000, whereas a year's supply of chlorpromazine might cost only $100. But while Sandoz could not promote the drug's use for patients other than resistant schizophrenics, in practice, the drug could be given to anyone whom a clinician thought it might benefit. Sales of clozapine grew dramatically following its relaunch in 1989, so much so that in the early 1990s it made more profit than any other psychotropic compound.

Clozapine's success led to new developments. As part of the terms of its license in the United States and some other countries, blood tests were mandatory. In several of these countries Sandoz established a Clozaril Patient Monitoring Service, which performed the blood tests, did the analyses, and reported back to the clinician as to whether treatment could continue. This expensive arrangement could be used by Sandoz to justify part of the cost of the drug. It also led to the collection of a great deal of data on the drug and its adverse effects that were potentially invaluable to the company. It gave Sandoz a clear idea of who was taking the drug and where.

But the cost caused a public outcry. During a symposium on clozapine being held at an American Psychiatric Association meeting, demonstrators burst in and demanded that the drug be made available at a price that was affordable by patients who were not wealthy. The public pressure was intense. Government programs and some insurers refused to pay for the drug. But the company was unyielding.[58] This selling of clozapine, and of the SSRIs, in the early 1990s led to the emergence of pharmacoeconomics, a field heavily supported by the pharmaceutical industry, whose practitioners appeared able to conjure equations that proved that one set of drugs costing forty to fifty times more than another set were in fact cost saving.

The price of clozapine set a benchmark for other companies to aim at, giving them a considerable incentive to penetrate this market. Any company that could produce a clozapine that did not cause agranulocytosis stood to make considerable amounts of money— so much that the cost of the drug threatened to bankrupt some state medical systems.[59] But the question remained: how precisely did clozapine work?

TARDIVE DYSKINESIA

The primary factor behind the survival of clozapine was its effects on tardive dyskinesia. Unnoticed in the 1950s, recognized in the 1960s, tardive dyskinesia by the 1970s was regularly portrayed as the greatest drawback to neuroleptic therapy. In the first years of chlorpromazine's use, clinicians saw and reported a number of odd jaw and tongue movements, which they regarded as dyskinesias of one sort or the other. As they became familiar with the idea that the neuroleptics could cause dystonias and dyskinesias and that these were drug induced rather than hysterical, they stopped worrying about them. They came to regard these neurological side effects as an inconvenience rather than a real problem.

The first report of dyskinesia involving the mouth and tongue that appeared to persist after discontinuation of treatment came from Sigwald and his colleagues and was published in a French journal in 1959.[60] Some German-language reports appeared around the same time. But the report that brought the phenomenon to the attention of the world came from an investigator in Denmark, Arbild Faurbye in 1960. In the first issue of *Psychopharmacologia*, Faurbye presented the first English-language report on tardive dyskinesia, based on a study of patients who had persistent involuntary abnormal movements. He illustrated the condition with a series of graphic photographs.[61]

One of the drugs Faurbye implicated in this condition was perphenazine, sold by Sterling. Sterling sought advice from Frank Ayd. Ayd had written the definitive English-language article on neurological complications of the antipsychotics for the *Journal of the American Medical Association*.[62] Sterling sent him to Denmark to see Faurbye and try to find out exactly what was happening with Faurbye's patients. Ayd recognized that among the cases, older women were more likely to develop tardive dyskinesia and that although many of the patients were taking a variety of medications, they all were taking perphenazine. He wrote to Sterling that in his opinion what Faurbye had described was a neurological complication, but whether it was related to drug treatment or something existing in the patients before treatment was less clear.[63]

In the 1960s, other reports on Faurbye's new syndrome, complete with photographs, began to appear.[64] The condition was particularly likely to occur after the discontinuation of drugs.[65] In the German-speaking world, R. Degkwitz drew attention to the problem of persistent abnormal involuntary movements. But there continued to be considerable skepticism that this was a drug-induced condition. In Philadelphia, William Winkleman, who had been one of the first to use the neuroleptics, presented an older woman exhibiting odd jaw, tongue, and cheek movements to a group of colleagues convinced that neuroleptics could cause these problems. He asked them for explanations and they said that the diagnosis was drug-induced persistent involuntary movements.[66] Winkleman asked the woman to leave the room; she came back in a few minutes with all the strange movements gone. What had happened? Outside the room she had been instructed to put her teeth back in and now there was no sign of the problem.

A further example illustrates the difficulties. Degkwitz discussed the problem at the CINP meeting in Washington, D.C., in 1966, where he presented details of the new syndrome. Challenged by skeptical clinicians, he volunteered to demonstrate the condition in the local psychiatric hospital, St. Elizabeth's. The next day, a group of clinicians duly set off for St. Elizabeth's, where Degkwitz drew their attention to a man who he thought showed classic features of the syndrome. The observers were impressed, until one of the nurses asked the man to remove the chewing gum from his mouth, and as soon as he did the syndrome "vanished."[67]

Throughout the 1960s, the phenomenon was often referred to as persistent dyskinesia, but gradually the term tardive dyskinesia, coined by Faurbye in 1964, caught on.[68] Despite initial skepticism, by the late 1960s opinion was beginning to accept that long-term treatment might cause the problem. Reviews by Frank

Ayd[69] and George Crane,[70] senior figures in the psychopharma-cology establishment, appeared confirming that drug treatment caused the condition.

Crane did more than anyone to raise the profile of the condi-tion with a series of reviews and studies.[71] But he faced a decade of difficulties and even hostility.[72] For fifteen years clinicians had looked to extrapyramidal effects as evidence that a drug was work-ing. Some, such as Haase in Germany, argued that an extrapyra-midal effect was necessary for therapy but that the patient should not be tipped into frank Parkinsonism.[73] But the opposite posi-tion was equally logical. If some extrapyramidal constraint was a good thing, even more would be better. If patients could be kept mobile with anticholinergic drugs, why not attempt to "choke off the oxygen" to their delusional and hallucinatory systems.

There was a further possibility. Perhaps neuroleptics did in-deed induce a problem, but what if the illness also caused it? When Crane presented his findings at meetings he drew hostile responses from Nathan Kline, Herman Denber, and Leo Hollis-ter, among others, who argued that the dyskinesias he was blam-ing on treatment could be demonstrated in untreated patients.[74] In 1968, the *American Journal of Psychiatry* published a supple-ment in which the protagonists laid out their positions.[75] The dis-cussions took a form that had characterized the debates about psychoanalysis previously and that has since characterized debates about Prozac and suicidality and abuse and recovered memories. Two positions typically are expressed. First, blame the disease not the treatment. Second, even if there are some problems with the treatment, there will be an even greater number of problems if patients are scared away from treatment. The field faces a calcu-lus. Do the challengers have evidence that warning about a new hazard will actually do more good in the long run? Ever since the development of anesthesia, taking the risk of injuring some while benefiting many has been an acceptable trade-off.[76]

Then ongoing research began to produce estimates that up to a quarter of patients on long-term neuroleptics might be affected.

It also became clear that tardive dyskinesia was a potentially irreversible condition. Initially described as emerging on withdrawal of treatment, the condition was then noted emerging during the course of treatment. When it became clear that some patients remained affected for several years after withdrawal of drugs, the problem became a crisis.

There was one solution: increase the dose. The dose escalation of the late 1960s may explain why the problem was slow to be recognized. Ironically, in the 1970s, the first formulation of a dopamine hypothesis, which when applied to schizophrenia was later to lead to the high dose regimes that did so much to create the problem, came from Daniel Tarsy and Ross Baldessarini in the form of a dopamine hypothesis of tardive dyskinesia.[77]

The FDA and the American College of Neuropsychopharmacology set up a task force to study the problem. It reported in 1973 that there could be a problem but that the medications could still "be used with confidence—the overwhelming clinical and objective evidence indicates that a majority of schizophrenic patients" should continue to receive medication.[78] But this report did not prevent legal action. Tardive dyskinesia provided psychiatric patients and their lawyers with a clear-cut case of drug-induced injury. In 1974, SK&F settled a claim for Thorazine-induced tardive dyskinesia.[79] Other lawsuits followed. There was research to support the claims and experts like George Crane were called to testify for plaintiffs.

Panic set in. The American Psychiatric Association set up a task force chaired by Ross Baldessarini to investigate the extent of and possible management of the problem. The resulting report acknowledged the problem, made recommendations about lowering the doses of drugs when possible, and outlined the role of the physician in consideration of the issues.[80]

In the early days of the antipsychotics, patients and their relatives, had they been asked, would in many cases have been willing to trade several years of life in return for the awakening from psychosis that the antipsychotics brought about. Had they forgotten so quickly? Tardive dyskinesia probably became a huge legal issue from the mid-1970s on for several reasons. First and foremost was the fact that it was visible. The patient could be put on the witness stand and sympathy could be elicited from jurors, who could see the obvious social problems of the patient. Anger was directed at the medical profession. Invariably, it was possible to show that the medical staff had either not reviewed the patient over the course of the preceding months or had done so cursorily. It was a simple matter to catalogue the details of medical arrogance, often resulting in a series of drug-induced problems, none of which might have attracted much notice except that one of them, tardive dyskinesia, could be demonstrated visibly on the witness stand.[81]

Although tardive dyskinesia could be as severe as Huntington's disease, it was in most cases a much less serious clinical problem than akathisia. Akathisia, however, remained invisible in court, whereas tardive dyskinesia was a clear symbol of the deficiencies of psychiatric treatments. It spawned enormous numbers of legal-liability cases and was a more potent factor in both drug and conceptual development than is commonly realized.

At the time, in the early 1970s, the antipsychiatry tide was lapping high against the walls of mainstream psychiatry. ECT was on the way to being marginalized in many states in the United States and countries, not because of any lack of efficacy but in great part because of its visibility.[82] This visibility, allied to the bad practices that were easily catalogued—lack of patient consent, incomplete explanations of how the treatment worked, and in all probability punitive administration of ECT on some occasions— made it a target for forces in society concerned about the practice of psychiatry. It was all too easily portrayed as being as barbaric as psychosurgery. It could accurately be portrayed as a treatment that had been invented to cure schizophrenia that had persisted despite the fact that it was generally thought not to help that condition.

Tardive dyskinesia was for similar reasons the Achilles heel of the antipsychotics. The growth of a significant legal problem in the 1970s led to a suspension of clinical studies with anti-psychotics. In places where clinical trials had flourished, they all but stopped.[83] Producing more antipsychotics, no matter how innovative and different, had become very difficult. If in the course of development, new agents showed a propensity to cause tardive dyskinesia, their development was likely to be aborted.[84] Even if clinicians were the first to be sued, ultimately blame was likely to fall on the pharmaceutical companies, as SK&F had found.

This situation led to series of meetings between the industry and the FDA concerning how to label the propensity of their compounds to cause tardive dyskinesia. These meetings have been portrayed by critics of psychiatry and pharmacotherapy as evidence of how much the FDA had become part of the medico-pharmaceutical complex.[85] This is almost certainly a highly exaggerated interpretation, but it is the case that far more than any clinicians appreciated at the time or still appreciate, the field was being driven by the problem of legal liability. Enter clozapine. Whatever the benefits of clozapine as far as clinicians or patients were concerned, from the industry's point of view its most significant feature was that it did not cause tardive dyskinesia.

There is another dimension to the tardive dyskinesia story. The freeze on drug development was not confined to the United States; it affected Europe also. Legal liabilities in the United States now had consequences for the development of drugs worldwide. The 1970s made it clear that the American market was the most important one for any manufacturer of a new technology, whether it was a new imaging device, such as a CT (computed tomography) or MRI (magnetic-resonance imaging) scanner, or a new drug. CT and MRI scanners were developed in Europe in the 1960s and 1970s, but they were initially used mostly in the United States. The less socialized medical system there, it seemed, meant that consumer demand made new diagnostic technologies available more quickly than in Europe.[86] This speed was apparent in the therapeutic as well as the diagnostic realm. The pharmaceutical industry had already begun to develop new drugs primarily for the North American market, which accounted for 60–70 percent of the world market in cash terms. Against this background the high cost of clozapine in 1988 was not going to deter sales, at least not in the United States. The 1980s, which had seen the emergence of almost no new neuroleptics, was about to give way to the 1990s, a decade in which the antipsychotics flowered.

FROM NEUROLEPTICS TO ANTIPSYCHOTICS

Risperidone

Launched in 1994, Janssen's risperidone was the first post-clozapine new antipsychotic. Its development and the marketing strategy underpinning it heavily influenced the approach of other companies. But not all was what it seemed to be in the case of risperidone, a prototype of which, pipamperone, dated back to 1964. Pipamperone had not been appreciated when first discovered but times had changed. In fact, the marketing of risperidone was much more distinctive of 1990s thinking than that of clozapine, which always remained somewhat of a sui generis compound.

Haloperidol had been developed in part as an antagonist to the effects of amphetamine in animals. Amphetamine was a known psychotogen but it was not the only drug to produce "psychoses" in humans. LSD did too, and the psychoses produced by LSD and tryptamine derivatives differed from those produced by amphetamine. It had been known since Gaddum's experiments that LSD acted on the serotonin system, and there were good grounds to presume that amphetamine was acting on a different system. Accordingly, Janssen set about screening for drugs that would block the effects of both amphetamine and the tryptamines.[87] His efforts led in 1961 to the development of fluoro-pipamide, later called dipiperone or pipamperone.

Pipamperone went into clinical trials in the United States in 1963.[88] Although it produced fewer extrapyramidal side effects than haloperidol, neither the McNeil nor the Searle pharmaceutical companies was interested in developing it. Haloperidol had just begun to make an impact in the United States, and McNeil thought that there wasn't room for two Janssen antipsychotics on the market. In addition, haloperidol was valued for its potency. Very low doses (5–10 milligrams) were effective, whereas pipamperone was effective only in chlorpromazine-like doses (200–300 milligrams). At a time when potency was becoming king, this was a drawback. Furthermore, the fact that the new drug produced fewer extrapyramidal effects was perceived as a drawback rather than a benefit.

Retrospectively, it is clear that developing a drug the way Janssen developed pipamperone would produce a compound that blocked both D-2 receptors and 5HT-2 receptors, but this was not clear at the time. There was no basis on which to sell the new compound. Although the development of pipamperone was sensible, in the mid-1960s it seemed entirely empirical. There was no way to portray it as a product of rational engineering. But it was essentially the same compound as the later risperidone.[89]

The capacity to develop drugs based on receptor profiling developed in the 1980s, following the introduction of radio-labeled binding technologies by Snyder (see Chapter 5).[90] In 1980, using these techniques, Peroutka and Snyder had distinguished between 5HT-1 and 5HT-2 receptors, making them a target of "rational" drug development. LSD, it became clear, acted on the 5HT-2 receptor.

Nowhere were the new receptor binding technologies used more enthusiastically than in the Janssen laboratories, where the techniques were used for screening purposes. Janssen's pharmacologists also made substantial contributions to the discovery of new receptors. Company chemists and pharmacologists targeted the 5HT-2 receptor and discovered a series of drugs that selectively blocked this receptor. The best known of these were ritanserin and ketanserin. These two drugs blocked the effects of LSD and mescaline, confirming that these drugs produced their psychotogenic effects by an action on the 5HT-2a receptor.[91] With further exploration of the effects of an action on 5HT-2a receptors, it became clear that drugs acting this way did more than just produce classic LSD effects: they blocked the microcirculation and they could produce convulsions and a range of extrapyramidal problems in rats, in addition to interfering with sleep. There seemed to be nothing good produced by acting on 5HT-2a receptors.[92] The Janssen experience agreed with findings at Eli Lilly, where it was becoming clear that giving fluoxetine, which made serotonin available at 5HT-2 receptors, could produce psychotic complications in patients without obvious psychoses.

There were good reasons to test ritanserin and ketanserin in psychoses. They offered the promise of producing antipsychotic effects completely different from those produced by traditional antipsychotics.[93] In clinical trials, however, they failed. There remains a compelling pharmacological rationale for supposing that using ritanserin or ketanserin along with haloperidol depot injections would produce significant therapeutic benefits. But arguments like this hold little sway with regulators. If the compound cannot be shown to be of benefit in its own right for treating a particular condition it cannot be brought to the market. Ritanserin and ketanserin remained orphan drugs.[94]

The only option seemed to be to build haloperidol and ketanserin into the same molecule. It was this that Janssen set about doing. He went back to the strategy that produced pipamperone, except now he screened for a drug that simultaneously blocked D-2 and 5HT-2 receptors. The chemists within the company came up with a new group of compounds, butyropiperidines. Out of this series came risperidone in November 1984. This had the desired S-2–D-2 blocking properties. The first of the serotonin-dopamine antagonists (SDAs), as they were later called, was born.

This development produced a template for further drug and market development. As regards drug development, no one knew how to develop another clozapine, but developing an SDA had by the late 1980s become an almost routine matter. Clozapine, it turned out, had significant 5HT-2 receptor blocking effects, leading Herbert Meltzer to argue that its particular benefits stemmed from the ratio of D-2 to 5HT-2 receptor blockage.[95]

An SDA effect became the molecular basis for what came to be called atypicality. Clozapine could legitimately claim to be atypical, on the basis that it was not a neuroleptic. It did not produce catalepsy in animals. It did not produce extrapyramidal side effects or tardive dyskinesia in humans. Everybody wanted another clozapine, another atypical. The semantics quickly became confusing. It was not possible for a drug to be an atypical neuroleptic because by definition neuroleptics produced extrapyramidal effects. If an antipsychotic was a drug that benefited psychoses without producing neuroleptic effects, the idea of an atypical antipsychotic was a tautology. But atypicality became shorthand for drugs that differed from haloperidol. It became the Holy Grail of market development in the 1990s.

The emergence and survival of concepts in both the business and academic marketplaces is often determined by the "slogan" value of the concept. Terms like schizophrenia and neurosis worked because they carried just the right level of ambiguity, so that disparate coalitions could muster behind them. The notion of atypicality was the ultimate marketing dream: a concept that contained its opposites within it. If it was not possible to make another atypical, the next best thing was to label your compound an atypical. Sales would follow. The association between SDA profiles and atypicality provided the means to effect this trick, a trick in the sense that risperidone and olanzapine, for example, did produce dyskinesias and catalepsy.

(-)-3-PPP

Morphine had been isolated from opium in 1806.[96] Subsequently, a range of other alkaloids such as codeine were extracted. Chemistry moved on to trying to improve on the natural compounds. In 1869, Mathieson and Wright treated morphine with acid. They ended up with apomorphine, a radically different agent with little functional similarity to morphine. For example, where morphine was anti-emetic, apomorphine produced vomiting.

In the 1880s apomorphine was shown to be useful in the treatment of movement disorders, including Sydenham's chorea and Parkinson's disease, although treatment was complicated by nausea, vomiting, and hypotension.[97] By this time, it had also been shown to be useful in treating nervous conditions.[98] Eugen Bleuler, among many others, was ready to endorse the benefits of the particular kind of sedation it produced. There was little understanding of these benefits at the time though, and apomorphine's use did not become widespread because its effects seemed short lived.

By the 1950s, it had been found that apomorphine was a useful screening test for antipsychotics. They blocked some of its effects. How could it be both antipsychotic and useful in screening for antipsychotics? The conventional wisdom was that it had a dual action on the dopamine system. It acted on presynaptic dopamine neurones to release dopamine and it acted also to block dopamine's release. These actions could be teased apart by varying the dose. In low doses, it shut down the dopamine system by an autoreceptor feedback mechanism discovered by Arvid Carlsson.[99] This finding raised the possibility that apomorphine might be antipsychotic and led to the rediscovery of its historical use in treating psychotic disorders. The combination of historical precedent and neurobiological rationale led Carol Tamminga and her colleagues in 1978 to give it to patients and rediscover that even a single dose of apomorphine could be significantly antipsychotic.[100]

Carlsson meanwhile had been involved in the discovery of (-)-3-PPP, later called preclamol. This proved to be more potent than apomorphine, more selective for dopamine autoreceptors, and freer of peripheral side effects. It showed up in animal screening tests as antipsychotic without inducing extrapyramidal side effects. If any compound was going to be a novel pharmacological agent, this surely was it. Tamminga linked up with Carlsson and from 1989 to 1992, they gave small groups of patients doses of preclamol with clearly beneficial effects through the first two weeks of treatment. These benefits later faded as tolerance of some sort set in.[101] Research continues in the effort to solve this problem, which if successful would lead to the production of a new compound distinctly different from others available. The examples of reserpine and tetrabenazine show that such problems can be solved. They show more: tetrabenazine, like clozapine, is an antipsychotic that does not cause tardive dyskinesia.

Sulpiride

In the 1970s, the blockage of dopamine receptors by antipsychotic drugs became the sine qua non of drug development. The name of the game was creating potent and selective dopamine antagonists. As fate would have it, a highly selective D-2 receptor antagonist existed long before anyone thought about inventing one. Quite mysteriously, however, it had properties that none of the proponents of the dopamine hypotheses could or indeed still can explain.

In 1958, the French company Delagrange, decided on a strategy that would move it away from licensing compounds and developing over-the-counter preparations to one that would focus on in-house research aimed at producing compounds that could be patented.[102] At the time a benzamide compound, orthochloroprocainamide, was used in radiology. In humans being X-rayed, this could be seen to cause an opening of the pylorus of the stomach and a slowing of intestinal movements. Maybe, the company thought, a similar drug could manage bowel disturbances, and there was certainly a big market for anti-emetics. In 1961, the company's chemist, Michel Thominet, developed from the benzamide nucleus metoclopramide, which company pharmacologists quickly realized was a very effective anti-emetic.

Licensed as Primpéran in France, metoclopramide was the pride of Delagrange's arsenal. Its success provided the basis for a subsequent merger as the senior partner with three other companies, Delalande, Robert and Carrière, and Dausse, to form Synthélabo, which by the 1990s had become one of the biggest European pharmaceutical companies. Metoclopramide appeared to have minimal side effects. But it did have one set of side effects that came to the attention of just the right people. It was used widely to treat gut disturbances, including such problems in psychiatric patients. In 1962, Pierre Deniker noticed that some patients in his clinic taking no antipsychotics but taking metoclopramide exhibited neuroleptic-type extrapyramidal side effects. Deniker wondered if, rare though the side effects were, metoclopramide might be a neuroleptic.[103]

The company took up the challenge and synthesized a range of related benzamides. The compound selected for antipsychotic testing was sulpiride. The first trials were conducted by Pierre Borenstein and a Parisian psychopharmacology research group, the Parisian counterpart of the CLRTP in Lyon. When given to psychotic patients, sulpiride had clear antipsychotic effects. On animal testing this compound was much less likely to cause catalepsy and in humans it seemed less likely to produce extrapyramidal problems.[104] As it later turned out, it was also much less likely to lead to tardive dyskinesia. It also seemed useful in treating a range of nervous states with neurotic depressions and anxiety states responding to low doses. It was widely used to treat neurotic and dysthymic states in both France and Japan during the 1970s and 1980s.[105]

Borenstein described sulpiride in terms that suggested it would produce less passivity and less chemical straitjacketing than traditional neuroleptics. To present the first clinical data at a meeting of the Académie française in 1968, he had, in a supreme moment of historical drama, to cross lines of students protesting about psychiatry. These were the students who derided the claims of Delay and Deniker that the antipsychotics had led to a silence in the asylums, preferring to view this silence as a silence of the cemetery produced by drugs that were nothing but a camisole chimique.

Had the dopamine hypothesis existed then, the mystery would only have deepened, because neuroleptic effects were later identified with D-2 receptor antagonism and the negative syndromes that neuroleptics could cause were later thought to stem from excessive D-2 receptor antagonism. But sulpiride was in fact the purest D-2 receptor antagonist there was and yet it produced fewer extrapyramidal effects, a fact that was inexplicable by conventional wisdom. It produced less tardive dyskinesia than other neuroleptics. This ran counter to accepted views that tardive dyskinesia was caused by a D-2 blockage. It was also a less potent and somewhat weaker antipsychotic, which was incompatible with the dopamine theory of schizophrenia. And in addition, it seemed less likely to produce negative syndromes.

These incompatibilities were not what led to sulpiride's relative lack of impact, although they almost certainly did not help. The significant factor was that Delagrange for a variety of reasons, one of which was a series of ongoing mergers, did not develop the compound for the U.S. market. By the mid-1970s, if a compound did not have an impact in the United States, even though it might be a best seller in Europe or Japan, in terms of theoretical impact it might as well not have existed.

Other European companies paid heed though. Roche developed another benzamide, moclobemide, as an antidepressant.[106] But it was Astra, which had previously developed the first SSRI, zimeldine, that took up the baton. Its research and development program led to the creation of remoxipride by Lennart Florvall in 1978. This could be marketed on the basis of its selectivity to D-2 receptors, since D-2 receptor binding had been discovered by the time remoxipride was launched.[107] Remoxipride came on the market just before the relaunch of clozapine and the emergence of atypicality. Like sulpiride, it had a relatively gentle profile of side effects. It had been launched in a number of European countries and was set for launch in the United States when Astra was jinxed. Zimeldine, a truly innovative development of Astra's, which in all likelihood would have relegated Prozac to a footnote in pharmacological history, had to be pulled off the market in Europe just before its launch in the United States by Merck after it was reported that in some patients it triggered Guillain-Barré syndrome, a life-threatening neurological condition. Remoxipride appeared in rare cases to trigger another potentially lethal disorder, aplastic anemia, and consequently it also was taken off the market.

Synthélabo subsequently developed amisulpiride. This too had few extrapyramidal effects. It also had sufficiently clear antidepressant effects in clinical trials to get a license in a number of European countries for use in treating dysthymia. But by the time of its launch in the mid-1990s, it had to make its way in a market dominated by companies extolling the virtues of atypicality. By the 1990s, nobody could conceive of a way in which atypicality could stem from selective D-2 receptor blockage, even though amisulpiride with its antidepressant effects came closer to meeting clinical criteria for atypicality than some other drugs marketed during the period. But it was not developed for the U.S. market and so remained a minor player on the antipsychotic stage.[108]

A New Clozapine?

From the mid-1970s on, several companies geared up to produce a clozapine that did not cause agranulocytosis. Their interest did not stem from anything distinctive in clozapine's antipsychotic profile, because this was still not clear. The efforts rather were driven by looming legal liabilities. Clozapine did not cause tardive dyskinesia. How could one reproduce this profile of action? One strategy was to look at the receptor profile of clozapine. It was then just becoming possible to distinguish between D-1 and D-2 as well as 5HT-1 and 5HT-2 receptors and others.

The stage was set for the reentry into the market of a Danish company, Lundbeck. Lundbeck had moved quickly into the antipsychotic market in 1958 with a chemical series called the thioxanthenes, from which came chlorprothixene, flupenthixol, clopenthixol, and zuclopenthixol.[109] Pfizer had managed to prize one thioxanthene from Lundbeck's grip: thiothixene. Chlorprothixene, a chlorpromazine-like agent, had been a well tolerated compound. The later thioxanthenes were increasingly potent.[110] From these drugs came most of the depot neuroleptics used outside the United States. After the eclipse of the benzodiazepines in the 1980s, flupenthixol became the best-selling neuroleptic in many European countries, where it was given in low doses as an alternative to Valium, until it was replaced by the SSRIs.

Under the influence of the new thinking in the late 1980s, Klaus Bøgesø and the chemists at Lundbeck, who had already developed the most selective of the SSRIs, citalopram, produced a new series of compounds, the phenyl-indanes. These were antipsychotic in preclinical tests. One compound, sertindole, was picked for further development. Compared with flupenthixol, sertindole was much less likely to cause extrapyramidal problems, very unlikely to cause akathisia, and seemed well tolerated by patients. It was active on D-2 as well as 5HT-2 and alpha-2 receptors. It resembled chlorprothixene in fact more than it resembled the later flupenthixol or clopenthixol. Many of the chlorpromazine generation of compounds had, it turned out, receptor profiles almost identical with the ones that chemists were now trying to reproduce in laboratories in new forms that would allow new patents and new market campaigns.

A remarkable thing happened in the course of developing sertindole. It was known from early on that this compound could cause some lengthening of the QT interval on the electrocardiogram. This was not notable because a majority of other antipsychotics had similar effects. There was less, it appeared, to worry about in the case of sertindole than for example in the case of thioridazine, which had caused fatal cardiac complications. Frank

Berger's wife, for example, died from a cardiac complication after being treated by Leo Hollister with thioridazine. As a precautionary measure, however, more than the usual number of ECGs were performed in the course of clinical trials of the compound.

Lundbeck and its licensee in the United States, Abbott Pharmaceuticals, had established a rapid development program. They had overtaken their competitors in the post-clozapine development field, Lilly and Zeneca. And sertindole was the first of this new generation of antipsychotics onto the market, being licensed in July of 1996 in the United Kingdom. But in the United States, in hearings before the FDA, Paul Leber asked what the lengthening of the QT interval meant.[111] He was faced with experts arguing on behalf of Abbott and Lundbeck that the lengthening was not clinically significant. But other experts claimed that there could be a problem, depending on the heart rate and the state of cardiac functioning of the patient. Lengthening of the QT interval could, in theory at least, lead to a fatal cardiac complication called torsade de pointes (a form of ventricular tachycardia). There had been a small number of deaths in the course of the Lundbeck trials. Were they related to the new compound? No one knew.

A potential legal liability loomed. This threat scuppered the launch of sertindole in the United States and led to its voluntary withdrawal from a number of European markets while further studies were undertaken to establish the nature of any problem. No clear results were forthcoming. But the problems with sertindole caused clinicians and companies to restudy all the antidepressants and antipsychotics they had been using, and they found that many of them caused significant QT interval changes. Nobody knew what the potential liabilities might be if a patient being treated with these drugs died shortly after significant QT interval changes had developed.

Every company producing any drug that affected the central nervous system had to include ECG recordings of the compound in the application for licensing. New compounds had to be devoid of significant QT interval lengthening. Many promising developments were almost certainly aborted or delayed because they could not meet this criterion, much as they once were at the first hint of extrapyramidal problems. Even though nobody could say with confidence that QT interval changes of the order of those found with sertindole and many other compounds were of clinical consequence, fear of legal liability retarded drug development. Particularly affected was Pfizer, whose compound ziprasidone, a risperidone analogue, was held in abeyance for almost four years by regulatory concerns. And although Lilly benefited initially because olanzapine had no early competition from sertindole, in the long run it too was impeded by concerns about QT interval lengthening and had to abandon the development of its successor to Prozac, R(-)fluoxetine.

Lundbeck and Janssen's receptor approach was one way to develop an antipsychotic as opposed to a neuroleptic. Another was to try to mimic the structure of clozapine. The difficulty here was to devise a structure sufficiently similar to get the benefits of clozapine that was at the same time different enough to allow the new compound to be patented. Several companies pursued this path. The most successful was Lilly, which came up with olanzapine. This was a compound similar in structure to clozapine with D-2, 5HT-2, and alpha-2 antagonist binding properties. It did, however, cause dyskinesias in both animals at relatively low doses and in humans. Olanzapine came onto the market in 1996 in the United States and in 1997 in other countries.[112] The clinical trials suggested that it was to be used in a 10-milligram dose. The price was extremely high for this first dose and doubled with every additional dose increment, and in practice it cost between $5,000 and $10,000 annually. The benefits were debatable and the cost high, but olanzapine had one of the most effective marketing departments in the pharmaceutical world behind it and sold well.

In the 1970s, Lilly had embarked on a policy of recruiting well-known figures from academic psychiatry. Among them were Steven Paul, Gary Tollefson, and William Potter. The roster of names suggested a respectable university department rather than a pharmaceutical company. This was a strategy that paid off when Prozac encountered problems, in the form of reports that it could precipitate suicide. In 1991, a meta-analysis of some of the studies undertaken with Prozac, which it was claimed laid the suicide question to rest, was published in the *British Medical Journal*.[113] This article did a great deal to tide the company over the crisis. It also marked a turning point. Until then, papers written solely by company personnel would never have been published in a leading journal like the *British Medical Journal*. This article cracked the dam that had separated the academic and commercial universes.[114] With the release of olanzapine, the water flowing through the crack changed from a trickle to a flood, as a series of reviews and comparative studies of this drug were published in the leading psychiatric and psychopharmacological journals.

A different strategy was adopted by the British company Zeneca. In 1976, Zeneca acquired a U.S. research base in Wilmington, Delaware, where it began to develop its research on drugs to treat central nervous system conditions. Zeneca hired a medicinal chemist, Edward Warawa, a behavioral pharmacologist, Bernie Migler, and a neurobiologist, Andre Salama.[115] The brief for the group was to develop a clozapine-like drug that did not cause blood problems.

Focusing on the receptor approach, as Janssen and Lundbeck had done, meant focusing on potential receptor systems and aiming at clinical efficacy rather than freedom from tardive dyskinesia. Focusing on the molecular structure, as Lilly had done, could lead to patent problems and gave little guarantee that the resulting molecule would not cause tardive dyskinesia. Zeneca's approach was to employ an animal model of tardive dyskinesia, and its research involved studying Cebus monkeys sensitized by haloperidol. All antipsychotics except clozapine produced dyskinesias in these monkeys. As olanzapine and risperidone became available, Zeneca tested them and then a range of compounds it synthesized. All caused dyskinesias.

One of the few compounds that did not cause dyskinesias was fluperlapine, one of Wander's other near misses. Warawa began to modify fluperlapine, and finally in March 1985 he discovered a new molecule, quetiapine. Seroquel, as it later became, was effective at blocking mouse climbing without affecting biting or gnawing. It did not cause dyskinesias in the monkeys. It had a profile of effects similar to that of clozapine but did not cause the blood cell problems. In clinical trials it reduced dyskinesia rates. By the time quetiapine came onto the market, however, the dominant view was that atypical drugs were atypical by virtue of acting on D-2 and 5HT-2 receptors. Seroquel was an SDA and this determined the way it was marketed, but it had not been developed to have 5HT-2 antagonist properties and no one in the company knew whether this effect was important or not.

None of the new compounds achieved acceptance as a new and improved form of clozapine, which still remained a mysterious entity out of researchers' reach. Throughout the 1990s, companies and laboratories invested huge amounts trying to determine what action or combination of actions made clozapine unique. When D-4 and D-3 receptors were discovered, research groups claimed that they were the sites where clozapine's unique benefits occurred. Despite lack of knowledge of specifically how clozapine acted, olanzapine, risperidone, sertindole, quetiapine, and ziprasidone were all portrayed as being significantly more effective than the older antipsychotics in combating negative symptoms, and researchers claimed that this was what made them atypical like clozapine.

But what was the mystery? If avoiding tardive dyskinesia was the solution to the mystery, the mystery had already been solved, even if no one knew exactly why neither clozapine nor quetiapine caused this problem. By 1996, however, the field had all but forgotten about tardive dyskinesia, and the mystery of clozapine supposedly lay, its advocates said, in its benefits in treating negative schizophrenia. It was the only drug, they said, that made a difference in treating this condition, a claim that demonstrated a lack of knowledge of the history of antipsychotic trials.

POSITIVE AND NEGATIVE SCHIZOPHRENIA

In the 1880s the British neurologist John Hughlings Jackson introduced the idea that a disease could have both negative and positive features.[116] Jackson's view was that a disorder, such as a stroke, causes a loss of function and this is the negative aspect of the disease. Typically, when higher functions are lost following the destruction of certain brain pathways, other phenomena are released that have previously been inhibited by these pathways. In the case of a stroke, for example, there are increased tone and reflexes and a range of altered behaviors. These, for Jackson, were the positive aspects of the disease.

When Eugen Bleuler developed his concept of schizophrenia in 1905, he was influenced by Jackson.[117] Whereas Kraepelin's dementia praecox was simply descriptive, Bleuler offered a model that made sense of the descriptions. He saw the primary disorder in schizophrenia as a disturbance in some thought processes leading to an inability to coherently present ideas in language or to execute willed actions. These were the negative features of the illness. A range of positive features stemmed from this primary loss, including delusions and hallucinations as well as ambivalence, ambitendency, and autism. For Bleuler, the negative features were at the heart of the disorder and the positive features were secondary release phenomena or reactions.[118]

This understanding of what was positive and what negative began to change in the 1960s with research on deinstitutionalization. One of the striking features of schizophrenia after the introduction of chlorpromazine was the emergence of high rates of relapse and recurrence. A revolving door syndrome had been set up that required investigation. There also appeared to be a number of patients who either failed to get well or who improved but not to a point where discharge seemed feasible. The Social Psychiatric Unit at the Maudsley Hospital in London began to investigate these issues, and in 1962 proposed the concept of an institutional neurosis.[119]

When schizophrenia was viewed in light of this idea, the positive symptoms—the illness—came first and committal to an institution led to the accumulation of secondary, or negative, problems. At this stage, there was a tendency to see the flattening of personality that had formerly been seen as the hallmark of schizophrenia as a hospital- or institution-induced flattening. These ideas fed straight into the antipsychiatric ferment brewing in Western psychiatry at the time.

Research on schizophrenia by psychologists produced another concept of positive and negative. The research of Jean Chapman and Andrew McGhie led them to propose the first of what are loosely describable as defective filter theories.[120] Defective filter theories stressed that the basic problem in schizophrenia is an inability to screen out incoming stimuli. The patient becomes overwhelmed, a state that is the positive aspect of the illness. In an attempt to cope, the patient retreats, trying to minimize incoming stimuli. This retreat constitutes the negative pole of the illness.

Into this growing confusion of terms came a proposal by Tim Crow of the Northwick Park Research Unit in London that there were positive and negative schizophrenic syndromes, which he called type 1 and type 2 schizophrenias. This proposal united the neurobiology and psychopharmacology of schizophrenia emerging in the 1970s in a way that both clinicians and nonclinicians thought they could understand.[121] Crow's proposal was that type 1, or positive, schizophrenia, involving delusions and hallucinations, came first and stemmed from abnormalities of the dopamine system. In some patients, another neurotoxic process, possibly caused by a virus, led to degenerative changes in the brain. This supposedly produced a ventricular enlargement in the brain, tardive dyskinesia, and type 2, or negative, schizophrenia, also called the defect state. This involved a flattening of personality, social withdrawal, lack of volition, and poverty of speech and thought. According to this formulation, neuroleptics should be effective in treating type 1 but not type 2 schizophrenia.

The genius in this proposal was that it neatly linked a certain amount of biological plausibility with other concepts in a way that everybody felt he could understand. Crow had a flair for formulating an idea, just as Eugen Bleuler had had seventy years previously when he coined the term schizophrenia. Positive and negative functioned as catch-alls in the same way that atypicality did. Crow's ideas quickly caught on. Few noticed that in fact all the substantial evidence ran exactly in the opposite direction.

Studies looking on the onset of schizophrenia had stressed that the condition began with negative features and that psychotic or positive features often appeared only a year or two after the recognizable onset of the illness.[122] Researchers commonly found that instead of beginning with positive features and moving on to a negative state, a schizophrenic disorder often reached its end stage in a floridly psychotic, or positive, state. Research in the nine-hospital study of chlorpromazine and subsequent research, moreover, had shown that (in low doses) neuroleptics had greater benefits in treating negative than positive states. This evidence, however, and the fact that Crow's use of the terms positive and negative were inconsistent with their use in the rest of the literature, had little impact on what was by then a prevailing belief in Crow's views.

By the time Study 30 with clozapine was undertaken, these concepts were well established. Clozapine's most interesting effects in this study appeared to be on what were now being called the negative features of schizophrenia. It promoted an increase in social contact, a reduction in passivity, and something of a warming of the personality. Clinicians as well as patients taking clozapine and subsequently other atypicals needed little convincing on this point. They saw or experienced the changes for themselves.

But there were, in fact, good grounds to question precisely what was going on. In Study 30, the effects of clozapine had been compared to the effects of chlorpromazine given in very high daily doses, in patients who had previously been on very large doses of conventional neuroleptics. The study reported in 1988, a time when more was still better. A majority of clinicians would not have been persuaded that superiority to doses of 5 milligrams of haloperidol per day or 200–300 milligrams of chlorpromazine a day was clinically significant. By 1990, however, research had made it seem quite possible that the only lesson to be learned from Study 30 was that administering clozapine was better than poisoning patients with drug cocktails or megadose therapies.

Quite aside from the findings of Baldessarini and Farde, there had in fact been grounds from the start to believe that the neuroleptics could induce negative states. The Lyon group became aware of the problem in the early 1960s. These psychiatrists took seriously the antipsychiatric critique that the falling decibel level within the asylums might in some cases be the silence of the cemetery.[123] Some of them convened a symposium at the Vinatier Hospital, where a consensus was reached among the pro and anti drug advocates that the drugs could produce a passivity syndrome. The introduction of depot medications made it even more clear that some patients who were sitting at home quietly were in a state that was not, as first thought, the calm tranquility of restored sanity but was rather a drug-induced withdrawal.

Oldrich Vinar in Prague noticed similar effects and commented on these to Arvid Carlsson in the early 1970s, wondering whether blockage of dopamine might be the cause.[124] Carlsson, committed to the view that it was abnormalities of the dopamine system that underlay the illness and that drug treatment corrected these, could not conceive of such an explanation.

Patients, however, were increasingly clear and vocal in their perceptions of the problems involved in drug treatment. There had been early comments from committed pharmacotherapists that the drugs could produce a beneficial indifference. Some practitioners, from Laborit on, had innocently labeled these changes a chemical lobotomy. These comments were now turned against psychiatry by its critics, who cited the fact that even the proponents of neuroleptic treatment referred to their effects as a chemical lobotomy.[125]

Whatever the merits of comparing the effects of doses of clozapine with the effects of high doses of traditional neuroleptics, there was no excuse for the clinical trials of the other atypicals, which came after the work of Baldessarini and Farde. The only studies that were properly designed were those done on sertindole, which compared the new drug to haloperidol in doses of 4, 8, and 16 milligrams per day. Sertindole was in fact no better than haloperidol at 8 milligrams per day, and both haloperidol at 8 milligrams per day and sertindole were better than haloperidol at 16 milligrams per day. The trials with olanzapine, quetiapine, and risperidone compared these new compounds to haloperidol in doses approaching 20 milligrams per day. Even so, they were not obviously more effective than haloperidol, except for their marginal benefits on negative symptoms. How would they have compared to haloperidol given in lower doses? Nevertheless, in clinical practice there was a wholesale switch from older to newer agents despite up to a hundred-fold increase in cost in some cases. In the United States within a couple of years, the "atypical" antipsychotics were taking up to 60 percent of the market share. Why?

The change stemmed from a mixture of wishful thinking and aggressive marketing. By the 1990s, pharmaceutical companies had discovered that patient activists were often the most effective lobbyists for the new treatments and they had allied themselves with some of the most aggressive patient groups of the 1960s. An advocate of low doses of traditional neuroleptics as an alternative to the expensive new agents was likely to be treated with scorn by patients and accused of attempting to save money at their expense.

But the changes that patients and clinicians were witnessing were often the consequences of changing from the equivalent of more than 5,000 milligrams of chlorpromazine per day to a dose of clozapine or a newer agent equivalent to 300 milligrams of chlorpromazine per day. There were obvious difficulties for clinicians in accepting that even part of the benefits they were witnessing with the new drugs might stem from the fact that they were not now poisoning their patients to the same extent as previously. These difficulties led to a need for myths to disguise what was happening, and marketing campaigns for the new treatments that used the concept of negative schizophrenia vigorously provided the required mythologies. As patients recovered from drug-induced negativity, the resulting benefits in turn seemed to validate the concept that atypicals had unique effects on negative states.

What was lost in the debate about the benefits of the atypicals was that it had largely been industry efforts to reduce legal liability by minimizing tardive dyskinesia that had led to the development of the new compounds. This was a worthy goal, but it should not have been confused with developments in psychopathological theory about the nature of schizophrenia. But confusion did ensue, and treatment-resistant schizophrenia had become a certain kind of negative schizophrenia that was essentially a creation of the pharmaceutical industry—a creation that was marketed vigorously, achieving among a younger generation of clinicians greater recognition than older terms such as hebephrenia or catatonia.

TWISTS OF FATE

Hebephrenia and catatonia had been the original forms of treatment-resistant schizophrenia. They did not respond to the early phenothiazines or haloperidol. In 1963, Frank Fish, categorized his patients according to criteria derived by Karl Leonhard from earlier work by Kahlbaum, and looked at the response of different subtypes of schizophrenia to pharmacotherapy. Up to 85 percent of paranoid schizophrenias responded. By contrast there was a 23 percent response in hebephrenia and less than a 1 percent response rate in some forms of catatonia.[126] None of the newer agents, not even clozapine, could show any improvement on these response rates.

The term hebephrenia was dropped from the fourth edition of the *Diagnostic and Statistical Manual* and replaced with the term disorganized schizophrenia. Where Kahlbaum had distinguished hebephrenia from other disorders, and modern pharmacotherapy appeared to support him, American and world psychiatry had gone Kraepelinian, as we shall see in Chapter 7, to the extent of eliminating any indicators that hebephrenia differed from schizophrenia, despite its almost complete nonresponse to antipsychotics.[127]

The fate of catatonia was even more dramatic. For younger clinicians it was almost a historical relic. The dominant assumption as of the year 2000 is that the advent of the antipsychotics led to the early detection and treatment of patients who were liable to catatonic developments and this meant that this form of schizophrenia simply didn't develop any more. Reduced rates of institutionalization are commonly thought to be one factor that has contributed to the declining numbers of catatonics. Other factors cited are an increase in the general health of patients and the availability of drugs like penicillin to treat the infections or fevers that sometimes precipitated catatonia.

But there were from the start compelling grounds to doubt this convenient story. Henri Baruk, Delay's most serious competitor for the chair of psychiatry at the University of Paris, had made his research reputation by demonstrating that experimental catatonia could be induced by bulbocapnine. By 1958, he had published a series of papers demonstrating that the phenothiazines could also induce catalepsy, a form of experimental catatonia.[128] From there on, he preached that the phenothiazines, far from being a treatment for schizophrenia, had been discovered in the management of mania, and that schizophrenia was a nonexistent disorder invented by Kraepelin, as evidenced by the fact that the phenothiazines could induce catatonia, supposedly one of the forms of this illness.[129] His was a voice crying in the wilderness, apt to be disregarded, with his concerns interpreted as a peevish effort to get back at Delay. Why worry about catatonia when it had vanished?

In 1962, Delay and Deniker described a syndrome they called syndrome malin des neuroleptiques.[130] A sprinkling of further cases were described in the world literature in the next twenty years. Then in 1980 Stanley Caroff wrote a review of neuroleptic malignant syndrome (NMS), isolating its typical features based on reported cases from Deniker's and Delay's onward.[131] Since the condition was caused by neuroleptic drugs, which blocked dopamine neurotransmission, Caroff and his colleagues recommended dopamine agonists as the mainstay of treatment.[132] Treatment seemed to work in only 50 percent of the cases, sometimes only after a week of intense anxiety about whether the patient would die. At a time of rising litigiousness, the lethal consequences and the potential for treatment of NMS conspired to thrust the "new" syndrome into general awareness. Awareness of the condition led to a recognition that it was not as rare as was once thought. Estimates of its frequency rose to 1 percent of patients being treated with antipsychotics.

In 1983, Gregory Fricchione, working at Massachusetts General Hospital, had a wealthy patient develop an apparent neuroleptic malignant syndrome. Extremely concerned, Fricchione called in his senior that night, Ned Cassem. Faced with a potentially terminally ill patient, they looked through the ward's medicine cabinet and decided on a lorazepam infusion. Very shortly after treatment, the patient sat up, declared he needed to go to the toilet, did so, and returned apparently coherent and well.[133] The improvement was sustained. Fricchione and Cassem had a new treatment for NMS, which not only flew in the face of theoretical models of what should work, but was much more successful than any predicted treatment.[134]

Fricchione joined Max Fink at Stony Brook Hospital in New York. Slowly the realization dawned on them and others that there were striking clinical similarities between NMS and catatonia.[135] They then remembered that catatonia commonly responded to barbiturates and accordingly tried both lorazepam and barbiturates in both conditions and found both worked. If this was the case, would ECT, which was dramatically effective in treating catatonia, also help NMS? It did. In fact it worked with virtually 100 percent efficacy. These experiences in turn led Fink and colleagues to rediscover that a cure for catatonia had been outlined decades before by W. Bleckwenn: barbiturates (see Chapter 2).[136]

Studies by Fink and his colleagues have since shown that catatonia exists to the same extent as before. The florid states of mute immobility lasting for months do not occur, but many of the other features of the syndrome do occur and can be observed if looked for.[137] Not only that, but while psychiatrists thought catatonia had vanished, neurologists were reporting on its relatively common occurrence and the overlap between it and NMS.[138] All of a sudden Baruk, who lived to the age of a hundred and two and was still repeating his message twenty years after the death of Delay, seemed vindicated.[139]

How could such a situation arise? How could anyone have thought catatonia had vanished when surveys in the 1990s showed rates of catatonic features in district general hospital psychiatric units of 5–10 percent?[140] The answer has to be that no company stood to make money out of encouraging clinicians to recognize these clinical features. The patent on lorazepam, which was remarkably effective in treating the condition, had expired. Did it make a difference that clinicians failed to recognize these features? Almost certainly yes: patients were losing their lives because of that failure. The only saving grace was that a widespread coadministration of benzodiazepines in many acute units was probably saving lives, but this was happening on a purely empirical basis at a time when companies and third-party payers were exhorting clinicians to practice medicine based on clinical trials.

One of the theoretical hopes with clozapine, which did not induce catalepsy in animals, was that unlike other neuroleptics it might have an impact on catatonia. It did not. In almost the reverse of the situation with animals, clozapine seemed even more likely to produce lethal catatonia in humans. This and not agranulocytosis had led to its failure on the Japanese market. This and not agranulocytosis had led Deniker to return it to Wander recommending that it never be developed. Shortly after the launches of risperidone and olanzapine, there was a stream of reports of NMS induced by these new "atypicals."[141] But the availability of effective treatments notwithstanding, the market development profiles of these new compounds were set in a manner that militated against any dismantling of the schizophrenic monolith that recognizing catatonia would have involved. And even knowledge that could save lives got nowhere in this new world without the backing of pharmaceutical companies.

By the year 2000 a number of academic centers were running studies randomizing patients who had not responded to clozapine or other "atypicals" to adjunctive treatment with standard neuroleptics—Study 30 in reverse. This development suggests that had haloperidol been withdrawn because of agranulocytosis, and clozapine-like compounds been left to dominate the marketplace, haloperidol might later have been rediscovered as a drug that, given in astonishingly low doses, could produce remarkable results in managing treatment-resistant schizophrenia.

Meanwhile a ghost left over from the reserpine era continued to haunt psychopharmacology. Reserpine had for a decade matched chlorpromazine in terms of scientific citations and then faded. It took with it an awareness of a mysterious problem it had caused: akathisia. Haloperidol and other potent neuroleptics also caused akathisia, but the megadose regimes of these drugs used in the 1970s and 1980s minimized the problem because in high doses these neuroleptics degraded the capacity to act on any of the murderous or suicidal impulses that akathisia can give rise to.

It was only in the later 1970s that the work of Philip May and Theodore van Putten again began to draw attention to the pernicious character of this side effect.[142] As late as 1980, the restlessness that akathisia could cause was commonly confused with tardive dyskinesia.[143] Senior figures in the field, however, readily agreed that akathisia and the dysphoria, which were part and parcel of the effects of neuroleptics on extrapyramidal systems, were a more frequently occurring and more subjectively distressing problem than tardive dyskinesia ever was. For many there was little doubt that akathisia led to a toll of suicides and violence.

This was the darkest side of the antipsychotics. Yet almost fifty years after the first reports of akathisia, no major organization worldwide had held a symposium on the nature of the problem. No one was making any efforts to minimize it. Akathisia was not a medico-legal problem for either the profession or the pharmaceutical industry. If patients complained of strange and unusual impulses, it would after all be difficult to persuade a jury that their difficulties stemmed from their treatment rather than their illness.

7

The Sorcerer's Apprentice

As you will recall, when Pavlov's St. Petersburg laboratory flooded in 1924, the differences in how his dogs weathered the flood appeared to hinge on their constitutional types.[1] In apparent confirmation of the constitutional differences between them, stimulants helped some while sedatives helped others overcome their traumatic neurosis.[2] This finding was to be replicated later in the century in animals by Jules Masserman and in man by Hans Eysenck, and the effects of drugs on conditioned reflexes were used by pharmaceutical companies to distinguish between the different groups of psychotropic drugs that emerged in chlorpromazine's wake. The distance between the thinking of Pavlov and the thinking of mid-century physicians using drugs to treat nervous disorders was not great. Nor was the distance between the dynamics of Pavlov's new science of conditioned (unconscious) reflexes and psychoanalytic psychodynamics. Furthermore, even Freud conceded that some pharmacotherapeutic method of manipulating internal endocrinology was likely to provide a way of treating psychoses.[3]

By the end of the century, however, therapeutic orientations in psychiatry were at loggerheads. How could this happen in a century when we were supposedly becoming more scientific? Science ordinarily resolves conflicts, finds points of agreement, and moves forward. The situation, however, had become so bad by 1998, that the leading journal of the time, *Archives of General Psychiatry*, invited two psychiatric grandees, Samuel Guze and Robert Michels, to diagnose the problem.[4] Guze was the former chairman of the psychiatry department at Washington University in St Louis, generally viewed as the home of DSM-III, the classification manual published in 1980 that was commonly portrayed as having reimposed order on American psychiatry. His orientation was unequivocally medical, as is shown by the title of one of his articles: "Biological Psychiatry: Is There Any Other Kind?"[5] Michels was the dean at Cornell Medical School, a prominent critic of DSM-III and one of the foremost advocates of analytic therapy, but also a man open to the insights that neuroscience might bring to therapy.[6]

Guze's concern was that the changes in medical service delivery brought about by managed care meant that psychiatrists were increasingly reimbursed only for making diagnoses and writing prescriptions, with social workers and others, because they were less expensive, actually delivering psychological therapies. This practice risked destroying the relationship in which therapy is delivered. It was a particular problem for psychiatry, where any talking with patients was itself, to a greater extent than in other branches of medicine, considered a form of therapy. Guze cited APA guidelines: "Treatment . . . is facilitated by a comprehensive understanding of the patient, including his or her needs and goals, intrapsychic conflicts and defenses, coping styles and strengths. The psychiatrist should attempt to understand the biological, interpersonal, social, and cultural factors that affect the patient's adjustment."[7]

Michels responded that he would not use the term psychotherapy for the kind of support Guze was describing. It should be reserved for "specific treatments that are based on a theoretical model of psychological functioning, its relationship to pathologic condition and subjective distress, and the way in which relationships and communications can modify it." He went on to argue that "there is a slippery slope from carving out psychotherapy for those with problems of living or less severe psychiatric disorders, to denying the importance of psychotherapy in modern psychiatric care of the seriously ill."

These exchanges embodied a set of dilemmas that faced late twentieth-century psychiatry. These dilemmas had their roots in the 1880s with the isolation by Robert Koch of the tubercle bacillus and with it ideas of disease and treatment specificity. Before Koch, diseases had been seen in terms of imbalances of humoral factors within the body or between the body and the environment, with treatments aimed at supporting the person and if possible correcting the imbalance. Advances in pathology in the eighteenth and nineteenth centuries led to an increasing crisis, as postmortems revealed discrete lesions in particular organs or even in specific tissues within an organ. But of what benefit was the new scientific knowledge if it did not lead to therapeutic advances? The old style of treatment, which involved reassuring support with which both practitioners and patients felt comfortable, even if it was based on an incorrect understanding of the disease, was surely still to be preferred.[8]

Koch's discovery changed everything. Within a decade acute respiratory and throat disorders, which had previously been seen as one disease, had begun to resolve into a range of different infectious diseases, with up to eighteen different throat infections recognized. Koch's opponents, the hygienists, protested that the isolation of specific bacteria made little difference. Nonspecific sanitary measures were still of greater importance than any other interventions.[9] But these protests faded when an antitoxin was shown to save lives threatened by one of the deadliest killers of children: diphtheria. No other throat disorders responded to this treatment. A premium was put on correct diagnosis and specific treatment.

Work by Koch's colleague, Paul Ehrlich, showing that each of the newly discovered microorganisms could be stained by a specific dye, raised the possibility that each might succumb to a magic bullet. A cure for the greatest scourge of the day, tuberculosis, appeared close at hand. But while tuberculosis could now be diagnosed specifically, no specific treatments emerged. Instead the first decades of the twentieth century were marked by a recognition that many of the interventions of the hygienists, which did not specifically treat established disorders, could now be reinterpreted as minimizing risks of infection and enabling the body to fight infections.

The pharmacological discoveries of the 1950s rekindled debates about the roles of specific and nonspecific interventions in the treatment of conditions from infectious disorders to schizophrenia. Notwithstanding chlorpromazine's dramatic effects in some cases, most clinicians initially viewed the drug as a relatively nonspecific intervention. The questions were to what extent did it work and could its effectiveness be convincingly demonstrated when cures were rarely if ever achieved. Could drug therapies be matched with particular syndromes or psychotherapeutic approaches to achieve the best possible outcomes? But there was a built-in default in the dynamic toward specificity. The new drugs were generally anti-something—antibiotic or antihypertensive. Why not antipsychotic? The nature of science favors a hunt for specificity, as the quotation from Michels suggests, but specificity, in addition, is, in health care at least, the best way yet invented to make money.

Central to these questions is measurement, the key feature of science. How do you measure whether therapies work? Since no one has ever had any reason to suppose that the magic of science should fail when it comes to psychiatry, there is little reason to suppose that methods that have served well in other scientific areas should not also work in the domain of psychiatry. But a lack of progress suggests that an uncritical adoption of traditional scientific methods has like the wand in the hands of the sorcerer's apprentice produced chaos and increasing bewilderment.

EARLY CLINICAL DRUG EVALUATION

The issue of what the new drugs could be shown to do achieved the greatest salience in the United States. Within a year of the introduction of chlorpromazine, a National Academy of Sciences grant led to a conference, chaired by Ralph Gerard and Jonathan Cole, aimed at establishing the appropriate evaluative methods for the new pharmacotherapies. The participants did not face entirely new issues. Concerns about psychosurgery had first raised questions about how to evaluate the impact of a biological therapy.[10] There was a recognition that rating scales and randomized controlled trials were needed.[11]

The conference gave rise to the NIMH's Psychopharmacology Service Center, which was run by Cole. The center got a $2 million grant from Congress to evaluate the new treatments and fund research on their mechanisms of action.[12] Cole instituted a grant program that capitalized biological psychiatry. He also set up the nine-hospital study of chlorpromazine, which firmly established the pharmacotherapy era (Chapters 3 and 6).

But further funds were forthcoming from Congress—more than could be utilized by the center. In addition, following the success of chlorpromazine, pharmaceutical companies flooded the market with copycat drugs and approached investigators to test them. These events led Cole to set up in 1959 a clinical committee chaired by Henry Brill to assemble interested clinicians in order to standardize evaluative methods in clinical studies and to avoid duplication of research efforts.[13] Brill recruited Leo Hollister, David Engelhardt, Al Kurland, Heinz Lehmann, Harold Williams, and Max Fink to serve on a steering group for what became the Early Clinical Drug Evaluation Unit (ECDEU). The unit's task was to study the safety of new drugs, to find their appropriate dose ranges, and to look for appropriate clinical niches. It was hoped that federal funding would confer independence on the investigators.[14]

Early ECDEU meetings involved Max Fink and Donald Klein from Hillside Hospital, Thomas Ban and Heinz Lehmann from the Douglas State Hospital in Montreal, Nathan Kline and George Simpson from Rockland State Hospital, Douglas Goldman from Cincinnati, Herman Denber from Manhattan State Hospital, Vernon Kinross-Wright from Texas, and a few others. The results of clinical studies were discussed, and out of these discussions came further research ideas that were communicated to pharmaceutical companies. Klein and Fink, for example, requested blinded samples of imipramine, chlorpromazine, and a placebo, which were given to patients admitted to Hillside Hospital regardless of their diagnosis.[15] This extraordinary study, which demonstrated the antidepressant properties of chlorpromazine and the benefits of imipramine in treating anxiety states, followed a scientific rather than a commercial agenda. It would never have fit a company's portfolio of studies. It would never have occurred to the "scientists" at NIMH to run such a study, because this was not how they did science.

Initially company representatives were not invited to ECDEU meetings. They were later permitted to participate as observers. As the program grew, so did company ambivalence. There was concern that the FDA might force companies to run their drugs through the ECDEU program if they wished to get a license.[16]

One of the major undertakings of the ECDEU group was the development of standardized clinical trial protocols, agreed methods of coding information, and rating scales such as Hollister and John Overall's Brief Psychiatric Rating Scale (BPRS). The global assessment scales, which have been a mainstay of clinical trials ever since, were developed by ECDEU. In collaboration with the NIMH, a centralized computerized system (BLIPS) was set up to collate information.[17] These efforts were aimed in part at controlling the potential excesses of the pharmaceutical industry. But there was also a hope that clinical trials could be channeled along development routes that would yield objective and reliable data that could benefit both clinicians and pharmaceutical companies. The main divisions within the ECDEU on clinical trial methods were between the advocates of large multicenter studies, such as Hollister, and those who thought that relatively small, single-center studies could yield reliable indications of the profile of a new drug.[18]

The ECDEU's program was radically empirical. For clinicians like Fink and Klein, the new drugs were an experiment that would lead to new observations. The trick was to remain open-minded enough to see phenomena that available theories did not predict. New theories to explain these new observations could be elaborated later. This was an almost new form of science, one that acknowledged that techniques drive progress as much as, if not more than, anything else—a form of science that was looked down upon by university-based scientists, for whom experiments were conducted to test already existing theories. No NIMH grant-giving committee would award research funds to the "fishing trips" that ECDEU investigators were engaged in. From the NIMH's point of view, what the ECDEU was doing was not science.

There has to be some marriage of theoretical input and practitioners' wisdom in therapeutics. Academia had emphasized theory and denigrated empiricism. For the first time, the ECDEU program and groups like the CLRTP in France put collectives of practitioners on an equal footing with the ivory-towered academics. It was an unheralded achievement that produced most of what was known early on about the new psychotropic drugs. The engine that drove progress was the clinical trial.

The first scientific efforts to use data from clinical practice for medical purposes were epidemiological studies in the nineteenth century. The advent of diphtheria antitoxin and other specific treatments brought with them an appreciation of the need for controlled trials.[19] The notion of a placebo control emerged in the late 1930s. The first placebo-controlled trial in therapeutics took place in 1939, when Dub and Lurie gave a mixture of depressed and schizophrenic patients amphetamine or a placebo in a cross-over design that demonstrated the benefits of amphetamines in treating depression but not schizophrenia.[20]

In Lurie's study, the patients acted as their own controls. This trial design can work for some conditions but it is not suitable for evaluating most psychiatric treatments. If patients cannot act as their own controls, the only option is to recruit a sample representative of the general population. This made clinical trials impracticable, until an appreciation of the power of randomization to overcome the difficulty led to a breakthrough. Randomization dramatically reduces the number of patients needed to run a controlled study. It was first used in a Medical Research Council study of streptomycin in 1947.[21]

The power of the new trial techniques lay in their ability to demonstrate when treatments did not do what they were claimed to do. The first randomized controlled trials (RCTs) in psychiatry in 1950 were designed to test claims that cortisone was useful in treating psychotic disorders. They demonstrated that it was not.[22] The first trials with chlorpromazine and reserpine in 1954 and 1955, in contrast, indicated that disinterested or hostile observers could not in good conscience claim that these drugs had no effect, whatever they might think about their overall benefits.[23]

But demonstrating that a treatment does something is a long way from proving that it is the right or the only treatment in the long term. In contrast to RCTs in other areas of medicine, RCTs in psychiatry evolved into something other than a means to working out the optimal package of care. Their convenient ability to demonstrate a treatment effect in small samples increasingly seduced companies, clinicians, and policymakers and ultimately changed the face of psychiatry.

RCTs changed the way psychiatrists look at patients. These types of trial works best where there is a homogeneous patient population. This fact favors fitting patients into categorical disease entities such as social phobia, generalized anxiety disorder, or panic disorder. A response of these seemingly discrete disease entities to a drug then creates an illusion of specificity that the more accurate "our drug is useful for a large range of nervous conditions, let's call it Largactil" does not convey. RCTs also require efforts to reduce inter-rater variability. This leads to the use of operational criteria and rating scales, which in turn add to the illusion that the disorder being treated is responding in the same way that cultures of bacilli on a Petri dish shrink when exposed to an antibiotic.

RCTs also changed the way we look at evidence. Many epidemiologists had misgivings about the capacity of randomization to produce results that generalized to real-life situations. This problem was aggravated by pharmaceutical companies, which in addition to recruiting small samples explicitly recruited patient samples of convenience. These are unrepresentative of the kinds of patients who will later get the drug being studied. Company RCTs are internally valid, in the sense of detecting a treatment effect, sufficient to register the compound with the regulators, but the external validity of these samples should have been an increasing worry. The early ECDEU investigators understood that their trials had the power to show that it was simply not acceptable to say that a drug had no effect, but they also knew that extrapolations to the actual effectiveness of treatment had to be based on clinical judgment rather than trial evidence. The ECDEU investigators, however, were not trying to sell products, and this understanding was to vanish when the ECDEU program fell apart.

The new drugs brought about a treatment effect rather than eliminated a disease. But how was this effect to be measured? The answer was rating scales. Even though this was an era in which clinical judgment was becoming suspect, with psychopharmacologists doubting the judgment of analysts and antipsychiatrists doubting the judgments of any establishment figures, these rating scales appeared to overcome the "subjective" aspect of evaluation. The limitations of these scales and the fact that they were mostly just selective checklists were no secret to their creators but were not apparent to many outsiders. (A revolutionary aspect of the use of these scales is explored in Chapter 8).

Finally, RCTs provide evidence on the possible treatment effects of a drug or a psychotherapy. Until such time as these interventions are delivered by computer, their ultimate effectiveness depends on whether the patient takes the treatment and that depends on the quality of the therapeutic act in which a treatment is embedded. The quality of the relationship between the patient and the therapist appears to be the greatest determinant of compliance, for therapy with antipsychotics or any other therapy, outweighing patients' attitudes toward drug treatment or their experience of side effects.[24] Conceivably, then, the quality of a treatment could improve dramatically but if a physician's capacity to do therapy decreased, there would be no overall improvement in outcomes for treatment of the disorder in question.

All of these factors were, at least implicitly, understood by clinical investigators in the early 1960s. But the thalidomide crisis, which led to the 1962 amendments to the Food and Drugs Act and support for RCT methods as a means of supposedly safeguarding the community against errors made by the pharmaceutical industry, was to change everything. All of a sudden an evaluative technology, whose strengths and weaknesses were being slowly worked out, was thrust into a central position in the war against disease. RCTs were to be the means of guaranteeing that specific treatments were delivered for specific diseases with treatment effects great enough to allow regulators and politicians to minimize the comparative risks of treatment. This was the hoop through which pharmaceutical companies had to jump if they wanted to make money. What could be wrong with forcing the financial camel through the eye of a scientific needle? Would there be any harm if pressure was also applied to psychotherapists to "prove" that their therapies worked too?

PSYCHOTHERAPY AND SPECIFICITY

In 1944, in a volume celebrating the centenary of the American Psychiatric Association, Thomas Moore wrote in his survey of American psychology: "Behaviorism must be viewed as essentially a historical development of the recent past . . . Of recent years the literature on behaviorism has dwindled into a barely perceptible stream and psychologists have grown weary of the very words."[25] Jules Masserman, a psychodynamic psychiatrist, following Pavlov's lead, had just induced neurotic behaviors in laboratory animals, and in some cases had been able to relieve these pharmacologically.[26] The work was dismissed as focusing "attention on certain minor therapeutic procedures" and offering "no help to the psychiatrist dealing with the major problems of truly human conflict."[27]

In 1952, Hans Eysenck articulated a view that became common later: that psychoanalysis was untestable and therefore inherently unscientific.[28] This statement ignited a war that lasted over four decades. Books later followed on the theme of the Decline and Fall of the Freudian Empire. But in 1952, Eysenck's idea of eliminating idols made little impact. There was no replacement for psychoanalysis. Then, astonishingly, behavior therapy was reborn. Joseph Wolpe, using the same models as Masserman, found that reintroducing a frightened animal to the fear-conditioning stimulus reversed the neurosis. This discovery laid the basis for somatic desensitization and subsequently reciprocal inhibition, which involved teaching the patient to relax or eat food or engage in other behaviors in the presence of a fear stimulus. These were the first steps in the evolution of a new therapy.[29]

Eysenck developed a theoretical structure for the new therapy.[30] But he did more than that: he set behavior therapy up as an alternative to analysis, as a properly scientific psychotherapy.[31] As the head of the largest British department of psychology, one that had a clinical psychology training program, he was able to train a cadre of behavior therapists. Behavior therapy would be a vehicle for clinical psychologists to replace psychiatrists. (Fascinatingly though, the development of behavior therapy in Europe was inhibited by perceptions that it was a profoundly materialistic and ungodly approach to human behavior.)

In the United States another form of behavior therapy developed. There, the work of B. F. Skinner and the development of operant conditioning had a greater impact than Pavlovian or classical conditioning. Skinner's work led to a therapy aimed at delivering rewards for appropriate behavior. In Skinnerian or radical behavior therapy, there was a denial of illness in general; the patient was considered to be suffering from a behavioral problem that could be corrected by a conditioning program. The Skinnerian approach was applied to the most severely ill patients living on the back wards of large hospitals. In these settings, American behaviorists laid the basis for a token economy approach to psychotic behavior.[32] This was radical behaviorism, which believed that all deviant behavior, including psychotic behavior, was a result of faulty learning. It was unqualified environmentalism practiced by behavioral engineers.[33]

In contrast, in British behavior therapy, there was some realization that patients could be mentally ill and that treatment might merely correct disabilities. The British approach was applied to the neuroses by therapists who had no contact with psychotic patients. It is, however, much easier to decondition neuroses of the introverted type—phobias —than it is to manage neuroses of the extraverted type—hysterias or psychopathic behaviors.[34] As behavior therapy evolved in Britain, it was a method of treating phobic disorders, particularly agoraphobia and OCD, rather than a method of managing hysteria. The token economy approach with its complete control of the environment was a much better method of managing hysterical and psychopathic disorders, but the application of these methods was problematic in treating informal patients.

Since behavior therapy was "properly scientific," in the sense of being derived from theory, Eysenck initially saw it as dealing with what was specifically wrong with the patient. Specifically distinct techniques would be needed for a range of specific disorders. As Michels later put it, the term psychotherapy should be reserved for specific treatments that are based on a theoretical model of psychological functioning which determined the relationship between the pathologic condition and distress. An emerging profession could aim at no less. Eysenck argued this point brilliantly and succeeded in establishing the importance of clinical psychology within mental health services.

Before World War II, psychologists who did clinical work were almost exclusively engaged in the psychometric testing of IQ, aptitudes, personality profiles, or other aspects of neuropsychological functioning.[35] In both world wars, there was a need for a cadre of therapists to treat shell shock and related conditions by psychological means. In 1914, this need had given rise to medical psychologists, men like William McDougall, C. S. Myers, and W. H. Rivers in Britain and a group led by Pierre Janet in France. Although the American Psychological Association had begun the process of training "clinical psychologists" in 1931, as of 1945, psychological therapy remained firmly in medical hands, especially in the United States, where psychoanalysis was an almost exclusively medical discipline.

Behavior therapy provided a vehicle for the entry of clinical psychology into this marketplace. It seemed different from "psychotherapy," a treatment intermediate between psychometric assessment and therapy. As such it escaped medical dominance. It was a treatment that "clinical psychologists" allied to medical teams might administer. In fact, clinical psychologists were more likely to take a humanistic or eclectic approach, but they now had a distinctive domain. As of 1962, there were only 198 psychologists working in the British National Health Service, and they were primarily engaged in making assessments. But both the United States and Britain saw an exponential rise in the number of clinical psychologists through the 1960s and 1970s, many of whom refused to perform IQ assessments, arguing that their mission was to do therapy. The continuing difficulties of psychoanalysis contributed to the opening in the marketplace, as did the increasing identification of physicians as prescribers.

Another therapy emerged in the 1970s. While the push toward community mental health had brought an increasing number of social workers into psychiatry, they had a minimal slice of the therapeutic cake. They were somewhat involved in social skills training but this was generic work that any mental health team worker could undertake.[36] The picture changed in the 1970s with the creation of interpersonal therapy (IPT) by Myrna Weissman, Gerald Klerman, and their colleagues. This was explicitly designed as a brief therapeutic intervention to be delivered by psychiatric social workers.[37] It focused on remedying the social disabilities suffered by patients as a consequence of their illness. It was almost entirely empirical in its orientation, with no claim to be theoretically based or specific.

The pragmatism of IPT mirrored developments within behavior therapy, a field in which Isaac Marks and others had begun to reframe behavior therapy's contributions in terms of its utility in remedying secondary disabilities—for which purpose nurses or even self-help manuals might be as effective as, and more cost-effective than, clinical psychologists. Far from being welcomed, this approach to behavior therapy led to its demise, a turn of events that surely indicates as almost no other can the complicated relationship between scientific evidence, clinical practice, and powerful interests. Behavior therapy was swallowed up by cognitive therapy.

Initially behavior therapists were hostile to the entire notion of cognition. Cognitions were internal mental events that could not be demonstrated to have a real existence and could not be tackled scientifically. The first example of what would later be called cognitive therapy was rational emotive therapy, developed in 1958 by Albert Ellis.[38] Then came the work of Aaron T. Beck. Beck was using a pragmatic form of psychoanalysis, which one of his trainees, John Rush, recognized was different from what psychodynamic therapy was supposed to be. As described by Beck in his first book, published in 1967, the method lay somewhere between a behavioral and a psychodynamic approach.[39]

Beck's approach was entirely empirical, but it spawned a vast industry as psychologists chased the results with theories that tried to accommodate his findings and predict what other therapies might be helpful. There were striking similarities in terms of faulty logic between the models constructed by academic psychologists to account for the efficacy of cognitive therapy and the catecholamine and dopamine theories constructed by academic psychopharmacologists to account for the efficacy of the novel psychotropic agents. The respective arguments were that since these therapies worked on certain cognitions or amines, therefore these cognitions or amines must be dysfunctional in the case of the disorders in question. This does not follow.

Cognitive therapy gained a foothold for a number of reasons. One was that the models erected to explain its efficacy appealed to notions of therapeutic specificity—it works because patients have faulty cognitions. A second factor was that it plugged a gap in the treatment market—the management of depression. Neither psychodynamic nor behavior therapies had focused on depression until then, in part because depressive disorders were thought to be rare while anxiety disorders were common. This was the era of Valium and Librium before the synthesis of Prozac and the invention of depression.[40] Advocating a form of therapy for depression, however, was welcome and by the time Beck's second book appeared in 1976 his procedures had begun to attract attention.[41]

A final factor was that by this stage a cognitive revolution was under way in psychology. After fifty years during which behaviorism had shunned mental events and psychoanalysis had downgraded mental events in favor of an appeal to the true meaning of those events, which only analysts were trained to determine, ordinary mental events—the stream of consciousness—were back on the scientific agenda. Work by Martin Seligman and others on learned helplessness challenged standard formulations of many of the learning theories on which behavior therapy was based.[42] But perhaps of even greater importance was the fact that this revolution and the new therapy shared a word in common—cognitive. Historical change is often driven by such trivial details.

In the hands of clinical psychologists, cognitive and behavior therapies merged to become cognitive-behavior therapy (CBT). This was anathema to card-carrying behaviorists, who described the term as an oxymoron.[43] There seemed in many respects little justification for using the name CBT other than as a political maneuver to encompass the largest number of positive study results under one rubric. But the fact that this merger could succeed indicated that an old order was giving way to a new one. This change put the question of diagnosis and accordingly the shape of the classification system in which diagnoses are embedded on the agenda. This was an issue of interest to all clinical trialists engaged in pharmacotherapy as well as to those engaged in the newly emerging disciplines of clinical psychology and psychiatric social work.

DEFINING THE SELF AND ITS DISORDERS

Jean Esquirol produced the first psychiatric classification system in early-nineteenth-century France. At the end of the nineteenth century, biologically oriented university psychiatry began to have an impact, especially in Germany. This is seen most clearly in the work of Emil Kraepelin. Kraepelin's 1899 textbook contained the hallmark of twentieth-century classification systems: the basic division of the psychoses into manic-depressive and schizo-phrenic. At the same time, a new psychodynamic approach to community nervous problems was being formulated by Freud and Janet that led to yet another way of classifying nervous problems.

Anglo-American psychiatry remained largely aloof from the influences of both university and psychodynamic approaches. It remained instead pragmatic and eclectic. Practitioners were generally uninterested in the nature of the disease entities afflicting patients. In the United States Adolph Meyer typified the approach. Rather than speak of diseases, he talked of ergasias and reactions. Where Kraepelin listed four types of schizophrenia—simple, hebephrenic, paranoid, and catatonic—Meyer outlined four types of parergastic reactions. Meyer argued that it was more appropriate to talk about reactions rather than diseases where the cause of a disorder was unknown.[44] Coughs and nausea, for instance, are common pathway reactions that occur in many different diseases, most organs having only a limited number of ways to react. Might "schizophrenic" reactions also occur in other diseases? Kraepelin conceded the possibility. In 1919, he asked his colleagues to assess the clinical pictures of several patients without knowing details of the illness course and found that many clear-cut cases of general paralysis of the insane (GPI) could not be distinguished from cases of schizophrenia.[45]

Meyer's other signature idea was the notion of psychobiology. He taught that clinical practice should aim at determining the significance of a particular reaction, occurring in a given individual with his individual constitutional type and life history, at a particular point in time. Having pinpointed that, the practitioner might have a clear idea of how to help the patient. This approach stood in contrast to the more neurological Kraepelinian orientation. Neurologists and Kraepelinians aimed to determine the nature of the disease, and if it was a disorder like multiple sclerosis or schizophrenia the patient might be left essentially untreated if there was no specific cure. In the Meyerian scheme of things, assessing the life history of patients or their social situation might reveal a great deal that could be done for them, even if there was no specific treatment for their disorder.

Meyer died in 1950, just as psychoanalysis was gaining a stranglehold on American psychiatry and at a time when the diagnosis of schizophrenia was becoming particularly common. In contrast to the emerging views, he argued that patients with manic-depressive disorders could have delusions and auditory hallucinations and that many so-called schizophrenic patients actually had manic-depressive disorders. The misdiagnosis of manic-depressive disorders, he thought, accounted for many of the so-called cures of schizophrenia. In 1952, DSM-I was published, the first major national classificatory system—a blend of psychoanalytic and Meyerian views.

Meyer left no school behind but through one of his pupils, Mandel Cohen, his legacy had an extraordinary impact on psychiatry later in the twentieth century. Cohen was born in Mobile, Alabama, in 1907.[46] He trained in medicine at John's Hopkins University and worked with Meyer. After training, Cohen moved to Massachusetts General Hospital in Boston, where he joined the Department of Psychiatry when it opened in 1935. Stanley Cobb, a former professor of neuropathology who might have been expected to view matters with a biological slant, was appointed the first professor. But in a testament to the force of the incoming psychoanalytic tide, Cobb became psychodynamically oriented and recruited to the department the analysts Eric Lindemann and Hanns Sachs as well as Helene and Felix Deutsch. Gradually the analysts took over departmental conferences.

Alienated from this new psychiatric department, in 1942 Cohen moved back into medicine at Massachusetts General Hospital. While there, he collaborated with Paul Dudley White, America's preeminent cardiologist.[47] Their first projects centered on a condition then called neurocirculatory asthenia, Da Costa syndrome, or effort syndrome by cardiologists and either anxiety neurosis or neurasthenia by psychiatrists.[48] Many of their patients would today be diagnosed as having panic disorder. Because of the profusion of names for and ideas about this condition, White and Cohen thought it necessary to define their patient group, and so they had to devise diagnostic criteria.

There were no philosophical precedents for this approach, although operational criteria had been introduced a decade before in physics by Percy Bridgeman to help physicists tackle questions where the object of their investigations remained obscure.[49] And an unselfconscious use of criteria to define patient samples was common practice in the rest of medicine, particularly in the treatment of cardio-respiratory conditions. For White and Cohen, criteria were a confession of agnosticism about the condition being investigated rather than a commitment to a notion of disease specificity.

Cohen and White's work was sponsored by the National Research Council, as part of war-related research. Many soldiers had effort syndrome during the World War I. The Americans and the British had had up to two million soldiers affected by war neuroses—more than were affected by any other condition. With the onset of the World War II, the hope was that research would discover the causes of the disorder and indicate possible treatments. Cohen and his colleagues were able to show that this disorder ran in families and that it had often existed before the war, although it may well have worsened during the war.[50]

Working on a group of patients with war neuroses, they noticed a pattern of abnormalities in response to challenges of various sorts. Subjects produced high blood lactate in response to carbon dioxide inhalations, but showed no abnormalities under basal conditions. The work led to the first experimental production of anxiety attacks, when Cohen gave subjects carbon dioxide inhalations.

After the war, Cohen and his colleagues went on to produce diagnostic criteria for manic-depressive disease[51] and hysteria. These foreshadowed those later published in DSM-III. Using the criteria for hysteria, they studied a group of female patients with over two hundred controls and described a condition that bore similarities to the condition described by the French physician Paul Briquet a century earlier.[52] While researchers with an analytic bent were describing cross-sectional aspects of single cases of hysteria, Cohen and his colleagues were describing common factors in large samples and discussing the longitudinal history as well as family backgrounds of the patient set (see Chapter 4).

One of Cohen's residents was Eli Robins. Under Cohen's supervision, he undertook the first studies of hysteria in men.[53] Robins later moved to Washington University in St. Louis, where Edward Gildea was head of psychiatry.[54] Gildea was an "old-style" biological psychiatrist who had studied thyroid function. The head of pharmacology at Washington University, Ollie Lowry, was famous for developing new technologies for measuring proteins in microscopic quantities. Robins, at this stage committed to a medical model of psychiatric disorders, thought that a biological approach was the way forward in psychiatry also.

Washington University, like every other university following the war, saw a vast increase in the number of returning medical personnel, many of whom were psychoanalysts. The university was unusual in having a strict full-time faculty rule, which meant that departments collected patient fees and used these as part of the departmental budget. The returning analysts, who had lost several years of their careers, were understandably keen to earn money rather than to contribute to a departmental budget. Eventually there was a showdown with Gildea. The university was not willing to change the system and accordingly most members of the psychiatric department went into private practice, contributing to the teaching program on a part-time basis. Aside from Gildea, only Robins, George Winokur, and Samuel Guze were left—a triumvirate. Critically, the psychiatry department at Washington University became the one department in the United States that had no analysts.

Having been influenced by Mandel Cohen, Robins would have found it difficult to be anything but skeptical about analysis, but he may also have been influenced by an episode he experienced in the army. His analyst thought he had hysteria. Robins went to see Raymond Adams, the head of neurology at Massachusetts General Hospital. Adams was certain that Robins had a neurological condition, although he was not able to specify precisely what it was. Robins may have been suffering from multiple sclerosis or an atypical post-polio residual syndrome. The illness reappeared and became chronic after Robins had succeeded Gildea as head of department.

The second member of the triumvirate was Samuel Guze, an internist with no initial interest in psychiatry. After the war, he returned to Washington University to complete his medical residency, only to find that all the posts were filled owing to a surfeit of returning trainees. He was placed temporarily with George Saslow, who had a liaison post between medicine and psychiatry. Saslow was biologically oriented and probably one of the few psychiatrists who would not have alienated Guze. Later, when Saslow resigned, Guze was appointed to succeed him.

The third member of the triumvirate was George Winokur, born in Philadelphia in 1925, who had come to do an internship at Washington University. He had planned to go back to private practice in Baltimore, but, influenced by Robins, stayed and became a critical figure in developing a training program that funneled Don Goodwin, Robert Woodruffe, Paula Clayton, Theodore Reich, Robert Cloninger, David Dunner, Denis Cantwell, and others into research.[55]

Winokur, Robins, and Guze worked out a new training program for medical students aimed at instilling in them the notion that psychiatry was a medical discipline and that psychiatric disorders should be approached in the same way as medical disorders—through a research program involving clinical studies, laboratory work, and epidemiology. The first articles embodying the new approach were studies by Guze of hysteria.[56] The first position paper outlining the Robins and Guze approach appeared in 1970.[57] A fuller statement of the new vision appeared in 1975 in a very influential book on psychiatric diagnosis.[58]

This approach was not, however, popular. The NIMH and other grant-giving bodies turned down all grant applications from Washington University.[59] To do research the new department had to harness the energies of its residents and supporters. In the process the department formed an in-group of trainees who saw themselves as standing apart from the rest of American psychiatry.

Another of Meyer's pupils, Aubrey Lewis, had become the director of the Institute of Psychiatry at the Maudsley Hospital in London, at a time when the first departments of psychiatry were being established around Britain. As the director of the institute that would supply the researchers who would chair these departments and by virtue of his political connections, he was well placed to influence appointments. He was determined to ensure that no analyst became head of a department in Britain. None did. Combined with the explosion of psychoanalytic influence in the United States and its effects on diagnostic orientations, this lack of analysts as heads of departments led to a widening gap between the apparent rates of schizophrenia in the United States and the United Kingdom.

The first person to draw attention to this was Morton Kramer, a biometrician at the NIMH. Kramer had begun comparative work on rates of schizophrenia in the United States and elsewhere and was struck by the differences.[60] There was apparently much more schizophrenia in the United States than in the United Kingdom, which had many more patients with depression. This was odd, since the two populations were similar. This finding led Kramer, along with Benjamin Pasamanick and Joseph Zubin, to convene an Anglo-American meeting on mental disorder classification at Somerset House in London in September 1962. Later meetings alternated between the United States and the United Kingdom, with the British delegation including Aubrey Lewis, Michael Shepherd, Robert Kendal, and John Cooper.

This initiative had a number of outcomes. One was a joint Anglo-American study during which Cooper and Kendal liaised with Zubin in the United States.[61] The question was whether these differences in rates were real or whether they were the result of different national diagnostic fashions. Film techniques had just developed to the point where cases could be recorded and shown to clinicians. A first study by Martin Katz produced a surprise: American and British clinicians systematically disagreed on the diagnosis of schizophrenia.[62] Subsequent studies made it clear that patients diagnosed as schizophrenic by American clinicians were diagnosed as depressed or neurotic by the British.[63] This finding left American psychiatrists exposed to the disdain of their European counterparts. This stung.[64]

Kramer had by this time linked up with the Washington University Department of Psychiatry through Eli Robins, who had discovered Child Guidance Clinic records dating back to the 1920s. Following up the children who had been seen at the clinic, she discovered that it was possible to produce operational criteria for defining antisocial personality disorder. The link with Kramer led to the inclusion of St. Louis in the Anglo-American study. And it turned out that there was one U.S. center that was in line with European diagnoses: Washington University in St. Louis.

In the meantime, the question of psychiatric classification had become an issue for the World Health Organization. After its foundation in 1948, WHO took over responsibility for the *International Classification of Diseases* (*ICD*), the sixth edition of which was scheduled to be published in 1948. This edition was the first to contain a section on mental disorders, which was later widely acknowledged as inadequate. It offered no codes for personality disorders or dementia and an inferior discussion of adjustment disorders. WHO convened a meeting in London to investigate standardizing psychiatric diagnoses and mental health statistics. Robert Felix and Aubrey Lewis chaired the meeting. The attendees agreed that there was a need for criteria for diagnoses and proposed a research agenda, which included an international comparison of diagnoses. Michael Shepherd organized a series of annual meetings, which proceeded systematically through the major categories of mental illness. John Wing and European epidemiologists who had spent time in Maudsley Hospital, such as Norman Sartorius, Assen Jablensky, and Jules Angst, played key parts in establishing the diagnostic criteria.[65] These criteria were subsequently embodied in the mental health section of the eighth edition of the *ICD*, which came out in 1968. The specification of criteria for the diagnosis of schizophrenia led WHO to undertake and publish the results of the International Pilot Study of Schizophrenia.[66] This study showed that the Americans and Russians were overdiagnosing schizophrenia, and put the onus on them to fall into line with the rest of the world and revise their concept of schizophrenia.[67]

Worse was in store. In a headline-grabbing study in *Science*, David Rosenhan reported that a group of healthy volunteers feigning the hearing of voices or other disturbed behavior had managed to get admitted to American psychiatric hospitals, where they were diagnosed as schizophrenic. The nursing and medical staff were apparently easily taken in. The only people who recognized the fraud were other patients.[68] American psychiatry was suffering a series of embarrassments.

While this was happening, the NIMH had funded the Psychobiology of Depression Collaborative Program.[69] This aimed to test Joseph Schildkraut's catecholamine hypothesis of depression, which proposed that depression was caused by a lowering of brain catecholamines.[70] The program kicked off with a conference in Williamsburg, Virginia, in 1969 involving Martin Katz, the program director, Eli Robins, Joseph Schildkraut, Gerald Klerman, Seymour Kety, David Hamburg, and many others.[71] The catecholamine hypothesis on one level seemed a simple matter to test. But the meeting at Williamsburg recognized that in order for any biological tests to make sense relatively homogenous groups of patients had to be collected. This required researchers to speak a common language, which meant that the program also had to investigate diagnostic criteria.[72]

Katz had a background in this area, having previously organized a meeting for the NIMH in 1965 to explore the interface between psychopharmacology and classification.[73] He now convened a working group involving Eli Robins, Jean Endicott, Robert Spitzer, and Joseph Mendels. Endicott and Spitzer were recruited because of their expertise in conducting structured interviews and Robins because Washington University was already on record as advocating the use of diagnostic criteria. In 1972, the St. Louis group had published a full set of its operational criteria. The group had a tradition of letting the person who produced the first draft of a paper be the first author, in this case a senior resident named John Feighner: and these criteria have ever since been referred to as the Feighner criteria.[74] The St. Louis criteria for depression, however, were inadequate for the purposes of the Psychobiology of Depression program: they contained too few distinctions within the depressive spectrum. The Spitzer-Robins brief was to improve on the Feighner criteria sufficiently for the purposes of the Psychobiology of Depression Collaborative Program. Endicott, Spitzer, and Robins's work led to the Research Diagnostic Criteria (RDC).[75]

This initiative attracted very little support or attention. One of the few supporters was Gerald Klerman from Yale, who had been involved in early work on the biochemistry of depression with Schildkraut and on the nine-hospital study on chlorpromazine with Cole. Klerman was persuaded that diagnostic criteria were important. He coined the term neo-Kraepelinian to characterize the new approach.[76] This was not welcomed in St. Louis, where it was thought an association with Kraepelin would be perceived as backward-looking.

Klerman had also characterized operational criteria as a Chinese menu approach to psychiatric diagnosis. This characterization fit with the psychoanalytic view of the time, which was that diagnoses made by selecting from a list—one symptom from column A and two from column B—did not require skilled physicians.[77] This was so superficial an exercise that it could be ignored, a carving by feathers rather than the carving by the joints of nature that real diagnosis was supposed to be.[78] It was conceded that criteria might be of some interest to biological researchers, but the use of criteria in clinical work was seen as such a retrograde step that the profession was hardly likely to waste much time with it, let alone adopt it. A majority of nonanalysts shared this view. Even observers from the biological research communities, in the period 1972–1978 when the new approach was taking shape, were of the opinion that although diagnostic criteria and the Washington University approach were interesting, they were not likely to be of much significance.[79] Few, if any, foresaw what was in store.

A parallel track with immense implications was developing. Before his involvement with the Psychobiology of Depression program, Spitzer had been working on structured interviews at the New York State Psychiatric Institute, where he had met Ernest Gruenberg. DSM-I had been published in 1952, and DSM-II was due out in 1968. Gruenberg, a chair of one of the DSM committees, coopted Spitzer onto one of the DSM-II panels. Spitzer was also interested in behavior therapy. Accordingly he attended a meeting on the behavioral treatment of homosexuality, one that was broken up by gay activists protesting against the diagnosis of homosexuality as a psychiatric disorder. One of the activists encountering Spitzer discovered he was a member of the DSM-II committee, which was responsible for labeling homosexuality a disease. This encounter led Spitzer to organize a symposium at an APA meeting to discuss the issue. This symposium and a personal hostility to the Columbia Psychoanalytic Center, which was in favor of maintaining the disease status of homosexuality, finally led Spitzer to the position that homosexuality should be decategorized as a disease.[80] His recommendation took effect in a revised version of DSM-II in 1973.[81]

In 1973, the DSM-II committee began getting drafts of the ninth edition of *ICD*, This was scheduled for publication in 1979 and was to reflect the findings of the International Pilot Study of Schizophrenia and related research. It seemed appropriate to try to harmonize the systems. This would mean a revision of DSM-II to produce DSM-III. The chair of the DSM committee fell vacant when Henry Brill retired from New York State Hospital in 1973. The successor was to be named by the president of the APA, who in 1974 was Judd Marmor. Marmor was among the few to publicly argue that homosexuality should not be considered a pathological condition, and therefore was in sympathy with Spitzer. He also knew that Spitzer was on the DSM-II committee and had an interest in diagnosis. There was little interest in the position of chair of the committee and as a consequence little lobbying for it. Marmor selected Spitzer and met no opposition.

Since classification was seen by most psychiatrists as a rather peripheral and unimportant exercise, Spitzer had a relatively free hand in selecting the other committee members. He chose researchers with a track record of interest in diagnostic criteria, such as Jean Endicott and Donald Klein from Columbia and a group linked to Washington University in St. Louis[82]—a group that was later labeled an invisible college.[83]

Klein, for example, had published a study while he was based at Hillside Hospital at a time when the analysts did therapy and liaised with "druggists," such as Klein, whose prescribing left the hands of the analysts unsullied. Nothing in the DSM-I or DSM-II description of diagnoses would stop an analyst from labeling schizophrenic any patients he thought displayed some schizophrenic symptom. The analysts accordingly diagnosed virtually all patients as having schizophrenia. Klein's research group, in contrast, was using criteria-based diagnoses, according to which some of the patients had schizophrenia but others were given alternative diagnoses. Patients who failed to respond to treatment were ordinarily transferred from Hillside to Creedmore State Hospital. Klein predicted that there would be a difference in the length of stay between those patients where there was agreement between the analysts and his group that the patient had schizophrenia and those patients where there was a difference of opinion. And there was a difference: the average length of stay for the agreed-on schizophrenic patients was nine months, whereas the average stay for the disputed patients was three weeks. Diagnostic refinements did count.[84]

In the two years preceding the publication of DSM-III, there was mounting concern among American psychoanalysts who had seen drafts of the new system in the course of fieldwork. One of the central difficulties was a proposal by the DSM committee to eliminate the word neurosis; this appeared, at the time, almost incredible.[85] Mystifyingly for many, the basis for the elimination lay in difficulties in operationalizing the concept. Analysts were appalled. Political skirmishing began that ended in open splits within the American Psychiatric Association. Delegations were sent to Spitzer to inform him that his proposals were not representative of American psychiatry. He was forced to coopt psychoanalysts but found analysts prepared to accept the notion of operational criteria. With a number of concessions, the manual was finally voted into existence and published in 1980. The crucial concessions were on the issue of neurotic depression, which was fast becoming the bread and butter of the office practice of psychiatry. Spitzer retained the concept of neurotic depression in parentheses, as a possible alternative to a name with less theoretical baggage that he had introduced—dysthymia. In the heat of a political crisis, Kahlbaum's creation of a century ago had been resurrected and put to work to save the entire DSM edifice.

The reemergence of dysthymia is striking for many reasons. Compared with the alternative, neurotic depression, it implied a more chronic personality-based condition. Moving it from a section of the classificatory system for personality disorders into Axis-1, the "disease entity" section, marks the initiation of a process sustained in the following editions of DSM and in clinical practice, a process whereby Kahlbaum's cyclothymia migrated from the personality realm to the disorder realm and avoidant personality disorder was transformed into social phobia.[86]

DSM-III was in fact Meyerian rather than neo-Kraepelinian in its use of the term disorders rather than diseases and in its willingness to codify a broad range of reactions and syndromes found in clinical practice. The one condition where these rules did not apply was catatonia. Although Freud's preconceptions had been cleared away, the same did not apply to Kraepelin's preconceptions, and catatonia remained locked within the schizophrenia complex, despite the rediscovery of its response to ECT.

DSM-III is widely regarded as marking a revolution in American and world psychiatry. Debates were later held at APA meetings through the early 1980s on the merits and demerits of the new system.[87] For many it seemed that a battle had suddenly been won by an army from nowhere, with the contest being over almost before anyone knew it had begun.

But what was at stake and why do so many people in the street now know of the existence of the DSM, while so few psychiatrists even knew about the existence of DSM-II? Why had the issue of classification, which had been of little interest to anyone previously, suddenly come to seem pivotal? Many have sought an explanation. Mitchell Wilson in a widely cited article put DSM-III's success down to the fact that it satisfied the needs of the insurance and pharmaceutical industries as well as the requirements of regulators.[88] Spitzer, in contrast, said the key point was that psychiatry had pulled back from a mission to save the world and was concentrating on a biomedical focus—pulling back from a mission that had brought the profession to the edge of extinction.[89] In Spitzer's view, the major innovation was the adoption of operational criteria and the reason the manual became quickly acceptable was that it included a range of diagnoses, which clinicians found reflected in their daily practice. The book also made money for the American Psychiatric Association.

None of these reasons, however, seems to capture fully the magnitude of the phenomenon. Commercial success for the APA was welcome to the APA but not a determinant of public interest.

Even the analysts could embrace operational criteria, although they found them superficial. Those who failed to do so risked being outflanked by the cognitive therapists, who were happy to jump on the bandwagon. The insurance and pharmaceutical industries had been content with DSM-II.

Unlike the psychiatry that gave rise to DSM-I, however, the psychiatry of the DSM-III era was part of the public domain. At stake were our very definitions of ourselves. The debates on homosexuality had prefigured broader attempts to define human beings. Psychiatry's definition of the self had become a public matter. Nothing in the text of the manual says this, but DSM-III's significance stems from and indicates the importance that psychiatry had assumed in the popular mind. Previously, psychoanalysis had been catering to the semi-spiritual needs of twentieth-century men and women and had been able to do so with very little reference to the rest of psychiatry. Now all groups within the mental health arena were yoked together and forced to hammer out agreements. It was as though the world's major religions were brought to the same negotiating table.

Unlike religion though, psychiatry had come from nowhere to be a major force in the public domain. Whereas before the 1950s and 1960s psychiatry had been solely concerned with serious mental illness, these decades saw the growth of the mental health industry. What had once been a classification used by a few alienists had now become the bread and butter of daily practice for a vast array of therapists. Freudian ideas had brought psychiatry into the arts and culture generally. In ways that Spitzer and his committee could not have imagined in 1980, new drugs like Prozac and older drugs like Ritalin were soon to push this process further. The restriction of these treatments to prescription-only status had removed from average people a major means of helping themselves. As a result, the way in which people's discontents were defined became a matter that deserved public scrutiny. DSM-III marks the point at which these processes were consolidated and a new psychiatry was born. The biomedical focus could never mean in the future what it had so recently meant to Spitzer. We were on our way to a new biomedical self.

BRAVE NEW WORLD

The operational criteria embodied in DSM-III were born into a world different from the one in which they were conceived. Richard Nixon's election in 1968 might have led to a demise of disinterested research in any event, but the administration also faced a health budget that was burgeoning alarmingly. The Vietnam War had led to an economic crisis in 1968, aggravated several years later by the oil crisis. The government began to cut back on funding for the National Institutes of Health. Sensing the change, Jonathan Cole left the Psychopharmacology Research Center (PRC) and returned to clinical practice.[90] The NIMH research budget declined by $5 million from 1969 to 1976. Grants from ECDEU came to an end in 1975. By 1980 state funds for research had dried up. Independent clinical research was over, although since "science" at the NIMH was untouched few realized it.

Forces operating on national and global levels were redefining the agenda. The community mental health center (CMHC) program launched in the 1960s came under question during the Nixon administration. This federal initiative was not in tune with Republican thinking and the new administration sought to eliminate federal support for CMHCs. In an odd echo of the antipsychiatrists, some questioned whether these centers were treating the seriously mentally ill or taking on a new clientele: the worried well.

In 1977, Jimmy Carter established a presidential commission on mental health.[91] This recommended greater attention to the psychiatric needs of children and minorities, support for research and in particular for epidemiology, the development of a specific

plan for treating the chronically mentally ill, and the establishment of methods for monitoring the performance of the mental
health services. These initiatives were embodied in the Mental
Health Systems Act, which was signed into law shortly before
Carter left office. This Canute-like bill faced a strong adverse
tide. Two months later, the new Reagan government recommended an interruption of all mental health grant programs in research and training. This Republican administration had come
into office committed to lowering taxes, deregulation, decreasing
federal control, and increasing the states' authority. The new act
was dismantled. Federal care and social security support for the
chronically mentally ill went into a sharp decline, and the continuing increase in health care budgets provided the matrix for the
birth of managed care.

The common perception in psychiatry during this period was
that placebo-controlled RCT methods had been used successfully
to evaluate the efficacy of psychotropic drugs since the 1960s and
that the elaboration of DSM-III could only enhance the quality of
the process. This seemingly sturdy scientific vessel came to be an
increasing source of comfort for psychiatry in the choppy post-
DSM waters. Whoever was calling the financial or ideological
shots, evidence would surely at the end of the day ensure the right
outcomes.

In fact, although there were some placebo-controlled trials of
psychotropic drugs from 1960 to 1984, the majority of trials involved a comparison between new and older drugs without a
placebo control. The vast majority of these trials did not show
whether any of the drugs tested actually worked. The regular inclusion of placebo controls in regulatory studies was not instituted until the mid-1980s, after the intervention of the FDA, and
it initially elicited dismay from the pharmaceutical industry.[92]

The crisis that arose may have contributed to the licensing
of Prozac. The plans to launch several antidepressants in the
United States were set back by the new requirement for placebo-
controlled studies, at a time when work on new antipsychotics

had all but ceased because of the legal liabilities associated with tardive dyskinesia. For a period in the early 1980s, there appeared to be a real risk that no new psychotropic drugs would emerge. Against this backdrop, in 1987, the FDA licensed fluoxetine, on the basis of its minimal superiority to a placebo and its inferiority to imipramine as a comparator and despite the fact that fluoxetine could not be shown to be beneficial in treating patients hospitalized for depression and was therefore in some real sense inferior to agents already available. Furthermore, many of the patients given fluoxetine were also prescribed benzodiazepines, to minimize the drug-induced agitation that had led a number of patients to worsen dramatically. In a population of mild depressives, it could not be assumed that these benzodiazepines were not working in their own right. It follows that fluoxetine alone had not been shown to work—and indeed has never since, in this sense, been shown to work.[93]

The Prozac story makes a number of points. One is that this absence of RCT evidence should not be taken as evidence against the effectiveness of psychotropic drugs in general or Prozac in particular. Rather, since a majority of clinicians had little doubt that their treatments were effective, it must be that clinical "knowledge" about what drugs really do comes from a source other than RCTs. None of the early antipsychotics, antidepressants, or anxiolytics, after all, had either been discovered in or shown to work by controlled trials. A second point is that the marketing of Prozac indicates that the evidence that counted now belonged to the pharmaceutical industry. Under the ECDEU system, no compound with an evidence base as weak as Prozac could have become the phenomenon that Prozac later became. The story of Prozac was not an isolated one. Throughout the 1990s, a succession of drugs with minimal effects on depression was licensed, in some cases with only two out of six trials showing a superiority to a placebo, with any trials that failed to show a differentiation from a placebo being termed failed trials.

The Prozac story shows something else. Although DSM-III did offer a new restrictive "Kraepelinian" concept of schizophrenia, it had in contrast moved from a restrictive concept of melancholic or endogenous depression to the looser concept of major depressive disorder. During the 1990s, when pharmaceutical companies were intensively marketing the SSRIs, this was to prove capable of leading to a vast expansion in the apparent frequency of depressive disorders. Whereas in the 1950s, less than 0.5 percent of the population had a depressive disease, the prevalence of major depressive disorder in the 1990s had risen over twenty-fold, to 10 percent of the population. Some studies reported that up to 25 percent of the population had a significant number of depressive symptoms—providing a vast market for the antidepressants. Depression had become a popular illness, and the existence of diagnostic criteria, it seemed, could do nothing to stop the estimates of its frequency from ballooning.

Finally, when it came to trials, an area in which psychiatry had once led the rest of medicine, the picture was also changing. In 1956, at the Conference on the Evaluation of Drugs, Nathan Kline had argued that drug studies should deal with overall treatment outcomes such as whether the patient left the hospital, got back to work, or moved from the back wards to open wards, rather than simply relying on rating scales.[94] The rest of medicine followed this path in the 1980s, engaging in large simple trials that focused on clear-cut endpoints such as mortality.[95] In psychiatry no such studies were conducted in the 1980s or 1990s. Small studies remained the preferred option for the by now almost exclusively industrial sponsors of trials.

The New Masters

By the mid-1970s the ECDEU program was failing. Funds had dried up. Out of the ashes of ECDEU arose a superficially similar body, the New Clinical Drug Evaluation Unit (NCDEU), but one with a very different character. This was a marketplace where companies hired clinical investigators. Previously researchers had told industry what needed to be done, but now companies did not have to approach investigators to design their trials for them, compile the statistics, or write the papers. The formulas for clinical trials that the ECDEU investigators had put together to contain the pharmaceutical industry became a petard on which psychiatry was hoist. Armed with off-the-shelf protocols, companies sought out those researchers who were prepared to do the work that suited a commercial agenda. A process had begun that led to the analysis of trial results within the company and thereafter to the writing up of the results by company personnel.[96] Senior clinical investigators now might be used as figureheads on papers or for presentations at academic meetings, but the clinical presence was increasingly becoming ornamental rather than substantial.[97] They were merely figureheads for studies conducted by relatively untrained nonmedical personnel and in some cases the patients did not exist.[98]

In the 1980s, a new phenomenon, satellite symposia, became increasingly frequent at national and international meetings. These were company-sponsored symposia. Between 1974 and 1988 there had been an increase from $6 million to $86 million in the amount of money spent by the major companies on these events in the United States.[99] In the 1990s, many senior clinical figures, some of whom were notional principal investigators on company studies, could be seen performing in both satellite and regular symposia at meetings, sometimes with a frequency that meant leaving one symposium before it ended to participate in another or in a press briefing.

The proceedings of satellite symposia were published in journal supplements. These were rarely peer-reviewed. Medical communication and public relations agencies sprang up, out-sourced from pharmaceutical companies. The writers in these agencies commonly wrote the drafts of articles that appeared in the journals, as well as producing the slides for speakers. In some cases, the contributions appearing under distinguished names were never even read by their notional authors.[100] Some of these articles gave the impression of producing new data but in fact republished already reported data, with the endorsement of a senior figure in the field. This process of multiple publication of studies with positive results led by one calculation to an overestimate of the benefits of risperidone of 23 percent.[101] To this must be added the nonpublication of studies with negative results and demonstrations that the identity of the sponsoring body is the greatest predictor of the outcome of a published study.[102] Some branded this state of affairs an abuse of trust and scientific misconduct.[103]

At the 1956 conference, Kline, Cassandra-like, had pointed out that a dependence on changes in rating scale scores ran the risk of producing a version of the rabbit out of the hat trick, which involved putting the rabbit in the hat to begin with. But even he could not have predicted the extent to which clinicians would be fooled by just this kind of trick in the 1990s. If rating scales are used, ideally a treatment effect should show up across a range of domains of measurement. The benefit of the drug, for example, should show on scales used by doctors as well as on self-rating scales used by patients, such as quality of life (QoL) scales. But where QoL scales have been used in trials of SSRIs, probably less than 10 percent of the data has been published.[104]

Add to nonpublication of data the fact that the distribution networks for these ghostwritten articles are far more efficient than the normal scientific channels for the dissemination of independent work and it becomes clear to what extent the control of information has become an industrial process.[105] Where once the psychopharmacology literature was invested with the authority of clinicians who knew at first hand what they were describing, by the end of the century an increasingly large amount of the literature had become the psychiatric equivalent of a Big Mac.

By the mid-1990s psychiatry meetings had reached mega-meeting status. In addition to bringing clinicians to these meetings, companies regularly brought journalists and held press briefings. What had once been forums for extraordinary intellectual debates had by the 1990s been transformed into little more than trade fairs.

Therapeutic Decline

The evisceration of the science of psychiatric therapeutics by pharmaceutical corporations went hand in hand with an increasing rhetorical dependence on "evidence-based medicine." If it is borne in mind that the evidence that practice is now supposed to follow is losing its credibility, the strains in the system are clear. The situation is arguably leading to a real therapeutic decline.

When haloperidol was given to the first patient to receive it, it was obvious that it worked. Straightforward clinical observation can also clearly show what a treatment is doing to help—it is sedating, or stimulating, or it has an anti-stereotypy action. In contrast, RCTs, like the epidemiological studies from which they are derived, aim at providing evidence of associations. But while studies, for instance, of smoking and lung cancer may show these to be linked, they do not explain how they are linked and they may indeed even obscure the linking mechanism.

In the case of haloperidol, there appears to be a specific anti-stereotypy action so that when given in low doses dramatic responses may be seen in Tourette's syndrome or certain paranoid disorders. There also seems to be a less specific tension-reducing effect, which produces a more diffuse benefit in a number of other psychotic disorders. Finally, there are a large number of schizophrenic states for which haloperidol and all subsequent antipsychotics are ineffective. On the basis of RCTs, however, the antipsychotics are portrayed as antipsychotics because in the aggregate they can be shown to make a difference in a group of patients with psychoses. This means they are now prescribed to patients simply because patients have a psychosis rather than in order to achieve a particular goal in treating the patients. In lieu of megadose therapies, therapists driven by an allopathic compulsion resort to increasingly complex combinations of drug cocktails, each individually justified on the basis of RCT data but none justified functionally.

Focusing on the RCT evidence that SSRIs can help treat depression, OCD, post-traumatic stress disorder, social phobia, panic disorder, and generalized anxiety disorder throws more light on what is actually happening. These positive responses can lead to two hypotheses. One is that that there is something wrong with the serotonin system in all these states and that drugs that act on the serotonin system are magic bullets. This is the favored view of pharmaceutical companies. The alternative is that SSRIs heal patients by reducing emotional reactivity, a serenic effect that cuts across a range of nervous conditions. If this is the case, some patients would be expected to respond to such a serenic effect, while others would not respond, with the degree and frequency of response sufficient to distinguish the compound from a placebo. This is exactly the state of affairs that best characterizes trials with SSRIs, which have been shown to have a modest treatment effect across this range of conditions, with striking clinical efficacy in some patients.[106] The clinical trial results are not compatible with the idea of a serotonin lesion or a magic bullet effect in any of these disorders.

Antabuse (disulfiram) provides another good example of the principles at issue. This agent obviously works in the sense of making a patient demonstrably sick after ingesting alcohol. On this basis it becomes useful therapeutically, an agent that can be adopted by a clinician faced with a case of alcohol dependence. When compared to a placebo in groups of alcoholics, however, Antabuse has been shown to be of only limited utility.[107] Nevertheless, when a physician has a patient impressed by the possibilities that Antabuse offers, it may be both legitimate and efficacious to prescribe Antabuse rather than choose a treatment that looks more efficacious on the basis of RCTs. Nobody suggests that alcoholism involves some brain disulfiram deficiency, but a similar effect is exactly what is suggested in the case of the antidepressants and antipsychotics.

Arguably, unless the prescriber knows what he wants the drug to do in order to get the patient well, he cannot prescribe rationally. A physician who prescribes on the basis of RCT evidence without a clear idea of what the drug does functionally is likely to invoke some biomythology if called upon to justify himself. This is a kind of prescribing that in the 1980s and 1990s handed over to pharmaceutical companies the power to decide when and for what drugs work rather than a prescribing that led clinicians to increasing clinical wisdom—a prescribing that transferred the magic of the therapeutic act from the healer to the brand name of the drug being administered by a technician.

This point also links to Pavlov's dogs, Masserman's monkeys, and later studies administering Eysenck's personality questionnaire to individuals being anesthetized. RCTs might show that a stimulant or a sedative on aggregate was better than a placebo for treating traumatic neuroses, but they do not say much if anything about what a particular animal or specific patient will respond to. In which cases does fluoxetine produce the dramatic responses that have probably been influential in persuading clinicians that it works? Can anything be done to make the process of matching the patient to the drug more rational? There are in fact studies showing that the personality traits of patients can predict up to 50 percent of their likelihood to respond to antidepressants acting on either the serotonergic or the noradrenergic system[108] and also to antipsychotics.[109]

Why aren't more studies like this done? A company that engaged in such trials would then only be licensed to claim that its drug worked in individuals with particular personality types. Such a claim would reduce the company's profits. This indicates what is really happening when RCTs are used in psychiatry. They provide data that coincide with the interests of the most powerful players in the therapeutic arena rather than data that inform clinical practice.

The compelling merit of the neo-Kraepelinian system for a pharmaceutical company is that it all but identifies psychiatric disorders as bacterial infections, with the implication that a condition will respond to treatment regardless of the psychosocial setting or the constitutional type of the patient. As a result there is a congruence of rhetorical interests between pharmaceutical and managed care companies that appears to be undercutting the abilities of psychiatrists to do therapy, as Guze lamented. Ironically, studies that have shown that temperament and personality play a role in drug responses have used Cloninger's Tridimensional Personality Questionnaire to measure personality profiles. This modified version of Eysenck's personality questionnaire originated in St. Louis, the supposed home of neo-Kraepelinism. In fact, there was never any belief in St. Louis that the disorders psychiatrists were attempting to clarify remotely resembled bacterial infections that could be hit specifically by the magic bullets of modern pharmacotherapy.

There are other trials not happening. Hypnotics and analgesics work in even more obvious ways than antipsychotics and may not require an RCT to show this. But the fact that they work does not mean that the patient will appreciate their use. An early study of hypnotics by Louis Lasagna showed clearly that although many patients may have been effectively sedated, some found the experience aversive.[110] Clinical trials could be designed to demonstrate the proportions of patients who are likely to find a particular therapy both beneficial and acceptable. But no such trials have been undertaken. If science means collecting a full set of data on any phenomenon, then despite its rhetoric, modern psychiatry would seem to be anything but scientific. But does this problem affect only pharmacotherapy?

The Psychotherapy of the Psychoses

Not until twenty years after the failures of Philip May's and Jack Ewalt's studies on the psychotherapy of schizophrenia (see Chapter 4) and the marriage of cognitive and behavioral approaches was life was breathed back into the psychotherapy of the psychoses. In the intervening years there was an emphasis in centers from the United States to Australia on the identification of early signs of relapse. The hope was that intervening with psychosocial measures and drug treatment early in the course of relapse might forestall a full-scale breakdown and the secondary disabilities that entailed.

In the mid-1980s, there were signs of a reemerging interest in psychotherapeutic approaches to psychotic symptoms, with Richard Bentall in Liverpool demonstrating that a range of behavioral interventions offered benefits for the treatment of hallucinations.[111] A sustained cognitive approach to the psychoses ensued, stimulated by reports of patients with delusions responding to cognitive interventions.[112] For the most part the outcomes were weak and unreplicated, but the data packed more punch than might have been expected owing to their identification with the professional fortunes of clinical psychologists. There was enough punch to lead a former president of the Royal College of Psychiatrists to wonder if psychiatrists in due course would be replaced even within the psychiatric heartlands of psychosis.[113]

Part of the force of the cognitive behavior therapy argument was the notion that this was a specific therapy, "specific" meaning logically derived from first principles. To be theory based even with weak results often appeals more to scientists than having the results on their side. The siren call of specificity in this sense can have a delusional intensity that overrides the evidence base. This kind of specificity is romantic. It persuades therapists they are doing the right and natural thing rather than just an artificial though useful thing. They are being physicians rather than surgeons. The hunters of specificity do not want just to let a sufferer get on with his life; they want to root out the original sin. The notion that they might be just managing disabilities is anathema to most pharmacotherapists and psychotherapists.

This style of psychotherapy of the psychoses was to run smack up against a psychotherapy propelled forward by another archetypal image of therapeutic specificity: the image of an environmental pathogen, in this case sexual abuse—the original sin. This virus had lain dormant since Freud abandoned his seduction theory in 1896. A combination of factors led to its reawakening.

One was the Vietnam War. In contrast to both world wars, in the Vietnamese conflict the role of army psychiatrists and psychologists was not necessarily to restore soldiers to the front line. A soldier's difficulties could be acknowledged and the blame could be linked rightly or wrongly to the horrors to which he had been exposed rather than the inadequacy of his personality integration. Shell shock had been a major threat to the nations involved in World War I and had nearly led to the execution of many sufferers. The sheer difficulties in executing thousands of men probably saved many from such a fate. This was not the case in Vietnam.

While the Vietnam War was being waged, the question of child abuse resurfaced in the work of C. H. Kempe and his colleagues on battered child syndrome.[114] They descried this syndrome after examining many X-rays of injured children that showed the presence of multiple, unsuspected healed fractures. It took two decades for clinicians and society to accept that non-accidental injuries of this kind might be occurring. The initial concern was with the physical consequences of the battering. At first, the quiet, timid, miserable, or sullen behavior of the children went unnoticed. As late as 1975, the *Comprehensive Textbook of Psychiatry*, a huge volume 2,707 pages long, contained no discussion of the mental states of abused children. Father-daughter incest was discussed without any indication that it could cause serious psychopathology. A time bomb was waiting to explode.

Also in the same *Comprehensive Textbook of Psychiatry*, John

Nemiah noted that the then prevalent view was that multiple personality disorders (MPDs) had become extinct in Western civilization.[115] But whereas neurosis had been airbrushed out of the psychiatric picture frame by DSM-III, MPD had been legitimized as a diagnostic entity by its appearance in the new manual.[116] In 1980 Eugene Bliss reported on fourteen cases of multiple personality disorder. Several series of cases were swiftly identified and by 1984 1,000 patients were thought to be in treatment, increasing by 1988 to 4,000 with estimates of prevalence rates of up to 20,000 cases across the United States alone. An increasing number of symposia were given over at APA meetings to assisting practitioners in making the diagnosis. To the skeptics, these clinical interview training sessions appeared to be methods for coaching patients in how to present themselves as having multiple personality disorder.

The descriptions of borderline personality disorder and multiple personality disorder in DSM-III gave a stimulus to a changing field. Using operational criteria for the latest syndromes, researchers demonstrated that up to 80 percent of patients with borderline conditions appeared to have been abused in childhood. Furthermore, up to 50 percent of patients diagnosed as schizophrenic appeared to have been abused during childhood also. It became clear that there was an overlap between Kurt Schneider's first-rank symptoms, often thought of as being pathognomic of schizophrenia, and the dissociative experiences described by Janet and others.[117] Either schizophrenia was being caused by trauma or clinicians were sloppily misinterpreting the statements of their patients. Either assumption fed straight into a long-standing and respectable tradition of interest in the possibility of an environmental precipitation of certain schizophrenias.[118]

Linkage of these syndromes to the emotive issue of child abuse brought together a set of combustible ingredients ignited in 1987 by Judith Herman's book on father-daughter incest.[119] Herman argued that father-daughter incest set up a massive repression in adult life, which might require the strenuous efforts of therapists to reverse. In 1988 Ellen Bass and Laura Davies published *The Courage to Heal,* which explained just how to reverse this repression and recover memories.[120] The book sold very well. This clinical issue quickly merged with wider feminist issues. To many there appeared to be some encouragement for women who had any relationship problems in adult life or with the medical services to reinterpret their experiences in terms of earlier abuse, even if details of this could not be recovered.[121] The recovered memory debate had become a political issue, with those accepting the validity of such memories suggesting that environmental trauma might be responsible for much of psychiatric morbidity.

Then came a backlash. In 1992, the False Memory Syndrome Foundation was set up in Philadelphia, and it soon reported that 18,000 people were seeking help. Similar societies sprang up in other countries. Recovered memory therapy took on a new meaning. Its critics argued that it created memories of abuse that had never happened. Families, it was claimed, were being torn apart by therapists who were pursuing their own agendas rather than putting the interests of their patients first. In 1993, the APA raised concerns about the possibility of false accusations of abuse based on memories recovered in therapy.[122]

The whirlwind sucked up many. Jules Masserman, who had kept working into his old age, became the subject of a legal action. Freud and Janet, had they been around, would have been equally at risk. There was an astonishing mix of competing visions involved in this controversy. Many recovered memory cases involved therapists who gave their primary allegiance to CBT, seduced by the ever more powerful vision of specificity that the abuse paradigm offered. Gone was any appreciation of Pavlov's and Eysenck's vision, which underpinned their work, that individuals differ biologically as well as in other ways. One of these differences was an individual's degree of extraversion; those who are extraverts handle their conflicts in the interpersonal domain and are exquisitely suggestible. CBT was a product of the RCT era. This seemed to mean for most psychotherapists that it—and psychotherapy generally—should work like a magic bullet, regardless of the personality type of the patient.

Many of those who recovered memories of abuse were young women, who may quite possibly have been abused, but whose reports of hearing "voices" had led to a diagnosis of schizophrenia. They commonly ended up taking megadoses of antipsychotics, as a failure of these voices to disappear led to ever increasing doses of antipsychotics, with the women themselves, for a variety of psychodynamic reasons, failing to protest and sometimes failing to survive (see Chapter 6). These megadoses fueled a great deal of the anger that propelled the psychiatric survivor groups that emerged to parallel the false memory groups arising in response to megadoses of psychotherapy.

One of the most influential and likely to be the most enduring of the groups hostile to all orthodox therapies was the Hearing Voices self-help movement, started by Marius Romme in Holland in the late 1980s.[123] Romme's contention was that auditory hallucinations were in fact common in the population, and particularly common after abuse during childhood. Rather than being specific indicators of an illness, they were nonspecific and they did not need treatment in their own right. Treatment would be the modern equivalent of the pathologization and forced treatment of homosexuality that had played such a big part in the politics of DSM-III. Romme's nonspecific approach to voices drew particular fire from the cognitive therapy establishment. The idea of letting people help themselves in such a nonsystematic way seemed horrifyingly dangerous.

EVIDENCE-BIASED MEDICINE

Clearly the psychiatric world is spinning more out of control than ever before. When RCTs were introduced in the 1950s, psychoanalysts argued that the processes being evaluated were too complex to be assessed by this method.[124] Recent history suggests that there may be more force to this criticism than is commonly conceded. The original trials of antidepressants and antipsychotics demonstrated a treatment effect in four to six weeks. But working in this sense meant having a measurable effect on scales like the BPRS or the Hamilton rating scale. It was assumed that such effects were likely to translate into effects of clinical significance. As rates of depression rise despite ever increasing levels of treatment and mortality rates for schizophrenia rise despite supposedly better and better agents, these assumptions have to be questioned.[125]

In the late 1990s, anticonvulsants, such as lamotrigine, gabapentin, and sodium valproate, were used increasingly to treat bipolar mood disorders without RCT demonstrations of efficacy for the bipolar syndrome. Clinicians seem to have been sufficiently impressed with the outcomes to continue this approach. Does this indicate a retreat to the bad old days when treatments were adopted on the basis of the authority of leading figures in the field? An alternative is that this development tells us that it is extremely difficult to prove by conventional RCT methods that any of these agents work rather than just have treatment effects. Have we underestimated the complexity of the clinical conditions involved? Consider the problems. No one rating scale can be used in assessing a condition that cycles from one pole to its opposite. If the criterion adopted was frequency of episodes, thousands of patients would have to be recruited across multiple centers and sustained within an experimental protocol for years in order to produce a convincing demonstration of prophylaxis. This cannot be simply done.

Clinical practice, however, can proceed in the absence of such demonstrations because there is a difference between proving something does not work and being unable to prove conclusively that it does work. Guided by patient responses, clinical practice readily adopts a host of procedures such as the use of trazodone in the management of SSRI-induced akathisia or sexual dysfunction without supportive RCT evidence. These examples suggest that

RCT-derived evidence affects clinical practice primarily in cases where trials fail to provide evidence of efficacy. Otherwise such evidence stands at one remove from clinical experience and, when available, is of primary use to clinicians not in deciding how to treat their patients but when facing legal or bureaucratic challenges or when engaged in ideological point scoring. Perhaps the most important use of such evidence today, however, is its rhetorical use by governments, third-party payers, or drug companies attempting to gain control of a market.

Further problems emerge if the nature of psychiatric treatments is scrutinized. The match between drug therapies and RCTs was based on the idea that a drug embodied one active principle, which had been isolated and could be delivered systematically. In the case of the antipsychotics, it is now clear that in addition to D-2 receptor blockage, actions on alpha, S-2, histamine, and other receptors may all be therapeutically useful. Far from being magic bullets containing one active principle, these drugs are cocktail compounds containing a number of therapeutic principles. In fact as a matter of simple chemistry, it is all but impossible to reduce current drugs to one active principle.[126] And this multiplicity of principles is complemented by a diversity of brain sites on which they may act, so that pure morphine may be antitussive, analgesic, hypnotic, and euphoriant as well as antidiarrheal, depending on which brain site it acts upon. This makes it even more difficult to judge from the results of RCTs exactly what is going on.

CBT is no different. Far from being a simple therapy that works only on cognitions, this therapy contains a number of therapeutic principles, including behavioral activation, cognitive restructuring, and problem solving. Studies in depression have revealed that all of these components may be independently active.[127] At the end of the century, Isaac Marks and his colleagues developed several computer packages that can systematically deliver the many different components of behavior and cognitive therapy. Pfizer funded their development program for a while.

Such a package potentially challenges many of the drivers in the current marketplace because it favors self-help rather than reliance on a professional and the programs are patentable and can be mass produced.[128]

In the 1990s, evidence-based medicine (EBM) became the dominant slogan. The enthusiasm for EBM suggests that for some "science" had come to be seen at some level as a means of dealing rationally with the values involved in medicine, if only by ensuring that effective treatments are made available. For others the economic efficiency of operating according to the "evidence base" was valuable in its own right. But from the preceding discussion it must be clear that psychiatry is far from being in a position to solve economic or value problems by appeals to the evidence base.

Consider the classic magic bullet language of main effects and side effects. By convention the main effect of antidepressants is taken to be on mood; other effects, for example on sexual functioning, are designated side effects. But in fact, sexual functioning may be more reliably affected by an SSRI than mood. Where up to two hundred patients may be needed to demonstrate a treatment effect for an SSRI in cases of depression, as few as twelve patients may be needed to demonstrate its efficacy in treating premature ejaculation.[129] Companies kept the evidence of the potentially beneficial effects of SSRIs on aspects of sexual functioning—useful for treating premature ejaculation—out of the public domain for two decades. This example should make it clear that deciding which is main effect of a compound is essentially an arbitrary decision, related to company economics and far from value free.[130]

The licensing system for drugs was put in place partly to constrain the claims that companies can make. A confusing intersection with clinical practice has come about since the 1962 amendments to the Food and Drugs Act, where the requirements for drug licensing moved from demonstrations of safety to demonstrations of effects in the treatment of particular disease conditions. This shift leads directly to the claims that imipramine is an antidepressant rather than a tonic, even though it improves appetite and sleep in the same way as tonics did. As a tonic, imipramine invariably works. As an antidepressant it is less clear that it works in many depressive syndromes. In the same way chlorpromazine and clozapine became antipsychotics rather than tranquilizers or sedatives.

With the restriction of drug treatments to disease states, companies have aggressively marketed medical disease models as a means of selling compounds. They market these models to clinicians, many of whom think that they can only prescribe compounds to treat the conditions indicated by the license. Clinical worries about prescribing off-license reflect an increasing lack of clinical confidence and confusion at this intersection between science and business.

All this would be of secondary concern if there were progressive developments in the caliber of the therapeutic arsenal. But as we have seen, either most agents now used were not properly evaluated by RCTs or, in the case of the antidepressants, there are good grounds to believe that RCTs have functioned to let onto the market agents that were in many respects less effective than older compounds. Furthermore, there is every reason to suspect that RCTs are now pushing good therapies out of health care. Psychiatric units, which once had active occupational therapy units, are now reduced to boring, sterile places. Patients are not exercised, or taken out to social activities, or involved in art, music, or other therapies. If they leave the hospital for a psychosocial reason, it is likely to be boredom.

This situation has developed because economically only treatments that have been shown to "work" can be justified. The problems of justification are made worse by the fact that demonstrations of specific efficacy, of the types that RCTs provide, also provide evidence that can be marketed. This makes it much easier to lobby for pharmacotherapies rather than nonspecific inputs to therapy. If funds were available for only one antipsychotic therapy, there can be little doubt that an antipsychotic drug should be chosen. If there are funds for two therapies, there may be a case for choosing two different antipsychotic drugs. But when the funding extends to a third therapy, or shortly thereafter, we reach a stage where a therapy other than a further conventional antipsychotic drug should be chosen, even though another antipsychotic may be demonstrably more effective than any nonantipsychotic drug or other nondrug therapy. To choose only antipsychotic drugs would be to impoverish the capacity to do therapy.

Feedback maneuvers or other therapeutic inputs such as sheltered work clearly make a difference. The fact that much of sports psychology is based on modulating performances in response to feedback demonstrates how, without the newspeak of the modern medical state, it is obvious to practitioners that these are powerful techniques. It is difficult to think of a condition in which feedback would not be of some help and relatively easy to think of cases which might resolve entirely with appropriate feedback. But feedback cannot be compared with a placebo—it is part of the placebo or nonspecific domain. Maneuvers like feedback or occupational work might not cure psychotic patients in the absence of anything else, but they might be expected to yield benefits once the patient has progressed beyond a certain threshold. However, because these interventions cannot be shown to work in the same way that drugs are shown to work, they will not be purchased by third-party payers—and this is setting up increasing problems for patients.

We have not yet devised evaluative strategies to assess the benefits of combining drug and nonspecific inputs to therapy. Three reasons may account for this. First, there is no one to market the evidence about feedback or work therapy. Second, we have reached the point where we believe that only RCTs deliver reliable evidence and every therapy, including music therapy, is forced through these rigid assessment procedures. Third, there is no professional group that stands to make a living out of combining treatments. As a consequence, as Guze warned, the capacity of any one therapist to deliver a full package of care to his patient has become increasingly circumscribed.

Another contemporary myth is that RCTs have helped control the furor therapeuticus. There is little evidence for this. In practice, on the basis of weak evidence of efficacy, a great deal has been done, for example, to detect and treat mild depressions, but little has been done to monitor whether treatment has in fact delivered the desired result. Because the SSRIs have been shown by RCTs to "work," primary care prescribers and others, besieged by the mass of community nervous problems and all but impotent to do much to treat these, have been trapped by the weight of supposed scientific evidence into handing out SSRIs on a massive scale virtually without warnings of possible adverse effects.

The first regulations on drug therapies in 1905 required companies to include a list of ingredients on the labels of their medicines. This reform was adopted in the belief that when consumers were informed of the opiate, cocaine, or 99 percent water content of some medicines they would stop buying. In fact, although the pharmaceutical companies of the time strenuously campaigned against regulation, they quickly turned the situation to their advantage, in some cases printing below the list of ingredients the rider "as approved by the Chemical Bureau." Arguably the 1990s has seen a modern version of the same trick. RCTs, which were developed to evaluate and control therapeutic enthusiasm, have been turned into a method used to justify the mass detection and close to forcible treatment of patients as all but a matter of public policy.

The evidence that companies provide to regulators is now commonly seen as supporting a company's claims, but in fact scientific methods refute rather than confirm. It can be shown that it is not correct to say that chlorpromazine has no beneficial effect on schizophrenia or fluoxetine has no beneficial effect on depression, but this is not equivalent to saying that fluoxetine is good for treating depression or chlorpromazine is good for treating schizophrenia. Historically, RCTs were set up to expose claims, not to produce evidence that can be marketed. Recently negative evidence from RCTs has fulfilled just such a role and has been used to rein in the enthusiasm for post-trauma debriefing, which, linked with the enthusiasm for recovering memories, was fast becoming all but a social movement.[131] Evidence-based medicine can indicate what should not be done. When it is used to tell clinicians what they should be doing, the evidence in question has invariably been produced for a purpose and carries with it a high risk of leading to evidence-biased practice.

Within therapy there is today a culture of the magic bullet. We want treatments to hit targets with specificity. At present the notion of equipping a physician with a range of therapeutic principles to be used judiciously would smack of a recipe to restore clinical arbitrariness. Within the realm of evaluation, we similarly have a range of evaluative methods that can be used judiciously but we appear to want a magic bullet method, which is arguably what we have made of the RCT. RCTs and EBM are functioning as a solution for complexity. This has been a solution with dramatic side effects.

The development of neuroimaging and pharmacogenetics may move us forward. Both of these technologies will put a renewed premium on producing models of diseases, which take into account the fact that particular therapeutic principles can in certain circumstances produce benefits in the treatment of certain syndromes against a background of particular constitutional types and psychosocial settings—a piece of obvious clinical wisdom that has become obscured in this RCT era. Both of these technologies will move us closer to "seeing" the mechanisms that underpin the associations visible in RCTs. Then an era dominated solely by the evidence from RCTs will look far from enlightened.

FIN DE SIÈCLE

One of the features of the rise of psychoanalysis was that a rootless patois of dynamic terms seeped into the popular culture to create a psychobabble. Another feature that is regularly cited was the way that analytic totalitarianism handled failures of patients to get well or of critics to be persuaded of the error of their ways. These were turned around and viewed as indicators of the psychopathology afflicting patients and critics respectively. Walter Reich, commenting on this in 1981, just after the launch of DSM-III, argued that this style was a defense against pessimism which stemmed, at least in part, from America's peculiar needs for solutions to complex problems. He predicted that the same dynamics would shape the evolution of the new biological psychiatry favored by DSM-III.[132]

By the 1990s, the rise of psychopharmacology and biological psychiatry was complete. The chances of a nonneuroscientist becoming a head of a psychiatric department in the United States or Europe were low. The standard textbooks were heavily neuroscientific in their approach. Annual APA meetings now generated millions of dollars, largely from the company-sponsored satellite symposia, of which there were forty in 1999 at approximately $250,000 per symposium. In addition, there were fees for exhibition space, registration fees for several thousand delegates brought to the meeting by pharmaceutical companies, and several million dollars per annum from sales of successive versions of the DSM.

DSM-III had been fiercely resisted in Britain, whose leading authorities had been the key figures behind the *ICD* classification. Michael Shepherd in 1981 dismissed the DSM: "serious students of nosology will continue to use the ICD."[133] But an empire was slipping from British hands. The World Psychiatric Association took as its banner for its 1996 meeting the slogan "One World, One Language." Few people, at least few attendees, thought this language was anything other than biological or neo-Kraepelinian.

The manual had strayed far from Kraepelin, however. After over a century of life the term hebephrenia, which immediately conjured up for most psychiatrists an utterly distinctive disorder, was replaced by disorganized schizophrenia. More bizarre for a manual supposedly following the evidence base was what happened to catatonia in DSM-IIIR, the 1987 revision of DSM-III, and DSM-IV. Work conducted in a variety of settings had shown that far from responding to supposed antipsychotics, this condition responded to benzodiazepines and ECT. This and evidence of catatonia's frequency should have guaranteed it a separate listing as catatonic disorder but it remained catatonic schizophrenia.

Compared with 1900, when Kraepelin and Freud were putting forward the ideas that would shape modern psychiatry, by 2000 there had been a fifteen-fold increase in rates of admission to psychiatric wards. There had also been a three-fold increase in rates of detention for psychiatric disorders. And psychiatric patients afflicted with schizophrenia or manic-depressive disorder, the disorders at the core of psychiatric business, were likely to spend more time in a service bed during their psychiatric illness than they would have done a century ago.[134]

Undaunted by these figures, by the end of the century, psychiatry had moved far beyond the treatment of psychosis. Where once the psychiatric concern had been for symptoms as these reflected diseases, the emphasis was now increasingly on the management of problems by biological means. The extent to which community nervousness stems from social problems rather than diseases is clearly uncertain, but where the best estimates of annual prevalence rates of depressive disease stood at between 50 and 100 per million in 1950, by the mid-1990s they had risen to 100,000 per million for depressive disorders as defined by DSM, with even higher rates for depressive symptoms. These facts caused American opinion leaders, despite a neo-Kraepelinian focus, to start arguing again that the profession faced disaster if it did not pull back to a medical focus and stop offering to solve social ills.[135]

Whereas once blame had been put on families, especially mothers, the 1990s became the decade of blaming the brain.[136] By the end of the decade, the psychobabble was fast being replaced by a newly minted biobabble. Tipper Gore, talking about her problems, told USA Today that "it was definitely a clinical depression, one that I was going to have to have help to overcome. What I learned about it is your brain needs a certain amount of serotonin and when you run out of that, it's like running out of gas."[137] The Guardian, Britain's leading broadsheet, ran a feature entitled "Oh no! We're Not Really Getting More Depressed Are We?" in which a psychologist, Oliver James, pondered whether the British had become a low-serotonin people.[138] Finally, an ever increasing emphasis on long-term treatment with psychotropic agents, along with difficulties with withdrawal from them, inevitably recalls Karl Kraus's quip about analysis becoming the illness it purported to cure. DSM-IV had, however, conveniently made it impossible to define dependence on SSRIs, antipsychotics, or benzodiazepines as a disorder.

The mass treatment of problems with psychotropic drugs could not help running into problems. A rising tide of suicides, homicides, and other distressing deeds committed by patients taking Prozac led Eli Lilly and the APA to adopt a strategy to manage criticism that had been pioneered by analysts: blame the disease, not the drug.[139] On 20 April 1999, two students took firearms into Columbine High School in Littleton, Colorado, and killed 12 students, one staff member, and then themselves. Within days of suggestions surfacing that one of the teenagers had an antidepressant in his bloodstream, the APA website carried a statement from the association's president, Rodrigo Munoz: "Despite a decade of research, there is little valid evidence to prove a causal relationship between the use of anti-depressant medications and destructive behavior. On the other hand, their [sic] is ample evidence that undiagnosed and untreated mental illness exacts a heavy toll on those who suffer from these disorders as well as those around them."[140] All that was missing was a "diagnosis" for the critics of the new establishment.

In 1985, the alumni of the Massachusetts General Hospital's Department of Psychiatry celebrated the fiftieth anniversary of the establishment of the department. At the meeting, Gerald Klerman spoke about Mandel Cohen's role as the originator within psychiatry of the concept of diagnostic criteria.[141] Cohen did not attend. He had been completely detached from the department for the preceding forty years.

In 1999, Cohen was still an unknown to most American psychiatrists. Even Robert Spitzer had never met him. Many of those who had known him did not even know whether he was alive. That year, at the age of ninety-two, Cohen was invited to the annual meeting of the APA in Washington, D.C., where he was honored with a lifetime achievement award. The president that year was a graduate of Washington University in St. Louis, one of the authors of the Feighner diagnostic criteria paper, and he saluted Cohen as the Moses that had led his people through the desert using diagnostic criteria as a guiding star. This was the same Munoz who had gone on record after the Colorado massacre with a "blame the disease not the drug" message.

In a multiply ironic coda to the century, however, Cohen saw DSM-III as a deeply flawed exercise and was concerned to avoid being called its father.[142] The approach that he, Robins, and Guze had pioneered evolved out of their belief that analytic approaches had oversimplified the problems of psychiatry. The strange and complex syndromes that we call manic-depressive disorder, schizophrenia, and multiple personality disorder are poorly understood and are likely to remain a puzzle for decades to come. Operational criteria emerged as a research tool to corral ignorance. They are a specialized tool that helps psychiatrists inch forward in certain areas, not an answer to the problems of complexity. Against this background, and in the face of the challenge managed care poses to psychiatry, professional calls to take a stand on the vast amount of scientific data that now forms the basis for psychiatric practice sound hollow.[143]

One of the peculiar things about the triumph of biological psychiatry has been that although biology is generally viewed as a science of natural variation, in psychiatry it appears to function more as a source of standardization. This gives the lie to the biological specificity that has been such a driver within psychiatry in this century. Even though the hunt for specific treatments for specific diseases has underpinned efforts to understand mechanisms of pathogenesis and drug action, specificity is often just a code for simplicity. Child abuse is a simple answer to the complexities of modern life. But in addition to being a code for simplicity, from the hopes of recovered memory therapists to the investments of shareholders, specificity is also a code for reimbursement.

At the 1956 Conference on the Evaluation of Psychotropic Drugs, Edward Evarts of the NIMH reminded his colleagues that but for an accident of history they would be discussing the use of the new tranquilizing agents for the treatment of dementia paralytica rather than dementia praecox. None of the rating scales, clinical trial methods, or animal models they were proposing to use to move the field forward would have helped them in any way to work out that penicillin rather than chlorpromazine or psychotherapy was the right answer to the problem of dementia paralytica.[144] Now that so many people earn a living out of chlorpromazine or psychotherapy, it is unclear how well we are placed to recognize right answers when they come along.

The neglected response of catatonia to lorazepam or ECT offers a sobering example to anyone who expects science to lead us closer to the truth by the shortest possible route. A superficial reading of this story might suggest the problem is a science corrupted by corporate business. The fact that similar dynamics have affected the field of psychotherapeutics cautions against accepting such an explanation too easily. An epidemic of prescribing of stimulants, antidepressants, and antipsychotics to preteen and even preschool children that cannot be simply be blamed on the marketing efforts of companies or therapists points to even deeper forces at work. It is to this, something closer to a basic force that marketing efforts shape and therapeutic establishments profit from, that I now turn.

8

Democracy

In 1968, in the aftermath of Henry Beecher's article on the lack of informed consent in research, Seymour Kety, among others, was called to testify before Congress at a set of hearings that it is now clear marked the birth of bioethics. Kety was questioned about the prospect that new psychiatric technologies would lead to an ever greater control of human behavior. He responded that "the manipulation of the brain by any of the biological techniques which can be developed in the foreseeable future would involve such drastic invasions of privacy, integrity, and the unalienable rights of the individual that in their application behavioral control would already have been achieved even if the electrodes carried no current and the pill were placebo."[1]

Almost as he spoke, students across the Western world were demonstrating against the behavioral control that the use of chlorpromazine and other drugs represented. The origin of this astonishing divide between Kety and the students lies in the world of Jean-Jacques Rousseau. In his *Confessions*, Rousseau had articulated some of the distinctive aspects of modern experience. The *Confessions*, however, appeared posthumously, and Rousseau spent the final twenty years of his life in retreat from a world that had rejected his major work, *The Social Contract*.[2]

The *Social Contract*, which appeared in 1762, articulated the political vision that lay at the heart of the Enlightenment, a period that that saw the execution of kings, the emergence of atheism, the dethronement of God, the rise of capitalism, and the rise of science. It was a period distinguished by a move away from tradition and from authoritarian, hierarchical, and patriarchal social arrangements in the direction of market-based individualism.

During the eighteenth century there was a growing realization that rulers ruled a people (a demos), not a land, and that democracy of some form would be the new political order. It was this vision that Rousseau articulated. Previously the world order had been one in which individuals occupied a particular place and had certain duties, a place ordained by God, that lay within a hierarchy at the apex of which stood the monarch and the church. Chaos resulted when things or people were out of place. Disease was one of the threats to what was seen as the natural order, and the role of physicians was to cure diseases in order to restore people to their place in that order. Mary Shelley's *Frankenstein* was a powerful parable about the perils of subverting this natural order. In this world, human engineering was the height of hubris.

The achievement of Rousseau and his contemporaries was to articulate a vision of a new order, a new means of government to replace the Will of God, or the natural order. In this new order the mandate for government would come from the governed. This would be an order in which individuals had rights as well as duties and the social arrangements in this new world were perceived as having an arbitrary or accidental quality, one that was open to medical interventions that might potentially enhance an individual's qualities or transform the social order.

There is no sense in which these new views were mystical. They stemmed from hard economic facts and they were paralleled by a growth in statistical thinking. Rulers have always needed to raise money to finance courts and campaigns. Success-fully raising money by issuing annuities and bonds requires knowledge of the people, their numbers and their rates of mortality, so that a rate of return can be offered that will encourage investment but will still prove profitable for the government. The need for knowledge of this sort led European states to begin to collect statistics. These were the first attempts to map the people rather than the land. The figures that resulted laid the basis for the development of the social sciences and epidemiology. The qualitative sciences of man, philosophy, and theology were supplemented with the positive or quantitative sciences of man. A further science, psychology, emerged at the end of nineteenth century, in which figures were used to map the range of aptitudes and attitudes of individuals. The first social scientists and psychologists set up a series of norms for behavior. These norms mapped out deviance and developmental aberrations where once we had seen sin and life's rich variety.

Mapping both the people and individuals like this intersected with the emergence of an understanding of probability.[3] Cultures outside the West had been populous and technically developed. They had explored, conquered, and exploited. So these factors on their own cannot account for the developments of the past two hundred and fifty years in the West. Other cultures had mapped their populations by taking a census. But no other culture had come to grips with the management of uncertainty in the way that Western statisticians did in the eighteenth and nineteenth centuries. The quantification of uncertainty that resulted introduced rulers and their people to the notions of predicting the future and in particular to the idea of predicting future problems and future risks. It introduced a market in futures. With this new market came a need for rulers and citizens to be seen to make some efforts to manage the problems and risks facing the people. This was particularly the case in the newly emerging market democracies, with their rule of the people by the people.

The example of Pascal's wager about God illustrates the shift in thinking. On the basis of a calculus of probabilities, Blaise Pascal, one of the mathematicians who created the new science, offered a radically different reason for believing in God than had ever been offered before. He argued that it still made sense to believe even if the chance was quite small that God existed, because if God did exist the consequences of not believing in him were extremely grave.[4] The new way of thinking created fundamentalism as its mirror image. The new thinking also shows how the government of the self and the people was becoming predicated on a management of future risks.

Managing risks in daily life was also important. This period marks the start of a new form of moral life, one where healthy living became desirable, indeed almost a civic duty, as part of an effort to reduce individual risks. The new thinking put a premium on maintaining health. Suffering became something to be avoided rather than welcomed as a means of storing up benefits in a future life. On a wider front, this new understanding gave rise to a moral movement that transformed health, including mental health.[5]

In this new world, changing social roles were altering the experience and understanding of the self. Fear, as in fear of God, had once been seen as a welcome reaction that helped maintain social order and gave shape to a human life, but now fear was replaced by anxiety, which in contrast was seen as a problem.[6] This process has now gone so far that social theorists can argue that we have moved beyond left and right and beyond class-based societies to risk societies, in which the central goods that are distributed are risks.[7]

Related changes can be seen within medicine. The old humoral therapies, which aimed at a restoration of harmony, were replaced around 1900 by the notion of a magic bullet. Although different from earlier treatments, magic bullets were understood as old-style medical agents that aimed at restoring order by eliminating the disruption caused by disease. Although the magic bullet remains the dominant therapeutic metaphor within medicine, in practice the best-selling medicines are drugs, such as the antihypertensives and lipid-lowering agents, that in contrast to magic bullets are used because they lower future risks rather than because they correct abnormalities. Similarly, antidepressants are prescribed to minimize the risk of suicide. Oral contraceptives and hormone replacement therapy are also tools to manage risks rather than treatments to restore harmony, but in managing certain risks they have contributed to a radical transformation of the social order. Plastic surgery, which began as an effort to return individuals to their former place in the social order, has become cosmetic surgery, a means of advancement in the social order.[8]

The interaction between emerging modernity and psychiatry came with the first confinement of lunatics to asylums. This brought nineteenth-century alienists face to face with aspects of humanity that they had simply been unaware of. As a result, the image of the raving madman began to give way to the image of chronically deluded patients. Among this new group of the partially insane were individuals whose behaviors were bizarre but not characterized by delusions. The deliriously mad and the chronically deluded were abnormal in the sense of laboring under an obvious defect of mind, but these newer groups came much closer to being abnormal in the statistical sense of lying at a distance from some ideal of regulated behavior.

Rousseau in his *Confessions* prefigured one of the new patient groups. There he had portrayed himself as playing different roles and having almost different selves to accommodate each of these roles. In the 1860s, the first cases of multiple personality disorder were noted in the asylums. This group of patients, which grew to include the fuguers and grand hysterics, had memory problems, and this put a premium on the emerging psychological sciences, one of whose domains was the study of memory. Studying memory in this extraordinary patient group rather than studying it, along with reaction times, in healthy volunteers, made psychology dynamic. This matrix of patients and new scientific approaches gave rise in the 1890s to the birth of the psyche and of psychodynamics.[9]

The appearance of psychodynamic psychotherapies, along with aptitude and personality testing, led to a growing involvement of psychology in both therapy and education. Psychology became involved in the governing of selves in the broadest sense of that word.[10] This was not a government by distant rulers but a government by market forces. Clients sought out therapists and parents sought out educational psychologists in an effort to improve their position or that of their children in society. Therapists and educational advisers easily accepted their new roles in formulating policy and guiding democracy. By the middle of the twentieth century it was not uncommon to find articles strongly arguing that if statesmen were analyzed properly world peace might be attainable.

The march of the new sciences reflected a heroic attitude, a belief in progress and a belief that although the old order had been abolished, a new rational order, one that could embrace religion, would arise to command the assent of citizens.[11] From this point of view the discovery of chlorpromazine and the psychotropic drugs that followed it marked one more step on the road to the effective government of the self, and the scientists behind these developments were the successors of the early scientists of the Enlightenment.

But chlorpromazine and its progeny were also drugs. We have a tendency to look at the actors on the historical stage when attempting to make sense of what has happened in history. This bias has been termed the fundamental attributional error.[12] It leads us to minimize the role of factors such as the availability of food or the occurrence of disease, like the Black Death or the smallpox that decimated the Aztecs.[13] Sex, disease, and drugs are among the major impersonal forces shaping the course of history. These three have always posed a challenge to the established order and our responses to them tell us much about individual and social values.[14] It is no coincidence that these three have been associated with the Romantic Movement that arose as a reaction to the rationalism of the Enlightenment.

Drugs have played an obvious role in history as commodities, with compounds such as poppies and cinchona bark traded vigorously. Humoral remedies from Galen on have provided enough business to power markets and underpin the distinctive trade of the apothecary and later the pharmacist.[15] This function continued until the nineteenth century, when the development of a patent medicines market did more than the development of any other set of commodity markets to establish the role of advertising in modern industry and to encourage the development of advertising techniques.[16] But in addition, under a new Romantic influence, from the nineteenth century on, artists celebrated a use of drugs as a means to enhance creativity and escape the constraints of rationality.[17]

Since the emergence of Western awareness of mescaline and related compounds, it has become possible for us to grasp the outlines of other areas in which drugs have influenced society. William James in his *Varieties of Religious Experience* was one of the first to tackle the new issues. He concluded that drug-induced experiences shed light on the nature of and broadly confirmed the validity of mystical experiences.[18] The advent of LSD raised new possibilities, namely that some religious thinking, particularly its mystical components, may have sprung from the taking of hallucinogenic substances. These hypotheses, which at first seemed incredible, have now achieved the status of respectability.[19]

These insights point to an uneasy relationship between drug taking and social order. Although hallucinogen intake seems to have been incorporated into the mainstream of some cultures, a range of other manifestations from the Eleusinian mystery cults in Greece to the witch hunts of the fifteenth and sixteenth centuries have reflected social unease at the potential of drugs to disrupt the social order.[20] Drug-induced states could cause peasants to forget their place in the natural social order. Recognized drugs such as henbane, used by midwives in fifteenth- and sixteenth-century Europe, could lead to such disruptive outcomes, as could unrecognized poisonings with for example ergot, which may have caused the grande peur of 1789 that immediately preceded the French Revolution.

If chlorpromazine was a further step in the enlightened government of the self and society, LSD and other psychotropic agents, which spilled from the very same laboratories and test tubes that produced chlorpromazine, were its mirror image. The threat to the social order that these embodied gave rise to a war aimed at halting the growth of underground movements whose members take drugs such as Ecstasy, phenylethylamines, tryptamines, and ketamine-like compounds that to this day are perceived as a potential source of disorder.[21]

FROM THE ENLIGHTENMENT TO CHLORPROMAZINE

The emergence of chlorpromazine and the struggles to define its place can be understood only against the backdrop of the Enlightenment. Delay's discovery was the discovery of a drug that restored order to the universe—an old-style medical discovery. Laborit, in contrast, discovered that the phenothiazines could cause an indifference that potentially could pose a threat to the social order; for example, within months of their first use these drugs were being blamed for causing taxi drivers to drive through red lights. The differences between the two men might have been a fine distinction if the treatment of a few psychiatric patients within the asylum walls was all that was at issue. But combined with a series of concomitant developments, chlorpromazine—and the cornucopia of new agents with effects on behavior that it gave rise to—led to a deinstitutionalization of psychiatry in a manner that made the differences between Delay and Laborit of concern to all of us.

A Rousseau exposing his genitals today would almost certainly be referred for a psychiatric assessment, and it is precisely the possibility of similar referrals that led to the uprisings of 1968, which also were trying to complete unfinished business left over from the Enlightenment. While God and kings had been dethroned from their former places in the public order of society in the eighteenth and nineteenth centuries, men, the older generation, and certain cultures still held a privileged place. The principles that underpinned the new social contract had not been extended to women, students, and all ethnic groups; their consent to be governed had not been sought. Against this backdrop the issue of whose interests were being served by the new methods of behavioral control, the new methods of government, was a very real one.

The battle over whose interests were being served was fought out against the backdrop of a full-blooded clash between rationalism and romanticism. Until 1960, science was still viewed as our best hope in the face of the perils of nature. The DuPont Chemical Company slogan "Better living through chemistry" was a credo for many. But in 1962, Rachel Carson's *Silent Spring* turned this world upside down. Science and humanity's employment of science became a problem, the answer to which was a retreat to a benevolent nature. Nature, which had so recently seemed red in tooth and claw, became a mother whose life was threatened by many entities, pharmaceutical companies among them. The parallels between the effects of and reactions to mesmerism, which contributed to the French Revolution and the rise of Romanticism, and those of LSD in the 1960s remain uncanny.[22]

No one ever assesses the impact of the development of psychodynamics in terms of whether Freud's treatment actually produced responses in patients. It is clear that the more important effects were on the culture in which we live. When it comes to chlorpromazine, however, all efforts at assessment to date have focused almost solely on trying to decide whether it contributed to an emptying of the mental hospitals or not. Whether it did or not is arguably as irrelevant to chlorpromazine's impact on modern civilization as efforts to determine whether Freud's patients got better or not. The social upheavals of the late 1960s coincided with a break in how we understand ourselves as great as the changes at the end of the nineteenth century that led to the birth of psychodynamics. In the 1960s a new biomedical self was being born, entailing a significant series of consequences for how we understand and indeed experience our selves. These consequences affect three domains: one domain involves changes in the populations being treated, a second concerns the changes in the nature of the therapeutic act, and a third concerns the issue of alienation.

One Flew over the Cuckoo's Nest

For some psychoses and for the delirious states that were the original form of madness, chlorpromazine was close to a penicillin of the mind. It and its successors produced an awakening from inaccessibility and a restoration to normality, often even when given in astonishingly low doses.

As regards the closure of the asylums, many in fact did close. This closure can mislead when it comes to assessing the larger impact of chlorpromazine, because it is unclear how much hospital closures were due to either the policies of political planners or the treatments of psychiatrists. In the United States, for example, there was a clear financial incentive to close mental hospitals. The hospitals were funded by the states. Their closure and the transfer of care to the community transferred the financial onus to the federal budget.[23]

In many other countries, the closures were almost accidental. In Britain a succession of asylum scandals during the 1960s had little effect even when they appeared on the front page of newspapers and led to official inquiries.[24] Finally, in 1967, a complaint that patients were being brutalized at Ely, a hospital for the mentally handicapped in Cardiff, precipitated action.[25] Probably this scandal led to action because it occurred during a brief time when the minister for health, Richard Crossman, was in favor of a change. Crossman could justify his decision to accelerate asylum closure on the basis of policy. Without the policy strand, the scandals would have had no effect; but without the appropriate minister, the policy strand alone would have produced little change, and without the scandal the semidormant policy of closing mental hospitals might well not have been activated.

But focusing on whether chlorpromazine cured any psychoses or emptied asylums completely misses the larger picture, even in countries such as Japan, where the asylum population grew dramatically during the chlorpromazine era. The important issues lie in the new realm of behavioral control that chlorpromazine opened up and the new mapping of social problems for which it laid the basis.

As health improved in the asylums and tuberculosis and general paralysis of the insane declined in the twentieth century, psychiatrists reconceptualized their mission as one of treating chronically psychotic patients, relatively unaware of a growing accumulation of other disorders in their domain. By the 1960s, with the deinstitutionalization that came about as a consequence of psychoanalysis, prescription-only status, and the new psychotropic drugs, psychiatry had become a discipline that primarily managed neuroses and personality disorders in community settings rather than psychoses in asylum settings.[26]

Although patients with personality disorders had not been released from asylums to create new problems of violence in the community, the changing circumstances led communities to map the different species of madness, the different forms of unacceptable behavior, in their midst. This was a mapping in which the media increasingly played an increasing part. The classic representations of madness in the nineteenth and early twentieth centuries had been the raving or the delusionally mad, but by the late twentieth century these had transmuted into psychopaths, pedophiles, and drug abusers.[27]

Whether physicians liked it or not, by the 1990s aggression, violence, and their management were being redefined as medical issues.[28] The slow trickle of patients with personality disorders into mental hospitals during the 1930s had led during the 1960s to the referral to asylums of ever larger numbers of young men and women with such disorders. Many were put on depot medication. Whereas the advertisements for antipsychotics in psychiatric journals in the 1950s and 1960s had portrayed the mute inaccessibility of untreated psychosis and its response to treatment, advertisements for the same drugs in the 1970s and 1980s showed threatened violence and antisocial behavior on the part of young males and females and were pitched explicitly as agents to control the behavior of patients with personality disorders.

Because these patients were given antipsychotics, many of them would have been diagnosed as schizophrenic. Treating them with antipsychotics may have contained a certain amount of social disruption. But some lives were undoubtedly blighted by the infliction of a drug-induced demotivation that interfered with the ability to obtain or hold down a job. Some patients surely exhibited akathisia-induced violence, while others displayed drug-induced tardive dyskinesia. But in the process everyone learned that the neuroleptics were reliably able to control behavior in a way that sedatives could not. This was even true of clozapine, an agent that later won favor because it was apparently not a camisole chimique. Although it does not immobilize people in the same way as neuroleptics do, clozapine has marked "serenic" effects. It makes people docile. This characteristic of the drug led to its widespread use in Europe in aggressive populations long before its resurrection in the 1990s.[29]

The 1990s saw a growing public demand for psychiatric involvement in the management of personality disorders. Psychiatric associations protested vigorously that their job was to treat mental illness and not personality disorders or violence. But if shown the typical case history of a psychopath and a schizophrenic and asked who was the madder, most laypeople would plump for the psychopath. Besides, notwithstanding the protests of psychiatrists, by the 1990s up to 40 percent of hospital cases involved personality problems rather than the old-style schizophrenic or

manic-depressive disorders.[30] More to the point, personality disorders, although not cured by neuroleptics, could be contained by
them. There was often public and political incomprehension of
psychiatrists' efforts to wash their hands of these "untreatable"
conditions.

During the last half of the century, forensic psychiatry was
born. Between 1967 and the end of the century, for example, the
number of forensic psychiatrists in Britain increased 250-fold,
driven in part by a series of high-profile psychiatric scandals in the
community—the Ely Hospital story turned out. These "scare in
the community" stories ranged from catalogues of the homeless-
ness and vulnerability of the truly psychotic to tales of pedophiles
or other dangerous patients being released without monitoring
into community settings. Like the scandal at Ely, these scandals in
turn led to the awakening of a variety of dormant policies in many
countries, with the resultant mushrooming of new facilities and
new confinement in hospitals of "newly" insane groups. The interface between psychiatry and government can be seen clearly
here: the alternative to confinement in mental hospitals has been
imprisonment and potentially capital punishment since the biology that underpins personality disorders is increasingly likely to
be viewed as a risk factor for future offending rather than as an
exculpatory factor.[31]

Many of these new patients are as untreatable as the delusionally insane were in the 1850s, but risk management rather than
cure has become the order of the day and antipsychotic drugs can
certainly contribute in this regard. These capacities for behavioral control will persist even if a new psycho-penicillin for psychoses unresponsive to chlorpromazine, such as hebephrenia, is
discovered.

Two conferences exemplify the changing scene. One was the
1967 Dorado Beach conference on genetics organized by Seymour Kety; this brought genetics and indeed biology back into
psychiatry (see Chapter 5). The second, organized by David

Wasserman, aimed to bring together key participants in a debate about the biology and management of aggression and urban violence.[32] Initially scheduled to be held at the NIMH in 1992, it was cancelled because of political pressure and then rescheduled to be held at the University of Maryland, and then finally held in eastern Maryland in October 1995. Some of the Dorado Beach participants such as Irving Gottesman were there.[33]

The meeting was disrupted by supporters of Leon Kamin and Richard Lewontin, critics of the new genetics, and by Peter Breggin, the most vocal anti-psychopharmacologist of the day. The protesters heavily influenced the media's portrayal of the meeting, warning about the chemical straitjacketing that a new behavioral genetics would supposedly give rise to. The science underpinning the genetic link to violence did not get a public hearing on that day, but the meeting nevertheless signaled a transition to a new era in which questions concerning the biology of aggression and violence had become respectable.[34]

The 1990s also saw the growth of the biologization of substance abuse, with widespread efforts throughout the West to treat it as a health problem rather than a criminal matter.[35] By the 1990s, the triumph of Alcoholics Anonymous over Antabuse in the early 1950s was forgotten as a series of new agents became available, such as naloxone and acamprosate, that were aimed at rationally engineering a reduction in craving and a control of addictive processes. A scientific establishment that had once emphasized the behavioral underpinnings of addiction switched to attempting to understand the molecular basis of the risk for addiction. The argument was that the addictions are diseases like any other, because they set up changes in brain pathways that endure long after an individual stops taking the substance in question.[36] The extraordinary aspect of this switch is the lack of a logical basis within the pharmacology of the drugs themselves to differentiate between good and bad drugs—between cocaine and methylphenidate or between alcohol and the antipsychotics—in terms of enduring post-discontinuation brain changes. What is happening can only be understood in terms of the post-1968 settlements within psychiatry (see Chapter 4).

The Norms of Behavior

By the end of the 1990s, the involvement of psychiatry in the control of behavior through medication extended well beyond the management of people with personality disorders. In the form of a mental health industry rather than a mental illness service, efforts to control behavior were aimed at the quarter to a third or perhaps even more of the population who had depressive symptoms or distress of one sort or another. These new patients were unlike patients with personality disorders because given the large number of them they simply could not be abnormal in the sense of being outside the normal range for personality variations or nervousness. But critically, as with the treatment of personality disorders, treatment of these groups was increasingly driven by a concern for enforcing behavioral norms that was new.

One of the major cultural phenomena of the 1990s was the rising use of Ritalin and SSRIs, such as Prozac, in treating younger and younger children.[37] This was front-page news.[38] And so were children who were acting violently and making schools ungovernable. The psychiatric treatment of children with drugs had until the 1990s been all but taboo, possibly a legacy of the psychodynamic hegemony in psychiatry. This taboo made it difficult for children severely afflicted with OCD, for instance, to receive drug treatment. Clearly some change was to be welcomed, but mass treatment on the scale that developed by the mid-1990s indicates a profound cultural shift. Extensive treatment of preschool children with psychotropic drugs cannot easily be viewed as the treatment of disease states as these have traditionally been understood. The media understood this, and it was common to read that parents and schools were just opting for a quick fix for behaviors that fell outside the norm. But why the change in the 1990s? Children had presumably always varied and Ritalin had been available since 1954. The reason almost certainly lies in a technical development that came into psychiatry with chlorpromazine.

Whereas the nineteenth-century mapping of new domains was largely qualitative (descriptive), twentieth-century mapping was quantitative. The quantitative mapping of IQ and other psychological functions powerfully introduced the notion of a norm and of deviations from that norm into considerations of behavior, giving rise in the process to new concepts, such as that of a personality disorder. Whereas qualitative approaches had targeted a limited number of patients, statistical approaches to psychological tests led scientists to claim that they could extrapolate from small samples to the population at large. All of a sudden large groups of people found out that they were abnormal. This new mapping of individuals quickly filtered through to the institutional level, initiating the establishment of child guidance clinics and the involvement of scientists in legal and educational forums, where their brief was to reduce future risks by adjusting outliers to a set of norms.[39]

Chlorpromazine drove forward a comparable mapping later in the century because it came complete with a set of evaluative methods such as the randomized controlled trial, which it shared with the rest of medicine, and a set of associated technologies such as rating scales and operational criteria that were distinctive to psychiatry. Just as the development of IQ scales led to an inappropriate reification of notions of intelligence,[40] the new evaluation technologies for psychotropic drugs have led to comparable problems. Evidence from randomized trials is not now interpreted as a demonstration that certain treatments can be shown to do something; it is interpreted instead as a set of results that can generalize to whole populations.

Underpinning the use of rating scales is a process of numericization. This numericization, however, conceals a problem. In the case of penicillin being used to treat general paralysis of the insane, RCTs and numericization are simply not needed. The use of and dependence on RCTs in modern psychiatry stems from the fact that the effects of the available treatments on many of the conditions for which they are being prescribed are nothing remotely like the effects of penicillin on GPI or indeed the effects of chlorpromazine or haloperidol on some psychoses and delirious states. This use of evaluative methods to quantify small effects is a specialized one that commonly obscures how the effects are being brought about. It does not therefore produce the same clinical outcome obtained when a clinician witnesses the relief of pain by an opiate or a bacterial culture shrink in a Petri dish. If the use of rating scales and other protocols had remained confined to the world of clinical trials, there would be little problem. Increasingly, however, in the 1980s and 1990s, clinical freedom became constrained by algorithms, and practitioners were encouraged to use instruments such as the Hamilton Depression Rating Scale (HDRS) in their daily practice. Far from these epitomizing a "scientific" approach to psychiatry, however, these new practices enjoin clinicians to fly blind or to immerse themselves in a virtual world. The behavior of clinicians is now progressively less likely to be based on knowledge derived from direct clinical encounters.

But some did recognize the limits of these practices. Jonathan Cole, who was influential in establishing the use of RCTs in psychiatry, saw their usefulness as limited. Austin Bradford Hill, commonly viewed as the father of the clinical trial, was clear that RCTs were a useful evaluative method that should be employed more than they had been before the mid-1960s. But he was also certain that if RCTs ever became the only method of assessing treatments the pendulum would not only have swung too far, but would have come off its hook.[41] Max Hamilton never used his own scale in clinical practice. Commenting on the impact of the new way of doing things, he noted that "it may be that we are witnessing a change as revolutionary as was the introduction of standardization and mass production in manufacture. Both have their positive and negative sides."[42]

Few if any of the clinicians now using these scales have any feel for the extraordinary implications of the unthinking use of such a simple checklist. A generation of older, analytically trained psychiatrists could feel the change in the "transference" relationships between them and their patients induced by psychotropic drugs. This led to discoveries such as the effect of antidepressants on OCD.[43] But later generations of clinicians have found it increasingly difficult to stand outside technologies such as the HDRS or the randomized controlled trial.

As a consequence, when minimal changes in behavior get "demonstrated" in clinical trials where children are given an SSRI, the clinicians have no basis from which to argue with the findings. In such circumstances, how can the public not respond, even when the direction of progress involves smashing through previous taboos on giving psychotropic drugs to children? The new figures—I use figures in contrast to knowledge—set up a market. The treatment option seems to offer the possibility of a better future for any child who according to checklists administered by teachers now falls outside some norm. If there is no intervention likely to make a difference, there is little harm, but when there are claims for some interventions, what parent can resist the possibility of reducing future difficulties for his or her child? Where is the evidence indicating that it would be wise to resist? If there were such evidence, who would market it?

This new form of behavioral control does not come from an authoritarian source but rather is driven by the market. This is the market force that underpins the efforts of pharmaceutical companies to develop their products, that puts wind in their sails. I have argued elsewhere that the market-development efforts of pharmaceutical corporations drive the psychiatric agenda far more than most people realize[44] and will amplify this point later in the chapter, but the mass administration of psychotropic drugs to children points to other forces, for the simple reason that pharmaceutical corporations have not marketed their drugs for children. The use of these drugs in children is furthermore not an old-style medical treatment of disease; it stems rather from a particular orientation to future risks and involves something much broader than medicine as it has traditionally been understood.

The Dynamics of Alienation

The emergence of both psychodynamics and psychopharmacology has given rise to much talk of alienation. It is not the aim of this book to analyze whether we are more or less alienated from some true nature we may possess. But talk of alienation is a marker for changes and putting the fact of that talk on the historical record and grappling with what the changes are is part of the purpose of this book.

An important facet of the discovery of the antipsychotics, which stemmed from research on reserpine, was the discovery of the functional importance of brain neurotransmitters such as norepinephrine, serotonin, and dopamine. The discovery of some of the mechanisms of actions of these drugs made it possible to produce variations on the original drugs. It also enabled researchers to describe some of the steps of drug development as rational and even to portray the entire process of drug development as rational.

Of greater importance though was the new vision of a particulate brain that slowly, over the course of twenty-five years, transformed our understanding of ourselves. Where before some sort of indivisible ghost had hovered in the cerebral machinery, we now came to understand our brains and ourselves as made of bits. This transformation was brought to a head by the marketing of Prozac. With Prozac, an understanding of ourselves as neurobiological entered popular consciousness. This was both articulated by and reflected in the success of Peter Kramer's *Listening to Prozac*, which in 1993 became an international bestseller, one of the few books dealing with psychiatry to do so since those of Freud and Jung.[45] It established a genre of psychobiological books, dealing with depression, ADHD, or other biomedical disorders of the self. Success on this scale suggests a significant shift in the tectonic plates of medical, psychiatric, and psychological culture. It helped set up a biobabble that had direct parallels with the psychobabble that had earlier stemmed from psychoanalysis.

Kramer's book introduced the notion of cosmetic psycho-pharmacology, an arresting juxtaposition of terms that immediately conjured up ethical and philosophical dilemmas. For many there was a disturbing sense that in some way alienation and spirituality had become grist for the medical and psychiatric mill and that viewing the unhappiness that stems from alienation as a psychiatric disorder was like thinking about the Eucharist in dietary terms.[46] The subsequent launch of paroxetine (Paxil) as an anti-shyness drug did nothing to allay these worries.

Far from being new, these concerns about the encroachment of therapies like Prozac on the "spiritual" domains of life are a re-play of the response of organized religion to the emergence of psychodynamic psychotherapies. With a long tradition behind them of awareness of a need to discern between good and bad spirits or impulses, the established religious orders of all faiths were among the first to employ dynamic therapists to sort out the wheat from the chaff. They did so while at the same time protesting, often vigorously, against the claims of the new therapies to map out the true wellsprings of human motivation. Along with the use of hypnosis, the practice of psychoanalysis was out of bounds to Catholics, for example, until the late 1950s. These bans were enforceable in small European countries such as Ireland but were quietly shelved in the face of an inability to enforce them in the pluralistic United States.

An awareness that dynamic approaches may liberate in some cases provoked anxiety that there might be efforts to reduce the problem of what all sides came to call alienation to a matter of psychodynamics. What might be gained in some areas would lead to losses in others. This insight was one that the religions shared with atheistic philosophers of Marxist persuasion, such as Herbert

Marcuse and others of the Frankfurt School who prominently argued during the 1960s that psychotherapy as it had evolved was a force for alienation rather than liberation.

Between 1945 and 1980, there was an expansion in the numbers of those seeking psychiatric therapy from 1 percent of the population, of whom the majority were treated as in-patients, to over 10 percent of the population, with most being seen in office practices.[47] These figures indicate that turn-of-the-century religious hostility to Freud had been based on a concern that his message that alienation was a matter of psychological adjustment rather than spiritual concern might end up being generally accepted. By the 1960s, however, Herbert Marcuse was taking aim at a widely entrenched public reality that had so changed the terms of the debate about alienation that many could not see any more how analysis could possibly alienate anyone from his or her true self.

The interplay between psychotropic drugs, the biologization of identity, and alienation sets up a similar set of conflicts regarding alienation. The possible ethical issues involved in the mass management of community nervousness with drugs began to be aired in debates about the benzodiazepines in the 1960s and 1970s. These debates gave rise to the notion of pharmacological Calvinism.[48] As framed by Gerald Klerman, this notion referred to the fact that treatments which made the taker feel good, without hard work being required, are commonly perceived to be morally bad and are likely to be accompanied by some form of secular retribution. In line with this, the histories of treatments in this domain typically have a moral tone as they chart a lineage of fashions from the opiates through the bromides, the barbiturates, the benzodiazepines, and now the SSRIs; initial medical enthusiasm for a quick fix is portrayed as ultimately leading to horror stories as successive generations become slaves to yesterday's miracles.

Chlorpromazine made Valium and Prozac inevitable and thereby brought the biology of alienation and spirituality into the health domain. Health is now an arena of obvious common interest but it has only become so astonishingly recently. Before the 1960s, governments did not have departments of health. The media did not cover health issues. The appearance of the health page in newspapers and later the emergence of health issues as front-page news owes a considerable amount to the controversies surrounding the widespread use of and dependence on the benzodiazepine tranquilizers.[49]

History is made when events change our understanding of ourselves, and a good indicator of the capacity of events to do this is whether they appear as lead stories in the print or televisual media. Whereas once politicians, wars, or natural events defined historical epochs, science and technology have increasingly become the arena in which history is created. New drugs and new events, such as the cloning of Dolly the sheep, create older sets of meanings, the world as it was before Dolly, or before chlorpromazine, Prozac, Valium, or Viagra. And as this list suggests, developments in genetics and psychiatry have a particular power to seize the public imagination. We seem to be moving from a theocracy through democracy to a sanitocracy. The vigor of the debates over DSM-III indicates that a new biomedical self had been born, and that how this self was defined and how its discontents were legitimated were matters of widespread importance.

It would be a mistake in any consideration of questions of alienation to see the new psychotropic drugs simply as forces for alienation. One of the consequences of the events of 1968 is that with the rise of feminism we have come to realize how much our attitudes and opportunities have been engendered, as well as how much these may be influenced by class and racial factors. Philosophers and historians have tackled issues of class from the nineteenth century on, but it took the rise of feminism in the 1960s to put biology on their agenda. The impact of this new perspective on historians has been enormous, with new disciplines emerging aimed, for instance, at establishing the role infectious diseases have played in history.[50]

Few would deny that the oral contraceptive has played a part in transforming relations between the sexes from the 1960s on and has had a huge impact on history as a consequence. But from many religious and ethical perspectives, the use of both oral contraceptives and hormone replacement therapy can be seen as profoundly alienating. Although once this alienation would have been keenly felt by wide sections of the population, it now needs a considerable effort of historical reconstruction to recapture a mind-set that can view the use of these agents as just as shocking as the idea of a heart transplant. A managing of the future risk of eternal damnation has been replaced by a managing of the much more immediate risk to a woman's future well-being of a pregnancy.

Beyond biological differences between the sexes, there lie differences in temperament, differences between introverts and extraverts, for instance. There is considerable evidence that such differences have a biological basis. Jerome Kagan has argued cogently for a recognition of the role of temperamental inputs to culture, even proposing that many of the world's major religions owe their distinctive features in part to the biology of those races that gave rise to them.[51] And it seems likely that a majority of philosophers and ethicists in Western cultures have been introverts. In these cultures, the brooding and melancholic Satan of Milton's *Paradise Lost* often seems a more substantial and heroic figure than God. How much has this cast of mind biased our ethical and philosophical systems? What would some of these figures have thought of the world if they had been made more sanguine by Prozac?

The interface between a pharmacological management of temperament of this kind and morality poses a set of interesting questions. On a practical level, society and medicine have been through this debate with the development of cosmetic surgery.[52] We appear to have plumped for some version of the concept of Moral Luck when handling the issues.[53] In brief, it is obvious that certain individuals possess benefits and resources that others do not have. It is also reasonably obvious that others are likely to attribute better moral qualities to an individual with a sunny and winning temperament than to someone with an irritable and obsessional personality. What is less obvious is that these attributions may in turn contribute significantly to, or all but determine, the morality of an individual's behaviors. Assessments of the morality of an individual's behaviors may therefore need to take into account the head start that some people have.

Now, take an individual in a stressful work environment. Should she struggle to change the environment? Many would argue she should, in part because some people do. Aside from the fact that this is likely to be a romantic assessment, it needs to be pointed out that changing such an environment will be easier for people who are less sensitive to interpersonal nuances than others. These fortunate individuals may not get this way by virtue of morally praiseworthy character building; they are commonly this way by virtue of their genes. The issues are the same as those facing subjects trying to hold onto work in a marketplace that rewards the physically attractive. Physical attractiveness does not derive from personal effort. But when the cosmetic means to enhance attractiveness become reliably available, the history of cosmetic surgery points strongly to the likelihood that these means will be eagerly embraced.

Are people likely to be alienated by such cosmetic interventions? Cosmetic surgery once was a symbol of alienation. Now, the growing acceptance of cosmetic procedures demonstrates just how potently markets can define the meaning of our experiences. That being the case, it is extremely important that we know what drug companies are up to and that we understand the consequences of the regulatory arrangements put in place to manage the production and use of drugs. As recently as the 1990s, the regulation of drugs was viewed as an industrial matter, differing little from the process of regulating and labeling foodstuffs, but it is now clear that much more fundamental issues are at stake—at least within psychiatry.

Rousseau was one of the philosophers who created the Enlightenment, but he stood at one remove from the main group, which included Voltaire, Diderot, and others. Another was Julien Offray de La Mettrie, who ended up as shunned as Rousseau and even more vilified as a proponent of atheism and materialism. But just as much as Rousseau, La Mettrie anticipated the outlines of the world into which we are now moving. In particular, he envisioned philosophical speculation withering once it became possible to intervene effectively at the biological level to change human behavior.[54] At this point, physicians would replace philosophers as the arbiters of human ethics. In 1750, his vision proved too extreme even for the set of philosophers who had done so much to create a favorable atmosphere for the development of both modern psychological attitudes and modern political philosophies.

A Loss of Equilibrium

The changing interplay between health, behavioral norms, behavioral control, and alienation during the course of the last century can be illustrated with a brief outline of the history of the eating disorders. Syndromes in which people, most commonly women, have starved themselves or eaten abnormally have been documented for centuries.[55] Before the Enlightenment, only saints and freaks starved themselves. For the most part, these starvations differed clearly from the modern syndrome of anorexia nervosa, which is conventionally seen as having begun its existence in the early 1870s. Descriptions by Charles Laségue and William Gull in 1873 are cited.[56]

Although several earlier descriptions of anorexia nervosa have since been noted, particularly those of Richard Morton in 1864, at the very least the descriptions by Gull and Laségue reflect an increase in frequency of the condition in the 1870s. Since then the syndrome has increased markedly in frequency, first in the 1920s and again in the 1960s, when new variants such as bulimia nervosa emerged.[57] These increases have given rise to a great number of theories aimed at accounting for both the nature of the eating disorder syndromes and the reasons for their increase. These theories have for the most part involved almost exclusively biological, psychological, or sociocultural views.

The first perspective to emerge was a purely clinical one, where the concern was to establish what family of disorders anorexia nervosa ultimately belongs to. Pierre Janet initiated this line of thought in 1903 by distinguishing between obsessional and hysterical types of anorexia nervosa.[58] The responsiveness of eating disorders to SSRIs, demonstrated in the 1990s, was seen as support for the position that there is an obsessive component to these disorders.

A biological perspective emerged early with the work of Morris Simmonds, who in 1914 proposed an endocrine input to syndromes involving anorexia. Subsequent work, however, distinguished endocrine-induced anorexia of the type outlined by Simmonds from anorexia nervosa of supposedly psychological origin.[59] There was a return of biological thinking about anorexia nervosa in the late 1980s, when all of psychiatry went biological, with a number of groups demonstrating that dieting can produce neurobiological changes, raising the possibility that the process could become self-sustaining.[60]

This biological turn seriously challenged the psychodynamic views that had become dominant during the 1950s and 1960s. In the 1950s, for instance, Joseph Waller interpreted anorexia nervosa as evidence of a rejection of a pregnancy wish. Others interpreted it as involving oral sadistic wishes and a reaction formation against incorporation wishes. Hilde Bruch focused on conflicts within the family between daughter and mother.[61] These psychodynamic views got the standard 1990s update when a possible contribution from childhood sexual abuse was noted.[62]

The emergence of bulimia nervosa and the explosion in the frequency of the eating disorders during the 1960s and 1970s de-emphasized intra-psychic theories and encouraged the development of theories that took into account the larger social and cultural picture. David Garner and Paul Garfinkel among others pointed to the role of sociocultural factors in shaping the syndrome, noting that dissatisfaction with body shape has become endemic to women in Western culture and that the tendency to diet consequent on this may trigger a vulnerability to eating disorders.[63] Such formulations focused attention on the role of women in Western societies, since for the greater part of the twentieth century the eating disorders appeared to be confined largely to Western societies.[64] This perception gave rise to arguments that the eating disorders reveal a form of contemporary control over the female body and that psychiatry as a Western discipline institutionalizes a mind over body ideology which is part of that control.[65] The Western psychiatric approach is commonly held to neglect the meaning of eating-related experiences in other cultures.[66] Where eating disorders have been found in nonindustrialized, non-Western societies, they have typically occurred among the daughters of a Westernized elite.[67] These perceptions fed directly into the powerful feminist movement of the latter part of the century.[68]

This brief overview of theories about the eating disorders suggests that a number of influences play a part in the generation of these syndromes. Fashion, pressures on women, whether overt or internalized, and what used to be termed neurotic difficulties as well as biological factors triggered by an initial fasting may all play a role in establishing and shaping the syndrome. The theories outlined above, however, have generally been mutually exclusive. Moreover, it is not clear that any one theory can explain the epidemiology of these disorders, their appearance in certain cultures at certain times, and their later transformation into syndromal variants. Nor is it clear that any one theory points to a unique factor that can stabilize these syndromes.

All theories to date, however, have neglected a development that occurred in parallel with the eating disorders. The first weighing scales for human beings began to appear in the 1870s.[69]

Their use in medical and other settings led to data which persuaded the insurance industry for the first time that obesity, which had formerly been seen as a sign of health, was actually a risk factor for future ill-health. This understanding led to increasing campaigns by insurers and physicians in which they extolled the virtues of thinness. It led to the establishment of norms for body weight and shape—one more set of norms to sit alongside the many different sets of norms that were emerging in the West at the time. The weighing scales also made it possible to know exactly whether a regime aimed at increasing or reducing weight was having the desired effect.

The 1920s saw the emergence of the first weighing scales that could be bought and placed in the home. These were too bulky and cumbersome to be found widely in homes but they often were placed in drug stores and other retail spaces. After World War II and particularly in the 1960s, small portable weighing scales appeared that could be placed discreetly in the bathroom. It became possible for most houses to have such a scale. The growth in the weighing scale industry in fact parallels the growth in the frequency of anorexia nervosa.[70] The weighing scale factor also neatly accounts for the apparent cultural distribution of the syndrome such that it appears first in Western settings and subsequently migrates to non-Western settings, being found first of all among wealthier classes. It also helps explain why immigrants to Western countries develop the syndrome so rapidly.

The power of the weighing scale as a behavioral reinforcer and as a feedback device should not be underestimated. It plays a role similar to that of the stopwatch in track events. But the really important aspect of the story is that, notwithstanding the fact that eating disorders may occur in the blind,[71] it is all but impossible to see how such disorders could mushroom to affect up to 30 percent of the population in the absence of weighing scales.

There are a several lessons to draw from this history. If it is conceded that the weighing scale is an important contributing factor to anorexia nervosa, this offers possibilities to marry biological, social, and psychological inputs in a way that is not possible without this kind of "behavior driver." Other factors are still needed to explain why this syndrome primarily affects women rather than men, and these may involve a mixture of social, biological, and psychodynamic factors. But without the weighing scale to organize these factors, it is hard to see how the disorder could have reached epidemic proportions in the West.

The eating disorder story points to the role of norms, and our responses to them, as a new factor in human behavior. It provides a dramatic metaphor for the problems of maintaining equilibrium once we establish a set of norms and step on the balance. It illustrates how certain feedbacks, which offer seductive possibilities of control, can become imperious and how subjects may lose the ability to contextualize these inputs into the rest of their lives.

Comparable difficulties have stemmed from our increasing capacities to measure environmental radiation and chemical pollution. As we develop the ability to detect these hazards and establish norms for appropriate ranges for them, our difficulties with these hazards seem to increase rather than diminish. These difficulties suggest that we may face further problems as our capacities to monitor brain functioning increase. These new capacities will set up further sets of norms and in the process will risk creating a large market for the use of physical interventions to keep individuals within norms.

The neuroses we end up with recall the experimental neuroses induced in animals by Jules Masserman in the 1940s and 1950s. In some of these studies, Masserman conditioned animals to expect rewards for correctly distinguishing between circles and ellipses. As the distinctions were made increasingly fine, the animals became unable to discriminate between the shapes and became neurotic.[72]

The problem is like our attempts to map economies. It is easy to gather statistics from industry, especially for bulk items such as cars and electronic goods, and from those numbers to construct the Gross National Product. But figures like these leave out the numbers of trees cut down and changes in the quality of life of a nation's inhabitants. These other domains could be brought into the marketplace but are not at present. In the meantime the figures that are available drive change, although in many cases the wisdom of those changes may be far from proven. The increasing application of a similar dynamic to the health domain suggests an updating of the notion that he who controls the means of production controls consciousness to a twenty-first-century version in which he who controls the production of key sets of figures controls consciousness.

PSYCHOTROPIC DIALECTICS

The developments there have been in the biological sciences and our increasing capacities to influence our biology should not stand in opposition to the development of psychology or sociology. Quite the contrary. Just as the discovery of germs helped explain many of the findings of the first socio-epidemiological surveys and led to a new flowering of epidemiology, so also the new genetics will inform the sociological and psychological investigation of many things, including religious and political beliefs. Brain imaging will make it clear that our brains are as social as they are biological and that being biological means having social arrangements stamped into our neuroendocrine systems.

Clearly, however, we are not faced with a static picture with social, psychological, and biological components; rather we are being driven forward in a dynamic process. This is a process that has the power to suck the cultural air out of our lungs and replace it with a new oxygen that can change our experience of ourselves as reliably as a slight rise in body temperature or a miniscule dose of dust containing LSD. In recent decades, social frameworks that held up for our emulation the values of sanctity, honor, and loyalty have been replaced by others that have cast authenticity in different terms, as the forces that swirled around Jean Delay illustrated so graphically.

It is a matter of personal importance for all of us then to come grips with the forces shaping psychopharmacology, forces that have led to a blurring of the distinction between the scientific laboratory and the factory. This is an issue that the chlorpromazine story illustrates perfectly. The antipsychotic story begins with the production of synthetic dyes, which led to the establishment of chemical companies. The current thinking is that there is little or no scientific knowledge about the latest generation of compounds other that what is provided by pharmaceutical companies. From 1950 to 1980, there was a certain amount of independent scientific information about the antipsychotics. This has been lost as part of what we can term the post-1960s settlement in society and the emergence of Big Science.

Although in the years since the 1960s there have been significant advances in completing the Enlightenment project of enlisting all the component groups of society in government, the period has also seen the growth of corporate power and governance, or what some have termed corporatism.[73] John Kenneth Galbraith referred to the emergence of a new industrial state, where corporations create markets for what they can provide rather than produce goods for which there is a demand.[74] Whether corporatism is the correct term or not for the post-1960s developments, the antipsychotic story shows very clearly that the clash of a rationalist psychiatry with a romantic antipsychiatry did not lead to the triumph of either but rather led to the takeover of both by a psycho-pharmaceutical complex. The dialectics governing the development of this complex can be seen in the careers of the best-known psychotropic drugs, in particular the antidepressants.

The introduction of chlorpromazine in 1952 marked a serendipitous breakthrough in the management of severe mental disorders. Within a few years its use, just like that of penicillin before it, had crossed frontiers and continents, regardless of ideological divides, demonstrating vividly how effective techniques propagate themselves in a way that acclaimed ideas, even in this information age, do not. Chlorpromazine crossed frontiers as quickly as few things except new weapons do. It was an engine of war.

The career of the antidepressants, introduced a few years later was strikingly different. When clinicians and pharmaceutical company executives surveyed the 1950s landscape, they could see no compelling rationale for "antidepressants."[75] The idea of an antidepressant was not a natural one that existed before this group of drugs was developed (see Chapter 2). The antipsychotics or ECT could be expected to ameliorate many of the most severe affective disorders. For treatment of the milder disorders, which merged into everyday misery, the new antidepressants could not compete with the minor tranquilizers. Clinicians used the antidepressants but did so sparingly—until the problem of dependence on benzodiazepines emerged in the early 1980s.[76]

Whereas the use of the antipsychotics, especially in depot form, could be extended to patients other than those who clearly showed a therapeutic response to treatment, the use of the antidepressants was far more constrained. With the antipsychotics behavioral control could be enforced through the barrel of a depot needle. In contrast the antidepressants, although they opened up the possibility of making some difference for an increasing number of people, were used only when clinicians and consumers could be persuaded that people needed this difference in their lives—persuaded, it could be cynically said, to use drugs in a manner that "would involve such drastic invasions of privacy, integrity, and the unalienable rights of the individual that in their application behavioral control would already have been achieved even if the electrodes carried no current and the pill were placebo."[77]

Against this background, consider again the impact of Kramer's *Listening to Prozac* in 1993. Its message that even sexual perversions might respond to pharmacological interventions appeared to open up a whole new world. But as early as 1958,

Roland Kuhn, the discoverer of imipramine, had noted that cases of sexual perversion responded to imipramine and that many patients, when they recovered after taking imipramine, felt "better than well." This result led him to state that an agent such as imipramine potentially posed significant philosophical and ethical issues.[78] Kuhn's language is now strongly suggestive of agendas laid out in *Listening to Prozac*, and encapsulated by Kramer in the term cosmetic psychopharmacology. But whereas Kramer's book became a runaway best-seller that seemed in some way to capture the mood of the moment or to articulate possibilities that many thought were within grasp, Kuhn's insights had minimal impact. No one was interested in imipramine in 1958.

What forces were at play in the transformation of worldview between 1958 and 1993? In the case of an engine of war, the developmental trajectory is largely determined by factors internal to the field. The response of delirious states to haloperidol, for instance, is so compelling as to brook no interference from regulators or company marketing departments. But in the case of the antidepressants, or Ritalin, the trajectory is more likely to be determined by external events and factors. The critical external event was the thalidomide disaster, which led in 1962 to the passing of amendments to the Food and Drugs Act. The critical factor is the development of a technological matrix capable of realizing the possibilities inherent in the discovery of imipramine.

The 1962 Amendments

The thalidomide crisis was an extraordinary event that dramatically changed health care worldwide. Surprisingly no history of it has yet been written. One of its consequences was that drug therapies suddenly became "risky" in a way they hadn't been before. In order to offset the risks of the therapies then available, the thrust of the 1962 amendments to the 1938 Food and Drugs Act was to channel drug development and drug availability toward disease indications where the risks of treatment would be offset by the prospective benefits.[79] There were changes in three areas. First, companies were encouraged to develop drugs targeted at specific disease indications. Second, it was confirmed that drugs would remain available only by prescription. This requirement placed the new agents in the hands of a set of individuals who by training would be inclined to make them available for diseases rather than problems of living. Third, the 1962 amendments endorsed randomized clinical trials. RCTs did a great deal to bring standardization into the field through the use of rating scales and operational criteria, in a way that the alternative, large simple trials, would not have done. But they are also expensive, and their use dramatically pushed up development costs, in the process forcing corporate development in the pharmaceutical industry.

The 1962 amendments put a premium on categorical rather than dimensional models of disease. Bacterial infections were the exemplar of a categorical disease state of the kind the 1962 amendments were aimed at. In contrast, within the mental health arena, until the psychopharmacological era, there had been a heavy emphasis on dimensional models of pathology. Psychiatric textbooks contained photographs of different constitutional types, the mesomorphs, endomorphs, and ectomorphs of the American literature or the schizothymes and cyclothymes of the European literature. Hans Eysenck had introduced a personality framework incorporating notions of inhibition and arousal into introversion-extraversion and neuroticism-stability dimensions. The first sedatives and stimulants appeared to map quite readily onto these dimensions. This is not surprising, since most biological functions can be mapped dimensionally. Given the antidepressants' rather minimal treatment effect on the various categories of depression and their more detectable effects on a range of other nervous disorders, it is far from clear that these agents would not be better conceived of as acting on some dimensional factor. It took the 1962 amendments to channel developments down a categorical route.

Increasingly since the 1960s, as thinking has become pharmacocentric, the FDA has ended up in a position rather like that of the magisterium in the Catholic Church. It acts to regulate claims that can be made. While not stating what is truth, by ruling out certain claims it provides a structure for the marketplace. It also sets up a dialectic between orthodoxy and heresy, so that in due course there may be a need for a taxonomy of medical heresies to parallel the taxonomy of medieval heresies.[80] But more to the point, what was once a process thought to involve the regulation of industrial products, not unlike the regulation of the labeling of dairy products or candy, is clearly now nothing of the sort. One stroke of a politician's pen could change the regulatory framework, in favor of a dimensional or over-the-counter use of psychotropic drugs, and thereby transform psychiatry. The gap between the DSM that appeared after such a change and the one that preceded it would be even greater than the divide between DSM-II and DSM-III.

One of the great hazards of reforms is that reformers often produce the opposite of what they set out to achieve. The 1962 amendments were passed as part of an effort to guard the people from the unfettered forces of capitalism. It is a moot point whether the reforms have fostered instead the growth of a psychopharmaceutical complex whose power to penetrate markets is now all but comprehensive. The "good" drugs are now difficult to access because they are available only by prescription, while the "bad" drugs, which prescription-only status was introduced to control, are widely available. These paradoxical effects of regulation are not new. Since the introduction of regulation into the medicines arena in 1906, there has been a clear dialectical interaction between companies and regulators.[81] Voices have been raised from the start protesting against this "conspiracy." There are probably no conceivable regulatory rules that will be acceptable to everyone, but what was not foreseen were the profound implications of arrangements of this sort for the understanding we have of our selves and our culture. Although regulation cannot be abolished, some effort by historians and human scientists to take its effects into account would seem to be needed.

The Technological Matrix

Penicillin was discovered in 1928 but, unlike the discovery of chlorpromazine, this discovery had no effect until a cooperative effort between the U.S. government and the pharmaceutical industry during World War II solved a number of technical problems having to do with producing it in usable quantities.[82] This demonstrates that creating a technology often requires more than devising a single technique or discovering a pharmaceutical agent. The capacity to transmit signals digitally, for instance, had been available for some time before a set of associated technologies and market opportunities was developed that made it worthwhile to bring the digital television to market. Even then, development required considerable state subsidization of the market.

In the case of the further development of the psychopharmacology revolution, it is possible to specify a number of the elements that the broader technological base will have to include. Among these are neuroimaging, pharmacogenetic, and genomic capabilities.

At the turn of the millennium, neuroimaging capabilities from the point of view of psychiatry remained rudimentary and essentially did not contribute to clinical practice. Despite this, the evidence of early CT (computed tomography) scans showing enlarged ventricles in patients with schizophrenia, which began to appear in the mid-1970s, generated considerable anticipatory excitement.[83] Clearly this excitement owed little to the results obtained, which have not been replicable or of consequence. The new techniques did, however, signal the possibility for future developments in the field. And right at the turn of the century a range of technical developments had led to a situation where a series of PET scan studies demonstrated variations in neurotransmitter receptor density that correlated with variations in personality.[84] It is expected that the next generation of machines will produce images in real time and achieve resolutions a thousand-fold clearer than those achievable during the 1990s. Issues central to the nature of psychosyndromes will then become open to reconceptualization on the basis of clear answers to the question of whether brain processing is distributed and dynamic (dimensional) or whether it operates on the basis of an if-then motor logic, subject to discrete lesions (categorical).

As with neuroimaging, developments relevant to the interface between psychopharmacology and genetics are underpinned by technical developments that are happening outside the field of mental illness. In this case, the underpinning comes from the Human Genome Project, which is one of the largest infrastructural developments ever undertaken, in terms of the investment of both public and private scientific and financial capital.

In the case of genetics, the need to establish precise pharmacogenetic responses to medications will drive the field forward. Once the technology to predict adverse responses to drugs becomes possible, product-liability issues will lead to its rapid deployment. In the case of psychiatry, these pharmacogenetic developments are quite likely to fracture the depressive and schizophrenic monoliths. Hitherto, companies have been able to target the whole of depression, but in the future they will only be able to count on usage by a proportion of depressed individuals, those with particular pharmacogenetic profiles. These profiles in turn will yield more information than simply the likelihood of an adverse effect. They will indicate temperament types, and these indications are likely to lead us back to conclusions that particular classes of antidepressants are more effective acting on certain personality dimensions than in treating a categorical form of depression.

Finally there have been a range of developments in the field of genomics and combinatorial chemistry that may shape the further evolution of the field of pharmacology. It is now possible to systematically produce compounds that will target a range of psychophysiological functions far more selectively than has been possible hitherto. Whereas once one new compound could be screened per week, companies can now screen more than 10,000 per day. The new methods of drug synthesis allow scientific leads to be transformed into market opportunities within months.

As outlined in Chapter 7, these developments will transform the therapeutics of serious mental illness and our assessments of whether or how drugs work. The likeliest psychosyndrome to benefit first is Kahlbaum's catatonia. This highly homogenous syndrome, involving clear ideo-motor disturbances that are very sensitive to specific interventions, offers the perfect opportunity for neuroimaging to demonstrate just what is going on during treatment. Catatonia also offers the almost perfect syndrome for discovering where the mind and brain connect, where the will and emotions get translated into action.

But the greatest impacts will lie in the management of community nervousness. The lack of a technological matrix for imipramine cut off all developmental avenues for the psychopharmacological engineering that was necessary for the development of the antidepressants. At some point soon, the conjunction of neuroimaging, novel drug-development possibilities, genetic techniques, and abilities to develop markets will realize the possibilities inherent in the antidepressant group of drugs that were hinted at in *Listening to Prozac*.

Market Development in the New Medical State

The 1962 amendments initially produced the outcomes intended. But as the years went on, the medico-pharmaceutical complex found ways to circumvent these restrictions. If drugs were to be made available only to treat diseases, it was perhaps predictable that there would be a mass creation of diseases.

When the antidepressants were first introduced, the general perception was that affective disorders were relatively rare— afflicting on the order of fifty people per million. In order to sell its compounds, the pharmaceutical industry has had to teach prescribers and the public at large to recognize depression. This educational campaign was so successful that no one now bats an eye at repetitions of the mantra that depression is a widespread disorder affecting over 100,000 people per million and that it leads to more disabilities and economic disadvantages than almost any other disorder, and in some cases to disastrous outcomes such as suicide. There is agreement that depression should be treated with antidepressant drugs, even though the evidence that antidepressants will be of benefit in treating a significant proportion of these depressive disorders is minimal.

The current prevalence of these ideas, however, conceals what actually happened. In the West, a 1980s crisis stemming from physical dependence on benzodiazepines led to the eclipse of the minor tranquilizers and indeed of the whole notion of anxiolysis.[85] This ushered in the antidepressant era. In contrast, in Japan there are fewer problems with dependence on anxiolytics. As a consequence, the anxiolytics remain the drugs most widely used to treat community nervous problems in Japan, while the antidepressant market remains a small one, with neither Prozac nor any other SSRIs available as antidepressants. In other words, depression as it is now understood both by clinicians and laypeople is an extremely recent phenomenon and one that is largely confined to the Western world.

The emergence of depression in this sense coincides with the development of the SSRIs, which in the mid-1980s appeared capable of being developed as either anxiolytics or antidepressants.[86] After the benzodiazepine crisis, the industry had a new set of compounds to sell, but its new offerings did not meet the demand from the marketplace. And indeed since their initial launch as antidepressants, various SSRIs have been licensed for the treatment of panic disorder, social phobia, post-traumatic stress disorder, OCD, and other anxiety-based conditions. Indeed, for some of the SSRIs, contrary to popular perceptions, it has simply not been possible to show that they are effective in treating classic depressive disorders.

In a pattern familiar from the story of depression, demonstrations that drugs active on the 5HT system could be useful for treating these other nervous conditions have led to marked increases in the estimates of their frequency. OCD has increased a thousand-fold in apparent frequency.[87] Panic disorder, a term that was not coined until the mid-1960s and that first entered diagnostic classification systems in 1980, has become one of the psychiatric terms most widely recognized by laypeople. Social phobia, which was all but invisible until the 1990s, now appears to affect the population in epidemic proportions, and this apparent growth in its incidence led to the launch of Paxil as an anti-shyness agent and a concomitant rise in the price of SmithKline Beecham shares.

Some of the mechanisms by which these changes have been brought about were outlined in Chapter 7. In brief, the pharmaceutical industry has highly developed capacities to gather and market evidence favorable to its business interests. Ideas and data are vigorously distributed. The techniques used to market information have developed to the point where significant changes in the mentality of both clinicians and the public can be produced within a matter of a few years. Increases in the incidence of conditions by a thousand-fold do not appear to surprise clinicians and the public has had a newly minted biobabble substituted for the psychobabble prevalent during much of the century.

These changes in popular consciousness are one thing, but when they are accompanied by an active suppression of information they are quite another. SSRIs can be shown to "work" through the use of clinician-based disease-specific rating scales. But when patient-based nonspecific rating scales, such as quality of life instruments, have been used in trials, the drugs cannot be shown to work, and this information has not seen the light of day. Current methods of estimating the side effects of drugs underestimate them, with only a third to a tenth of side effects detected in trials. SSRIs have been sold on the basis of a suicide rate for people with depression of 600 per 100,000; but this is the rate for people with severe depression for which the SSRIs are ineffective. In contrast, the annual suicide rate for those with nonhospital depression is probably less than 35 per 100,000, and in these populations suicide rates of 189 per 100,000 have been reported for patients taking SSRIs. Thus there are good grounds to believe that some of these agents may trigger as many suicides as they prevent.

Far from recommending that pharmaceutical companies investigate drug-induced suicidality, their lawyers may have given them advice that echoes that given to tobacco companies: that any investigation of these issues may increase claims of product liability.[88] From this vantage point, a drug such as Prozac might seem a symbol of the alienation that large corporations can visit on people rather than a symbol of the potential personal enhancement that a psychotropic agent can bring about.

There are a number of problems here. One is a set of corporate practices. Another is that the selling of Prozac has stretched to breaking point a disease-oriented framework that channeled all drug development through the prescription-writing power of medical practitioners. This framework operates on the tacit assumption that the legal advice given to other corporations would not be a factor in the relations between doctors and pharmaceutical corporations, but it is no longer clear that this assumption holds. A further issue is the concentration of care-giving that has occurred since 1945. There has been a vast increase in the use of mental health beds, which is probably best interpreted as a funneling of health-seeking behavior toward a limited number of legitimate providers.[89] The fact that treatments are solely available by prescription is another manifestation of just this.

Diseases and Lifestyles

Part of the promise of fluoxetine, at least the public perception of it, as shaped by *Listening to Prozac*, was that this drug had supposedly been developed through a process of rational engineering. The notion of rational engineering entails the implication that the effects being produced could easily be reproduced. The implication was that drug development had passed a certain quality threshold. Quality in this context refers to the reproducibility of an industrial process—not to the delivery of treatments with sensitivity and humanity.

A concern with this kind of quality is a pervasive aspect of peri-millennial life that plays a huge role in service industries from restaurants to educational and health care institutions. While therapy depends to a significant extent on input from another human being, the quality standard that can be achieved from an industrial point of view is limited. As the health marketplace in the Western world changed in the late decades of the twentieth century, managed care organizations in the United States and other health care providers in Europe have placed increasing emphasis on offering quality services. But this emphasis refers to the interest these organizations have in constraining clinicians, by means of algorithms and rating scales, and forcing them to produce reproducible outcomes where risks are controlled. It does not refer to any interest in producing the best possible encounter between two human beings.

The drug element of therapy is the point where issues to do with quality in this sense come into the clearest focus. Until the year 2000, it was not possible to offer any guarantees as to the quality of the therapeutic outcome. This does not matter in the therapeutics of severe disorders where the patients are in danger, and even doing something risky is, by general consensus, preferable to doing nothing. (Although the treatment of serious mental illness with antipsychotics has not been characterized by a predictability of recoveries, if psychiatry's mission is interpreted in terms of behavioral control rather than simply the treatment of disease, the outcomes with antipsychotics have been of a very high quality standard in this sense.) Poor outcomes have been much less likely to be tolerated in the management of the less severe mental conditions, where companies and clinicians have run into opposition in part because of the lack of consistency in outcomes.

A disease model has until now offered companies and clinicians an escape from the quality standards that apply to other industries. In a famine, no one is going to sue a food provider if the quality of the goods falls short of accepted standards. A further benefit of a disease model is that it has functioned as a means of managing equity in the access to health resources. Since World War II, people have protested at the inequities in access to health services more than they have protested, for instance, at inequities in the access to stereos, digital TVs, or computers. Finally, a libertarian element also emerges with the disease portrayal of disorders; there is something of a moral onus on the individual to get a disease treated. This onus does not exist when it comes to benefiting from an enhancement technology or a cosmetic intervention.

Given this analysis, it should be clear why the antidepressant story at first could not develop in any way other than the way it did. The technological matrix was simply not there to guarantee quality outcomes. But it should also be apparent that the technical base is developing rapidly and in a manner that is likely to release a range of other possibilities in the near future. The combination of selective drugs, pharmacogenetic profiling, and neuroimaging assessment of drug effects brings dramatically closer the possibility of offering quality outcomes of the type Kramer's book hinted at. Of critical importance in this area is not the notion that new agents will be more effective than older ones, as *Listening to Prozac* suggested, but the notion that the reliability with which certain responses can be elicited will approach quality standards found elsewhere.

Consider what happened when Viagra hit the market. It produced much more reliable responses than the antidepressants do. It quickly came to be seen as a lifestyle agent rather than an old-style drug to be used to treat a disease. This perception owed everything to the reliability with which responses to Viagra could be elicited. When a drug produces the claimed outcome more than nine times out of ten, a disease model is no longer needed.

Far from being the first of a new group of agents that will slowly have an impact on the field, Viagra is just one more in a long line of agents whose cumulative weight is leading to a wide-scale change away from therapeutics to something closer to lifestyle modulation. We have in fact been living with a number of anomalies for some time. The development of and provision of oral contraceptives on a prescription-only basis is notionally underpinned by the same model that underpins the treatment of infections—that is, an understanding that these agents are being used to treat a disease. This is faintly ludicrous, not least because of the quality of the outcomes these agents deliver. Similarly, hormone replacement therapy cannot truly be regarded as treating a disease. It is much better seen as an enhancing technology or a cosmetic intervention, and although it seems a good idea to have medical practitioners available as a source of advice, the idea that these agents should be available only by prescription is difficult to defend. These examples all indicate that the field of therapeutics is comprised of a series of domains, many of which may be far removed from the treatment of disease.

In fact, the public had been kept in the dark for two decades about other drugs with reliable effects on sexual function. The SSRIs have weak and unpredictable effects on depression, but they can delay orgasm reliably and other agents can advance it. We have had capacities to "engineer" sexual performance for some time, but these have not been marketed by companies, owing to uncertainties about the acceptability of establishing a market for lifestyle agents.[90] The SSRIs and Viagra both produce effects on sexual functioning that allow a manipulation of that function relatively immediately, for defined periods of time, and at an acceptable cost in terms of adverse consequences.

There already are treatments for baldness, agents to reverse age-induced skin changes, anti-obesity agents (Xenical), and there are a range of other lifestyle agents waiting in the wings. All of these raise in an acute form the question of what constitutes a disease. In recent history a disease has been thought of as an entity established by an underlying biological lesion. Before that illnesses were defined as anything that made an individual feel less well, a definition which led to the treatment of halitosis. Lately, the emergence of agents that can modify natural variations in hair loss or ejaculatory latency push us closer to making explicit one of the currently implicit definitions of disease, which is that in practice diseases are things whose treatment costs third-party payers will reimburse. But there are clearly limits to what third-party payers can pay. If some of these new agents are to come to market, it may have to be into another market funded in a different way—a lifestyle market.

The interplay between the social impact of psycho-pharmaceutical technologies, potential markets, and political will as expressed in regulations is a key factor in what will happen. The power of pharmacological agents to transform social consciousness is difficult to deny in the face of the transformation of social and work relations that followed the development of oral contraceptives. The prospect of "smart drugs" gives some glimpses of similar social and political impacts to come.

In general, when used in animal populations, smart drugs offer more benefits to less bright, less able, or aged animals than to younger, more able animals. In our current society, discrimination on the basis of sex, age, race, or religion is unlawful, but discrimination on the basis of intelligence remains legitimate. Clever children go to college and receive subsidies to do so. They end up with the better-paying and more prestigious jobs because of this advantage.[91] This advantage, however, stands to be eroded by smart drugs unless, for instance, the use of these drugs is confined to diseases such as age-associated memory impairment (AAMI). The political influence of the 1962 amendments to the Food and Drugs Act that channeled developments in particular directions can be seen clearly in the case of the possible restriction of cognitive-enhancing drugs to the treatment of AAMI.

But the effects of the 1962 amendments applied just as much to the antidepressant market. Before 1962, tonics flourished along with treatments for halitosis and a range of other agents targeted at everyday problems rather than diseases. Cyproheptadine, a tricyclic agent that has since been shown to have antidepressant efficacy, was widely used as a tonic. Just like imipramine, it increases appetite and improves the quality of sleep (see Chapter 2). In many ways, the use of imipramine and other tricyclics as tonics, a usage underpinned by centuries of practice, might have been much more acceptable to laypeople than their use as antidepressants, a neologism that quickly became associated in the public mind with risks of addiction and other problems.

The tonic effects of imipramine can, in fact, be produced much more reliably than any depression-resolving effects. And these tonic effects can be produced consistently enough to come close to meeting the quality standards that modern markets require. How many debates would there be about alienation and antidepressants if it were over-the-counter tonics rather than prescription-only antidepressants that were involved? Or if there were a debate would the public take it seriously? St.-John's-wort probably acts very much like Prozac. It is sold over the counter in many countries as an agent to reduce stress or burn-out. It is not necessary to be made diseased or to have someone else sit in moral judgment upon you in order to get it. How much does the regulatory framework create disease?

This example helps crystallize one set of dilemmas raised by cosmetic psychopharmacology, as framed by Kramer. As the use of Prozac for cosmetic purposes has been portrayed in the media, it has posed moral problems for the physician, who is called upon to decide whether it would be a good thing for society to reduce the extent of melancholia in the community, with the consequent loss of spirituality or creativity that that might entail. Should alienation be treated? These dilemmas would be transformed if the power to make such decisions were returned to the consumer. We are not alienated when choosing St.-John's-wort. We are not alienated when choosing our own cars but might well think we were if it were the prerogative of the automobile salesmen to decide which brand of vehicle we should buy. Some of the difficulties therefore stem from the current regulatory and disease framework rather than from the drugs themselves

Why should a physician with no ethical training have the ability to decide whether taking a pill that makes one less sensitive to work-related stress is a good idea? Clearly, taking a pill will be an escape for some, who might be better advised to build character, but equally clearly it seems possible that character building is more likely to proceed beneficially for some after cosmesis. Should a personality glitch be a given any more than shortsightedness, a hooked nose, or a flat chest are? Inducing brazenness in the timid may in fact make workplace transformations more rather than less likely.

Will psychotropic agents remain available only on prescription? Current agents are safer than the barbiturates and other drugs that were available over the counter before the 1960s. Many psychotropic drugs are safer than the H-2 antagonists that have been regraded from prescription-only to over-the-counter status in many countries.[92] Redesignation of agents as over-the-counter medicines would have a number of consequences. It would save on health service providers' expenditures, while at the same time maintaining the drug industry's incomes. It would also call into being powerful new consumer agencies, which would more vigorously scrutinize pharmaceutical company claims than psychiatrists have done. These consumer groups would by inclination be more likely to approach the issues from the point of view of quality standards rather than disease models. The advent of the Internet is of huge significance both in terms of facilitating access to information and of facilitating the purchase of medicines available only in other countries. It has already made possible the availability of Viagra and Xenical outside a medical framework, in the process making talk of a lifestyle or cosmetic market much more conceivable than might have seemed likely less than a decade ago.

THE SHAPE OF PSYCHIATRY TO COME

There is a palpable sense at the start of a new millennium that humanity is on the verge of great changes. The Internet is billed as a communications revolution as great as the development of the printing press. The fruits of the Human Genome Project will transform the futures marketplace and accordingly the government of our selves. Government, education, and health care will all need to be rethought. To believe that we will remain the same people despite changes on this scale is unrealistic. For all Marxism's failures as an economic system, the essential Marxist social science insight that "in adopting new productive forms, men change their mode of production and in changing their mode of production, they change their way of being—they change all of their social relations," seems likely to hold true. But the new revolution will go beyond anything dreamt of by Marx, because not only will changing social relations change our selves but changing technical capacities will allow us to change even the biological basis of our selves and our societies.

Science is about measurement technologies. Industry is about standards. The dominance of simple checklists such as the Hamilton Depression Rating Scale or the Positive and Negative Schizophrenia Scales within such a complex area as the psychopharmaco-therapeutic arena suggest that these have functioned more as standards than as measurement technologies.

There are other measurement technologies tapping into dimensional and personality-based aspects of psychopathology, such as the Cloninger Tridimensional Personality Questionnaire (TPQ)[93] and computerized repertory grid techniques that can tailor the rating of change to the precise state of each individual.

As with Apple and Microsoft, or Betamax and VHS video systems, development trajectories within an industry become established when a field settles on a standard, even though that product may be inferior to its competitors. Combined with pharmacogenetic and neuroimaging technologies, the adoption of repertory grid approaches or the TPQ would be likely to lead to an accelerating set of developments. The question then would be whether novel dimensionally oriented psychopathologies would become the new standards within psychiatry or whether the manipulation of temperamental variables would escape the disease domain entirely.

Unless someone can see a way to make a living out of these possibilities for development nothing will happen. Making a living in this new world will require a certain amount of predictability as regards outcomes. Making a living out of something today also means operating at a corporate level. Individual entrepreneurial activity makes little difference. But technologies once they develop support new sets of livelihoods and compromise older ones. For this reason, the use of drugs in other than medical settings will generate hostility on the part of medical practitioners unless some form of medical input to the new technological domain is negotiated or medicine as it has functioned until recently withers away—as many alarmed at the encroachments of managed care would argue is happening.

It seems likely that developments will follow the trajectory of cosmetic surgery. Plastic surgeons initially attempted to restrict the new specialty to the domain of reconstructive work. This had the benefit of escaping from the quality standards imposed on other areas of engineering. But once the possibilities of intervening effectively and reliably became available, the profession has had to come to terms with the public demand for cosmesis.[94]

Cosmetic psychopharmacology will not emerge onto an empty stage. A public basis for the emergence of such an approach has existed since the 1950s and 1960s, which saw the widespread and increasing use of a range of psychotropic compounds, such as LSD, Ecstasy, cocaine, and cannabis, along with the use of growth hormone, erythropoietin, steroids, and other agents to enhance physical performance. There are substantial markets for all these and related agents, whose very reliability has led to their unorthodox use as enhancement technologies rather than therapeutic agents. This market is currently estimated to be as large as the licit pharmaceutical market.[95]

Indeed, the current relation between society and drugs bears many resemblances to the nineteenth-century interplay between society and sex. Then the question of the regulation of sexual activity became explicit, with only certain forms of activity being deemed legitimate and many aspects of sexuality being controlled or repressed. Until the twentieth century drug use was largely uncontrolled and unregulated. But increasingly since 1900, there have been efforts to demarcate legitimate from illegitimate use and efforts to establish societal control over drug-related activities.[96] In the process certain drugs and the awareness of what some drugs have meant and can do have been repressed. At the start of the twenty-first century, however, the extent to which controls on sexuality have been relaxed would have astonished Freud. Few taboos remain. Will twenty-first-century drug use follow a developmental trajectory similar to that of twentieth-century sex?

From the pharmaceutical industry's point of view, the problem drugs are not the opiates or cocaine but the hallucinogens, the drugs so indelibly associated with the 1960s. The problem is not that these drugs could tell us a lot about ourselves and this knowledge might foment revolution, although these do seem to be possibilities. The problem is that with each dose every individual is likely to have a different experience. This is the very antithesis of quality as corporations currently define it. It seems difficult to see how the hallucinogens can be brought into the arena of standardization. There may be good reasons for banning their widespread use, but the current position of effectively prohibiting all research on such drugs is extraordinary. These are agents that may provide insights into the influence of both visions and biology on religious thinking and on the possible interface between having visions and being moral. Charting the use or nonuse of the hallucinogens therefore may yield critical indicators of what is happening in our societies.

In the case of any technical development, there is an issue about the willingness of particular societies to go down a new route. Western societies in recent centuries have appeared prepared to utilize new technologies almost regardless of possible societal consequences. This may not be the case for all societies. A fundamentalist reaction in some societies to psychocosmetic technologies is not inconceivable.

There is also the fact that technologies develop relative to the level of wealth in a society. It takes a relatively wealthy society to fund widespread provision of treatment for a mental illness such as schizophrenia, where the sufferers have very little money of their own with which to make the purchases. To date, societies for the most part have not sustained programs where treatments for severe diseases are available only to a few. The development of cosmetic agents, however, may escape the need for societal decisions on the question of whether they will be made available to an elite only or shackled to programs that would make them available throughout the society. Maybe the decision can be left to the marketplace, and people can decide whether if the new agents work reliably they can afford not to have them.

The development of a market ethos in the West arguably put a premium on an individual rather than a group ethos. This provided a stimulus for capitalism and for the development of technologies of production. We have at present moved from a relatively simple market into one that is dominated by corporations with industry standardization being a key feature of development programs. Until recently medicine was a simple business with a multitude of independent providers offering care in a completely nonstandardized way. Predictions of change date back to the 1980s: "Physician surpluses and escalating medical care costs have fostered an alliance among government, corporate America, and health insurers that has inspired medicine's industrialization. These same forces will transform psychiatry into an industry where prospective payment, automation, salaried employment, and central control of clinical activities threaten to become the dominant form of medical practice."[97] Managed care has realized those predictions and in the process has astonishingly left American physicians, who trusted to the marketplace more than the Europeans, possibly more circumscribed as regards their clinical freedoms than physicians in socialized medical systems.

This orientation toward the marketplace, toward the future, is Western in origin. It has given rise to global agreements on trades and tariffs and more recently proposals for global agreements on trade in services. One of the few things that seem capable of derailing this process is a rise in sea levels sufficient to force groups, even nations, to work together to solve the problem. By the time any such scenario was enacted GATS agreements, which permit for-profit managed care to move into countries other than the United States,[98] may have dramatically changed the character of health service delivery throughout the world, for better or for worse.

Should for-profit managed care spread in this manner, the splits within medical therapy are likely to grow, and nowhere will this be seen more acutely than in psychiatry. Just as psychiatrists develop capacities to reliably and quickly modify the input of constitutions and personalities to psychosyndromes with pharmacological approaches, and capacities to modulate transference relationships that psychoanalysts could only dream about, mental health services and the training that equips physicians to practice within those services are producing a set of physicians almost completely insensitive to these aspects of the exchanges between themselves and their patients. In the bad old days of psychoanalysis, Gershwin's analyst could inform his family that George was falling off his piano stool because he was hysterical, when in fact he had a brain tumor, but now we have physicians who have comparable blind spots for the psychosocial consequences of the physical interventions they make.

We have jumped out of the frying pan into the fire just when the emerging possibilities go beyond either of the positions outlined by Guze or Michels in the previous chapter. It will soon be possible not only to offer support while physical therapies are administered or to do traditional psychotherapy but to intervene in a manner that transcends this old dichotomy. To do this, however, will require skills from both sides of the traditional divide. The capacities for really effective interventions will not be realized in situations where one person prescribes and another, cheaper, therapist untrained in the new possibilities does the listening.

As the modulation of personality comes within the psychiatric remit, it will also become clear that a significant proportion of distress remains psychosocial in origin. Ironically, the completion of the Human Genome Project may do more than anything else to make this clear. Once the contribution of genetic factors is established, it will become clear that many things that have previously been explained socially have a predominantly biological basis— perhaps even some of the religious trappings of religions. But it will also become much more clear what proportion of our predicaments and disorders are epigenetic in origin. At that point an insistence on treatments that are solely biological may become oppressive.

Hitherto debates on these issues have been characterized by extraordinary antipathy between the nature and nurture camps. The nurture camp plays the card of genetic and biological determinism. In contrast, the nature camp, from Jean-Jacques Rousseau onward, has portrayed nurturing as a potent set of repressive societal forces aimed at colonizing the human mind. But recent twin studies have shed light on new aspects of our historicity. It would appear that one of the greatest determinants of our identities is the choices we make in response to the accidents that befall us. These choices and accidents cut across both nature and nurturing.[99] Given that there must be a real question as to how much of what may appear to be our deliberate choices are actually ours rather than apparent choices determined by societal introjects, it makes sense that the choices we make in response to accidents are the ones that truly shape our histories.

When it comes to the larger question of the choices that psychiatry makes, the extent to which the psychiatric mind has been colonized by the pharmaceutical industry is an increasing issue. The engine of colonization has been prescription-only arrangements. In contrast to what happens in other areas of clinical practice, there has been an absence of inputs into psychiatry from nontherapy-based disciplines such as bacteriology and pathology. The "hard" sciences input has come almost exclusively from pharmacology, and psychiatric thinking has accordingly become pharmacocentric. The development of neuroimaging or a change in the regulatory status of drugs from prescription-only status might change this.

But as we move into the twenty-first century, the mission of psychiatry is changing. Increasingly it involves the management of personality. In the not too distant future, the idea that psychiatry was once about the management of psychoses will be as distant a memory as the memory now is that it was once about the management of delirious states. This is not to say that psychoses will have been eliminated any more than delirious states now are. But even now people with psychotic conditions often come to a hospital only because they have particular problems at that point in time, and as with any other medical conditions the fact that these conditions pose a problem when they do is heavily influenced by the personality of the patient and the interaction of that personality with a particular psychosocial situation. Extensive medical service usage almost by definition indicates a personality disorder.

The typical professional response to psychiatry's current problems is to argue that the profession's future lies in neuro-psychiatry, with social problems being left to nonmedical psycho-therapists or social workers.[100] Neuropsychiatry may well flourish, but the more the neurobiological underpinnings of the disintegrative psychoses such as Kahlbaum's hebephrenia or disorders like Alzheimer's dementia are established, the more likely it is that the physicians managing these conditions will see themselves as neurologists rather than neuropsychiatrists.

One of the most fascinating conditions will be manic-depressive disease, which in its classic form, a form likely to have a discrete neurobiological underpinning, is in fact quite rare. When the basis of manic-depressive disorder becomes clear, psychiatry will be faced with a number of problems. For the most part, modern psychiatry is sold as a success story based on apparently good responses to treatments for its supposedly core disorders: manic-depressive illness and schizophrenia. But in fact the success rates in these conditions are much less impressive than they are commonly portrayed to be, with a greater number of bed days spent by a patient now and a greater number of detentions than in the pre-psychopharmacological era.[101] Truly effective treatments for these conditions will raise in acute form the issue of continuities between a hard core of neuropsychiatric disorders and a range of other, personality-based disorders. In so doing, these new treatments will shed light on whether psychiatry has been leading the pharmaceutical industry for the past fifty years or following it.

In the meantime, disorders of the personality from Kahlbaum's paranoia, now renamed delusional disorder, to his cyclothymia and dysthymia will remain. And if the most effective way of managing them is biological, as seems almost certain, psychiatry will remain in some form. We seem at present, in fact, to be in a position where these disorders are being redefined as conditions treatable with pharmacotherapies.[102] If psychiatry retains the management of these conditions, it will function as it always has to some extent, although it may completely reject the characterization, as an arm of government. Its function will be to control certain behaviors in order to minimize future risks for the sake of both the patients and the community. Paranoid states, paranoid personalities, and paranoid reactions, along with the explosive and impulsive personality disorders, which are increasingly being reconceptualized as having dysregulated affective states at their core, are among the disorders most likely to pose risks to the future of others.

Psychiatry can perhaps look forward to being increasingly faced with problems of the type posed by Jean-Jacques Rousseau, a part of whose personality led him to expose his genitals. Should this happen, any future Rousseau should be able to try the interventions of twenty-first-century psychiatry in a setting that will enable him to decide freely whether they have anything to offer him. If the technological capacities remain in medical hands, some form of scrutiny by others of what is being done will be needed. Every designation of a state as a disease involves a value-laden act. The ethics of such acts are relatively uncontroversial when urgent interventions to save a life are involved. In these circumstances the paternalism inherent in nineteenth- and twentieth-century medicine works to the advantage of the patient. In other circumstances, the values become more complex, and the need for genuineness and scrutiny increase. This will be the case in many domains of twenty-first-century practice, but will be of particular importance in areas involving children, where future interventions may have more to do with our government of our selves than with anything resembling the medical practice of an older era.

We can imagine some future Rousseau contemplating the possibilities of facing "treatment" and finding a dramatic tension in Paul Ehrlich's notion of a magic bullet—how it came in the twentieth century to mean hitting a target specifically with a minimum of nonspecific collateral damage. This understanding is quite different from the magic Ehrlich saw in antibodies. Unlike ordinary bullets, which had to be aimed at a target, antibodies, Erlich thought, borrowing an idea from Carl Maria von Weber's romantic opera *Der Freischütz*, were both magic and life saving because they found the right target without being aimed at it. Rousseau's contemporary Adam Smith had invoked the notion of the Invisible Hand to explain how the new market democracies would govern themselves. This powerful metaphor has suffered from the perception that the Invisible Hand may work to favor some rather than others. As the economic and health domains fuse in the twenty-first century, the hope must be that developments will bring a reappearance of the original understanding of a magic bullet.

Notes

INTRODUCTION

1. Cited by W. Malamud, "The History of Psychiatric Therapies," in J. Hall, ed., *One Hundred Years Of American Psychiatry* (New York: Columbia University Press, 1944), 285.

1. STRANGERS IN A STRANGE LAND

1. J. -.J Rousseau, *Confessions* (1782; Oxford: Oxford University Press, 2000), 86–88.
2. J. Goldstein, *Console and Classify: The French Psychiatric Profession in the Nineteenth Century* (New York: Cambridge University Press, 1987).
3. E. Kraepelin, *One Hundred Years of Psychiatry*, trans. Wade Baskin (London: Peter Owen, 1962); J. Reynolds, *Grangegorman: Psychiatric Care in Dublin since 1815* (Dublin: Institute of Public Administration, 1962); N. Tomes, *The Art of Asylum-Keeping: Thomas Story Kirkbride and the Origins of American Psychiatry* (Cambridge: Cambridge University Press, 1984).
4. J. McManners, *Death and the Enlightenment* (Oxford: Oxford University Press, 1981).
5. Reynolds, *Grangegorman.;* Tomes, *The Art of Asylum-Keeping.*
6. D. Healy, M. Savage, P. Michael, M. Harris, D. Hirst, M. Carter, D. Cattell, T. McMonagle, N. Sohler, and E. Susser, "Psychiatric service utilization: 1896 and 1996 compared," *Psychological Medicine* 31 (2001): 779-790.
7. E. Clarke and L. S. Jacyna, *Nineteenth Century Origins of Neuroscientific Concepts* (Berkeley: University of California Press, 1987); D. Healy, *Images of*

Trauma: From Hysteria to Post-Traumatic Stress Disorder (London: Faber & Faber, 1993).

8. R. K. French, *Robert Whytt: The Soul and Medicine* (London: The Wellcome Institute for the History of Medicine, 1969).

9. G. E. Berrios, *The History of Mental Symptoms* (Cambridge: Cambridge University Press, 1996).

10. J. C. Prichard, *"Moral Insanity"* (1835), *History of Psychiatry* 10 (1999): 117–126; G. E. Berrios, "J. C. Prichard and the concept of moral insanity," *History of Psychiatry* 10 (1999): 111–116.

11. J. E. D. Esquirol, *Des maladies mentales considerées sous les rapports médical hygienique et médico-legal* (Paris: Baillière, 1838); trans. by E. K. Hunt as *Mental Maladies: A Treatise on Insanity* (1845; New York: Haffner Publishing Co., 1965).

12. D. Healy, *The Antidepressant Era* (Cambridge, Mass.: Harvard University Press, 1997), chap. 1.

13. A. Bayle, *Traité des maladies du cerveau et de ses membranes* (Paris: Gabon, 1826).

14. M. Lanczik, H. Beckmann, and G. Keil, "Wernicke," in G. E. Berrios and R. Porter, ed., *History of Clinical Psychiatry: The Origin and History of Psychiatric Disorders* (London: Athlone Press, 1995), 302–323. See also C. Perris, *"Leonhard and Cycloid Psychoses,"* in ibid., 421–430; and G. Ungvari, "The Wernicke-Kleist-Leonhard school of psychiatry," *Biological Psychiatry* 34 (1993): 749–752.

15. P. Pichot, "The birth of the bipolar disorder," *European Psychiatry* 10 (1996): 1–10.

16. Berrios, *The History of Mental Symptoms*, 424–429.

17. B. A. Morel, *Etudes cliniques sur les maladies mentales* (Paris: Nancy, 1852).

18. P. Pichot, "The diagnosis and classification of mental disorders in French-speaking countries: background, current views, and comparison with other nomenclatures," *Psychological Medicine* 12 (1982): 475–492.

19. D. Pick, *Faces of Degeneration: A European Disorder, 1848–1918* (Cambridge: Cambridge University Press, 1989); R. Huertas, "Madness and degeneration. 1. From fallen angel to mentally ill; 11. Alcoholism and degeneration; 111. Degeneration and criminality," *History of Psychiatry* 3 (1992): 391–412; 4 (1994): 1–22; 4 (1994): 141–158.

20. S. Krueger, "Karl Ludwig Kahlbaum," address at the meeting of the American Psychiatric Association, Washington, D.C., 15 May 1999; P. Braunig and S. Krueger, "Karl Ludwig Kahlbaum," *American Journal of Psychiatry* 156 (1999): 989.

21. S. Krueger and P. Braunig, "Ewald Hecker," *American Journal of Psychiatry* 157 (2000): 1220.

22. K. Kahlbaum, *Die Gruppirung der psychischen Krankheiten und die Eintheilung der Seelenstorungen* (Danzig, 1863), part of which has been translated by G. E. Berrios as "The relationships of the new groupings to old classification and to a general pathology of mental disorder," *History of Psychiatry* 7 (1996): 167–181.

23. E. Hecker, "Die Hebephrenie," *Archiv fur pathologische Anatomie und Physiologie und fur klinische Medizin* 25 (1871): 394–429, part of which was translated in M. J. Sedler and M.-L Schoelly, "The legacy of Ewald Hecker: a new translation of "Die Hebephrenie," *American Journal of Psychiatry* 142 (1985): 1265–1271.

24. K. Kahlbaum, *Katatonie oder das Spannungsirresein* (Berlin: Kirschwald, 1874), trans. by Y. Levij and T. Pridan as *Catatonia* (Baltimore: Johns Hopkins University Press, 1973); M. Lanczik, "Karl Ludwig Kahlbaum and the emergence of psychopathological and nosological research in German psychiatry," *History of Psychiatry* 3 (1992): 53–58. For a contemporary American reaction to the syndrome and descriptions of cases see J. G. Kiernan, "Katatonia: a clinical form of insanity" (1877), reprinted in *American Journal of Psychiatry* 151, sesquicentennial supplement (1994): 103–111.

25. D. Healy, "One hundred years of psychopharmacology," *Journal of Psychopharmacology* 7 (1993): 207–214.

26. E. Kraepelin, *Psychiatrie: Ein Lehrbuch fur Studierende und Aerzte*, 5th ed. (Leipzig: J. A. Barth, 1896). See also P. Hoff, "Kraepelin," in Berrios and Porter, ed., *History of Clinical Psychiatry*, 261–279, and G. E. Berrios and R. Hauser, "Kraepelin," ibid., 280–291.

27. C. G. Jung, "The Content of the Psychoses," in *Collected Works of C. G. Jung*, trans. R. F. Hull (London: Routledge & Kegan Paul, 1960), 158–178; C. G. Jung, "On the psychogenesis of schizophrenia," *Journal of Mental Science* 85 (1940): 64–1011.

28. E. Bleuler, *Dementia Praecox or the Group of the Schizophrenias* (1911), trans. Joseph Zinkin (New York: International University Press, 1950).

29. M. Shepherd, "Psychopharmacology: Specific and Non-specific," in Healy, *The Psychopharmacologists*, vol. 2, 237–238.

30. P. Pichot, "The diagnosis and classification of mental disorders in French-speaking countries," 475–492.

31. The story of Janet and Freud's contribution to the redefinition of the psyche is outlined in Healy, *Images of Trauma*. The larger forces at play in the period are outlined in I. Hacking, *Rewriting the Soul: Multiple Personality and the Sciences of Memory* (Princeton: Princeton University Press, 1995), and N. Rose, *Inventing Our Selves: Psychology, Power, and Personhood* (Cambridge: Cambridge University Press, 1998).

32. Quoted in J. M. Masson, *The Assault on Truth: Freud's Suppression of the Seduction Theory* (Harmondsworth, Eng.: Penguin Books, 1984), 46.

33. For seminal accounts of the work of Charcot and Janet see H. Ellenberger, *"The Discovery of the Unconscious: The History and Evolution of Dynamic Psychiatry* (New York: Basic Books, 1970).

34. Healy, *Images of Trauma*, chap. 5.

35. I. Marks, "Marketing the Evidence," in Healy, *The Psychopharmacologists*, vol. 2, 543–560.

36. O. Fenichel, cited in M. R. Trimble, *Post Traumatic Neuroses: From Railway Spine to the Whiplash* (Chichester, Eng.: John Wiley, 1981), 49.

37. K. Schneider, *Psychopathic Personalities* (1923), 9th ed., trans. M. W. Hamilton and E. W. Anderson (London: Cassell, 1958).

38. Healy, *Images of Trauma*.

39. P. Mazumdar, *Species and Specificity* (Cambridge: Cambridge University Press, 1995); N. Tomes, *The Gospel of Germs* (Cambridge, Mass.: Harvard University Press, 1998).

40. B. H. Kevles, *Naked to the Bone: Medical Imaging in the Twentieth Century* (New Brunswick: Rutgers University Press, 1997).

41. G. Le Bon, *The Crowd* (1896; London: Benn, 1952).

42. See D. Healy, "The Role of Irish Members in the Medico-Psychological Association: Plus ça change," in G. E. Berrios and H. E. Freeman, ed., *150 Years of British Psychiatry* (London: Gaskell Press, 1991), 314–320.

43. G. N. Grob, "The Severely and Chronically Mentally Ill in America: A Historical Perspective," in S. M. Soroff, ed., *Handbook for the Treatment of the Seriously Mentally Ill* (Seattle: Hogrefe & Huber, 1996), 27–44.

44. J. Raftery, "Decline of the Asylum or Poverty of Concept," in D. Tomlinson and J. Carrier, ed., *Asylum in the Community* (London: Routledge, 1996), 21.

45. Healy et al., "Psychiatric service utilization," 779–790.

46. S. R. Belenko, *Drugs and Drug Policy in America* (Westport, Conn.: Greenwood Press, 2000); D. F. Musto, *The American Disease: Origins of Narcotic Control* (New York: Oxford University Press, 1987); S. B. Karch, *A Brief History of Cocaine* (Boca Raton: CRC Press, 1998).

47. Healy, *The Antidepressant Era*.

48. American Medical Association, *Nostrums and Quackery* (Chicago: American Medical Association Press, 1912).

49. Healy, *The Antidepressant Era*.

50. P. Temin, *Taking Your Medicine: Drug Regulation in the United States* (Cambridge, Mass.: Harvard University Press, 1980).

2. THE DOCTORING OF MADNESS
BEFORE CHLORPROMAZINE

1. C. Pogliano, "Pharmacology in the Nineteenth Century," in A. Zanca, ed., *Pharmacy through the Ages* (Parma, Italy: Farmitalia Carlo Erba, 1989); W. H. Brock, *The Fontana History of Chemistry* (London: Fontana, 1992)

2. C. Ginsburg, *Ecstasies: Deciphering the Witches' Sabbath* (London: Hutchinson Radius, 1990).

3. S. Plant, *Writing on Drugs* (London: Faber & Faber, 1999).

4. S. Garfield, *Mauve* (London: Faber & Faber, 2000).

5. C. A. Russell, *The History of Valency* (Oxford: Leicester University Press, 1971).

6. D. Healy, *The Antidepressant Era* (Cambridge, Mass.: Harvard University Press, 1997), chap. 1.

7. K. Menzi, "Geschichte der Chemie in Basel," *Schweizerische Zeitschift fur die Chemische Industrie*, 5 (1983): 15–30.

8. J. Swazey, *Chlorpromazine in Psychiatry: A Study in Therapeutic Innovation* (Cambridge, Mass.: MIT Press, 1974).

9. P. Mazumdar, *Species and Specificity* (Cambridge: Cambridge University Press, 1995).

10. F. J. Ayd, "The early history of modern psychopharmacology," *Neuropsychopharmacology* 5 (1991): 71–84.

11. E. Shorter, *A History of Psychiatry: From the Age of the Asylum to the Era of Prozac* (New York: John Wiley, 1996).

12. J. T. Braslow, *Mental Ills and Bodily Cures* (Berkeley: University of California Press, 1997); J. Pressman, *Last Resort* (Cambridge, Mass.: Cambridge University Press, 1998). Pressman's book massively details the story of psychosurgery in the United States.

13. S. B. Woodward, "Observations on the medical treatment of insanity" (1846), *American Journal of Psychiatry* 151, 6, suppl. (1994): 220–230.

14. T. Koppanyi, "Sleep and Hypnotics," in *Discoveries in Pharmacology*, ed. M. P. Parnham and J. Bruinvels, vol. 1 (Amsterdam: Elsevier, 1983), 423–446.

15. O. K. Linde, "Chemie und Schlaf—Hoffnung und Hilfe für die Psychiatrie," in O. K. Linde, ed., *Pharmakopsychiatrie im Wandel der Zeit* (Landau: Tilia Verlag, 1988), 56–79.

16. P. Bodoni, "Dell'azione sedativa del bleu di metilene in varie forme di psicosi," *Clinica Medica Italia* 38 (1899): 217–222.

17. Shorter, *A History of Psychiatry.*

18. W. Allexsaht, "The use of methylene blue in the treatment of catatonic dementia praecox patients," *Psychiatric Quarterly* 12 (1938): 245–254.

19. G. J. Naylor, B. Martin, S. E. Hopwood, and Y. Watson, "A two-year double-blind crossover trial of the prophylactic effect of methylene blue in manic-depressive psychosis," *Biological Psychiatry* 21 (1986): 915–920.

20. Swazey, *Chlorpromazine in Psychiatry.*

21. J. O. Cole, "The Evaluation of Psychotropic Drugs," in D. Healy, *The Psychopharmacologists*, vol. 1 (London: Arnold, 1996), 239–263; G. E. Simpson, "Clinical Psychopharmacology," in D. Healy, *The Psychopharmacologists*, vol. 2 (London: Arnold, 1998), 285–306.

22. F. N. Johnson, *The History of Lithium* (Basingstoke, Eng.: MacMillan Press, 1984). Diathesis roughly means vulnerability.

23. C. Lange, *Om periodiske Depressionstilstande og deres Patagonese* (Copenhagen: Jacob Lunds Forlag, 1886); Johnson, *The History of Lithium*; M. Schou, "Lithium," in Healy, *The Psychopharmacologists*, vol. 2, 259–283.

24. W. A. Hammond, *A Treatise on Diseases of the Nervous System* (New York: Appleton, 1871);. V. K. Yeragani and S. Gerson, "Hammond and lithium: historical update," *Biological Psychiatry* 21 (1986): 1101–1102.

25. Johnson, *The History of Lithium.*

26. M. Schou, N. Juel-Nielsen, E. Stromgren, and H. Voldby, "The treatment of manic-psychoses by the administration of lithium salts," *Journal of Neurology, Neurosurgery, and Psychiatry* 17 (1954): 250–260.

27. Schou, "Lithium," 259–283; M. Shepherd, "Psychopharmacotherapy: Specific and Non-specific," in Healy, *The Psychopharmacologists*, vol. 2, 237–258.

28. I am indebted for the following account to a lecture by John Crammer in North Wales in March 1999.

29. Shorter, *A History of Psychiatry*.

30. L. Kalinowsky, "Biological Psychiatric Treatments Preceding Pharmacotherapy," in F. J. Ayd and B. Blackwell, ed., *Discoveries in Biological Psychiatry* (Philadelphia: Lippincott, 1970), 59–67.

31. J. Braslow, *Mental Ills and Bodily Cures* (Berkeley: University of California Press, 1997).

32. R. Kuhn, "From Imipramine to Levoprotiline: The Discovery of Antidepressants," in Healy, *The Psychopharmacologists*, vol. 2, 93–118.

33. See Healy, *The Antidepressant Era*, chap. 3, for some of the thinking behind the conventional view.

34. M. Fink, R. Shaw, G. Gross, and F. S. Coleman, "Comparative study of chlorpromazine and insulin coma in therapy of psychosis," *Journal of the American Medical Association* 166 (1957): 1846–1850.

35. B. Ackner, A. Harris, and A. J. Oldham, "Insulin treatment of schizophrenia: controlled study," *Lancet* 2 (1957): 607–611.

36. Such reactions to ICT were caught on a film made in the Vinatier Hospital in Lyon in 1955 by the Comité Lyonnais de Recherche en Thérapeutique en Psychiatrie.

37. See R. E. Thayer, *The Origin of Everyday Moods* (New York: Oxford University Press, 1996).

38. M. Lurie, "The Enigma of Isoniazid," in D. Healy, *The Psychopharmacologists*, vol. 2, 119–133.

39. Healy, *The Antidepressant Era*. For the dictionaries see *Websters Third New International Dictionary* (Springfield, Mass.: G. & C. Merriam, 1966); *The Random House Dictionary of the English Language*, 2nd ed. (New York: Random House, 1987).

40. D. Healy, P. Michael, M. Harris, M. Savage, D. Hirst, M. Carter, and D. Cattell, "The burden of psychiatric morbidity," *Psychological Medicine* 31 (2001): 779–790.

41. There are many claims that the medicinal use of opiates to treat nervous conditions goes back to antiquity. The claims I have depended on are G. Young, "Opium in Melancholia and Mania" (1753), in R. Hunter and I. MacAlpine, *Three Hundred Years of Psychiatry, 1535–1860* (New York: Carlisle Publishing, 1982), 395–398; M. M. Weber and H. M. Emrich, "Current and historical concepts of opiate treatment in psychiatric disorders," *International Clinical Psychopharmacology* 3 (1988): 255–266; S. B. Woodward, "Observations on the medical treatment of insanity" (1846), *American Journal of Psychiatry* 151, suppl. 6 (1994): 220–230; R. Kuhn, "The Discovery of Imipramine," in F. J. Ayd and B. Blackwell, ed., *Discoveries in Biological Psychiatry* (Philadelphia: Lippincott, 1970).

42. N. Tomes, *The Art of Asylum-Keeping* (Philadelphia: University of Pennsylvania Press, 1984).

43. See Healy, *The Antidepressant Era*, chap. 1.

44. R. Lawson, "A contribution to the investigation of the therapeutic actions of hyoscyamine," *Practitioner* 17 (1876): 7–19.

45. Woodward, "Obervations on the medical treatment of insanity."

46. A. Norton, "Depression," *British Medical Journal* 2 (1979): 429–430.

47. M. Lurie, "The Enigma of Isoniazid," in Healy, *The Psychopharmacologists*, vol. 2, 119–134.

48. P. Hoch and W. Mauss, "Atropinbehandlung bei Geisteskrankheiten," *Archiv für Psychiatrie* 97 (1932): 546–552; A. Herz, "Central Cholinolytic Activity and Antidepressant Effect," in D. Bente and P. B. Bradley, ed., *Neuropsychopharmacology*, vol. 4 (Amsterdam: Elsevier, 1965), 404–407; D. Loew and M. Taeschler, "Central Anticholinergic Properties of Antidepressants," in Bente and P. B. Bradley, ed., *Neuropsychopharmacology*, vol. 4, 404–407; S. Kaspar, H.-W. Moises, and H. Beckmann, "The anticholinergic biperiden in depressive disorders," *Pharmacopsychiatry* 14 (1981): 195–198.

49. R. P. Greenberg, R. Bornstein, M. D. Greenberg, and S. Fisher, "A meta-analysis of antidepressant outcome under 'blinder' conditions," *Journal of Consulting and Clinical Psychology* 60 (1992): 664–669; S. Fisher and R. Greenberg, *From Placebo to Panacea* (New York: John Wiley, 1979); J. Moncrieff, S. Wessely, and R. Hardy, "Meta-analysis of trials comparing antidepressants with active placebos," *British Journal of Psychiatry* 172 (1998): 227–231.

50. Healy, *The Antidepressant Era*, chap. 1.

51. S. B. Karch, *A Brief History of Cocaine* (Boca Raton: CRC Press, 1998).

52. C. Leakey, "The Long Road for a Drug, from Idea to Use," in F. J. Ayd and B. Blackwell, ed., *Discoveries in Biological Psychiatry* (Philadelphia: Lippincott, 1970), 68–84.

53. L. M. Dub and L. Lurie, "Use of Benzedrine in the depressed phase of the psychotic state," *Ohio State Medical Journal* 35 (1939): 39–45. In histories of the randomized controlled trial this trial is never mentioned. Louis Lurie was the father of Max Lurie, whose original discovery of the antidepressants also slipped from view.

54. C. Bradley, "The behavior of children receiving Benzedrine," *American Journal of Psychiatry* 94 (1937): 577–585.

55. L. Panizzon, "La preprazione di piridil-e piridilarilacetonitrilie di alcuni prodotti di transformazione," *Helvetica Chimica Acta* 27 (1944): 1748–1756; R. Meier, F. Gross, and J. Tripod, "Ritalin, a new synthetic compound with specific central stimulant action," *Klinische Wochenschrift* 32 (1954): 445–450.

56. L. Eisenberg, R. Lackman, P. A. Molling, A. Lockner, J. D. Mizelle, and C. K. Conners, "A psychopharmacologic experiment in a training school for delinquent boys," *Journal of Orthopsychiatry* 33 (1963): 434–447.

57. R. J. Chiarello and J. O. Cole, "The use of psychostimulants in general psychiatry," *Archives of General Psychiatry* 44 (1987): 286–295.

58. D. Healy, "The marketing of 5HT: anxiety or depression," *British Journal of Psychiatry* 158 (1991): 737–742.

59. G. Claridge, "The psychopharmacology of individual differences," in Healy, *The Psychopharmacologists*, vol. 1, 441–462.

60. Healy, *The Antidepressant Era*, chap. 5.

61. S. R. Belenko, "First Federal Law against Depressants and Stimulants, July 15th 1965," in *Drugs and Drug Policy in America* (Westport, Conn.: Greenwood Press, 2000), 260–262.

62. A. Chettle, *Problem Drugs* (London: Zed Books, 1995), 172–175.

63. Mirtazapine is sold as Remeron, trazodone as Desyrel in the United States and Molipaxin elsewhere, nefazodone as Serzone in the United States and Dutonin elsewhere.

64. J. Delay, R. Laine, and J.-F. Buisson, "Note concernant l-action de l'isonicotinyl-hydrazide dans le traitment des états depressifs," *Annales Médico-psychologiques* 110 (1952): 689–692; H. M Salzer and M. L. Lurie, "Anxiety and depressive states treated with isonicotinyl hydrazide (isoniazid)," *Archives of Neurology and Psychiatry* 70 (1953): 317–324.

65. T. Ustun and N. Sartorius, *Mental Illness in General Health Care* (Chichester, Eng.: John Wiley, 1995).

66. J. Thuillier, *Les dix ans qui ont changé la folie* (Paris: Robert Laffont, 1980), trans. by G. Hickish and D. Healy as *The Ten Years Which Changed the Face of Mental Illness* (London: Martin Dunitz, 1999).

67. H. Maudsley, *The Pathology of Mind* (1895; New York: St. Martin's Press, 1979).

68. M. M. Glatt, "The abuse of barbiturates in the United Kingdom," *Bulletin of Narcotics* 14 (1962): 19–38; R. Balme, "Early medicinal uses of bromides," *Journal of the Royal College of Physicians* 10 (1976): 205–208. Actual usage was undoubtedly more extensive than the number of these prescriptions indicates.

69. M. C. Smith, *A Social History of the Minor Tranquilizers* (New York: Haworth Press, 1991).

70. J. W. Meijer, H. Meinardi, and C. D. Binnie, "The Development of Antiepileptic Drugs," in M. J. Parnham and J. Bruinvels, ed., *Discoveries in Pharmacology* (Amsterdam: Elsevier, 1983), 447–480.

71. E. Fischer and J. von Mering, "Uber ein neue Klasse von Schlafmitteln." *Therapie der Gegenwart* 44 (1903): 97–101; M. J. Clarke, "Chloral hydrate: medicine and poison," *Pharmaceutical Historian* 18 (1988): 2–4.

72. This rather than Librium or Valium was probably what the Rolling Stones took.

73. E. M. Tansey and D. A. Christie, "Drugs in Psychiatric Practice," in E. A. Tansey, D. A. Christie, and L. A. Reynolds, ed., *Wellcome Witnesses to Twentieth-Century Medicine* (London: Wellcome Trust, 1997); R. Rushton and H. Steinberg, "Mutual potentiation of amphetamine and amylobarbitone measured by activity in rats," *British Journal of Pharmacology* 21 (1963): 295–305.

74. A. Jenner, "Catatonia, pink spots, and antipsychiatry," in D. Healy, *The Psychopharmacologists*, vol. 3 (London: Arnold, 2000), 135–166.

75. Franz Halberg originated the term "circadian" in 1968.

76. M. Fink, "Meduna and the origins of convulsive therapy," *American Journal of Psychiatry* 141 (1984): 1034–1041.

77. L. Meduna, "Autobiography of L. J. Meduna," *Convulsive Therapy* 1 (1988): 43–57 & 121–135.

78. L. Meduna, "Versuche uber die biologische beeinflussung des ablaufes der schizophrenie: campher under cardiazolkrampfe," *Zeitschrift fur die Gesamte Neurologie und Psychiatrie* 152 (1935): 235–262; L. Meduna, "New methods of medical treatment of schizophrenia," *Archives of Neurology and Psychiatry* 35 (1936): 361–363.

79. U. Cerletti, "Electroshock Therapy," in F. Marti-Ibanez, A. M. Sackler, M. D. Sackler, and R. D. Sackler, *The Great Physiodynamic Therapies in Psychiatry* (New York: Hoeber-Harper 1956).

80. M. Fink, "Neglected Disciplines in Psychopharmacology: Electroshock Therapy and Quantitative EEF," in Healy, *The Psychopharmacologists*, vol. 3.

81. G. Bush, M. Fink, G. Petrides, F. Dowling, and A. Francis, "Catatonia: rating scale and standardised examination," *Acta Psychiatrica Scandinavia* 93 (1996): 129–136.

82. W. J. Bleckwenn, "Production of sleep and rest in psychotic cases," *Archives of Neurology and Psychiatry* 24 (1930): 365–375.

3. EXPLORATIONS IN A NEW WORLD

1. I. G. Farben, or Interessengemeinschaft der Deutsche Teerfarbenfabriken, was a group of German companies established in 1925 that included BASF, Bayer, Agfa, and Hoechst.

2. E. Shorter, *The Health Century* (New York: Doubleday, 1987).

3. D. Bovet, "Introduction to antihistamine agents and antergan derivatives," *Annals of the New York Academy of Sciences* 50 (1950): 1089–1126.

4. C. H. A. Walton and J. A. Kristjansson-MacDonell, "Antihistamine drugs," *Canadian Medical Journal* 56 (1947): 162–169. J. Swazey, *Chlorpromazine in Psychiatry: A Study in Therapeutic Innovation* (Cambridge, Mass.: MIT Press, 1974); B. Halpern, "Recent advances in the domain of the antihistamine substances: the phenothiazine derivatives," *Bulletin of the New York Academy of Medicine* 25 (1949): 323–330.

5. Antergan, Benadryl, Phenergan and other products from this period are still available.

6. R. Stephenson, "Receptor and classical pharmacology," in D. Healy, *The Psychopharmacologists*, vol. 3 (London: Arnold, 2000), 175–188.

7. R. Domenjoz, "From DDT to Imipramine," in Healy, *The Psychopharmacologists*, vol. 3, 357–370; A. Broadhurst, "Before and After Imipramine," in D. Healy, *The Psychopharmacologists*, vol. 1 (London: Arnold, 1996), 111–134; L. Cook, "Pharmacology, Behaviour, and Chlorpromazine," in D. Healy, *The Psychopharmacologists*, vol. 2 (London: Chapman and Hall, 1998), 17–38.

8. P. Guiraud and C. David, "Traitement de l'agitation motrice par un antihistaminique (3277RP)," *Comptes Rendues du Congrès Médicale des Alienistes et*

Neurologues du Langue Français 8 (1950): 599–602; Comité Lyonnais Recherches et Thérapeutiques en Psychiatrie (hereafter abbreviated as CLRTP), "The Birth of Psychopharmacotherapy: Explorations in a New World, 1952–1968," in Healy, *The Psychopharmacologists*, vol. 3, 1–54.

9. O. Vinar, "A Psychopharmacology That Nearly Was," in Healy, *The Psychopharmacologists*, vol. 3, 55–79.

10. J. Thuillier, *Les dix ans qui ont changé la folie* (Paris: Robert Laffont, 1980), trans. by G. Hickish and D. Healy as *The Ten Years Which Changed the Face of Mental Illness* (London: Martin Dunitz, 1999); J. Thuillier, "Naissance de la psychopharmacologie ou 'une histoire de nez,'" *Urgences* 1 (1994): 21–22.

11. D. Macht and C. F. Mora, "Effect of opium alkaloids on the behavior of rats in the circular maze," *Journal of Pharmacology and Experimental Therapeutics* 16 (1921): 219–235.

12. Swazey, *Chlorpromazine in Psychiatry*; Cook, "Pharmacology, Behaviour, and Chlorpromazine," 17–38.

13. Unhappy with the weak effects of imipramine, a compound very similar in chemical structure to promazine, the German company Geigy in 1958 chlorinated it in the hope of dramatically transforming it into a more useful agent. The resulting compound, chlorimipramine, turned out to be just another antidepressant, it seemed, not worth significant market development. Not until thirty-two years later did this drug, now recognized to be the most potent of the antidepressants, reach the U.S. market. See D. Healy, *The Antidepressant Era* (Cambridge, Mass.: Harvard University Press, 1997).

14. Swazey, *Chlorpromazine in Psychiatry*.

15. See Cook, "Pharmacology, Behaviour, and Chlorpromazine," 17–38.

16. H. Laborit and P. Huguenard, "L'hibernation artificielle par moyens pharmacodynamiques et physiques," *Presse Médicale* 59 (1951): 1329; H. Laborit, P. Huguenard, and R. Alluaume, "Un nouveau stabilisateur végétatif (le 4560 RP)," *Presse Médicale* 60 (1952): 206–208.

17. Swazey, *Chlorpromazine in Psychiatry*.

18. Ibid.

19. CLRTP, "The Birth of Psychopharmacotherapy," 1–54.

20. J. Hamon, J. Paraire, and J. Velluz, "Rémarques sur l'action du 4560 R.P. sur l'agitation maniaque," *Annales Médico-Psychologiques* 110 (1952): 331–335.

21. See L. Meduna, "Autobiography," *Convulsive Therapy* 1 (1984) for a good example of the standard psychiatric response to the idea that schizophrenia is treatable.

22. L. Cook, "Pharmacology, Behaviour, and Chlorpromazine," 17–38.

23. E. F. Domino, "History of modern psychopharmacology: a personal view with an emphasis on antidepressants," *Psychosomatic Medicine* 61 (1999): 591–598.

24. P. Pichot, "The diagnosis and classification of mental disorders in French speaking countries," *Psychological Medicine* 12 (1982): 475–492.

25. CLRTP, "The Birth of Psychopharmacotherapy, 1–54.

26. P. Pichot, "The discovery of chlorpromazine and the place of psycho-pharmacology in the history of psychiatry," in Healy, *The Psychopharmacologists*, vol. 1, 1–21.

27. Thuillier, *Ten Years That Changed the Face of Mental Illness*; R. M. Palem, *Henri Ey: psychiatre et philosophe* (Paris: Rive Droite, 1997).

28. H. H. de Jong, "Die experimentelle Katatonie," *Zentralblatt für die Gesamte Neurologie und Psychiatrie* 139 (1932): 468 ff.; also in H. H. de Jong, *Experimental Catatonia: A General Reaction Form of the Central Nervous System and Its Implications for Human Pathology* (Baltimore: Williams & Wilkins, 1945).

29. H. H. De Jong and H. Baruk, *La catatonie expérimentale par la bulbocapnine* (Paris: Masson et Cie, 1930). See "La catatonie expérimentale bulbocapnique," in H. Baruk, *Précis de psychiatrie* (Paris: Masson et Cie, 1950), 190–222, for the full details of the experimental catatonia story up to 1950.

30. See Thuillier, *Ten Years That Changed the Face of Mental Illness*.

31. H. Baruk, "Henri Baruk," in T. Ban and O. Ray, ed., *A History of the CINP* (Brentwood, Tenn.: J. M. Productions, 1996), 195–196.

32. F. L'Hermitte, "Nécrologie: Jean Delay (1907–1987)," *Revue Neurologique* 144 (1988): 77–78.

33. Thuillier, *Les dis ans qui ont changé la folie*; Pichot, "The discovery of chlor-promazine and the place of psychopharmacology in the history of psychia-try," 1–21.

34. He was subsequently killed in a mountaineering accident, which makes it impossible to know his precise contribution to the story.

35. J. Delay, R. Laine, and J.-F. Buisson, "Note concernant l'action de l'isonicotinyl-hydrazide dans le traitement des états depressifs," *Annales Médico-Psychologiques* 110 (1952): 689–692. See Healy, *The Antidepressant Era*. Had Buisson's and Lurie's discoveries registered, the amine theories of depression would never have taken hold, and generations of drugs like Prozac might not have been developed. Buisson later went into private practice. In part this may have been because the opportunities for advance-ment were limited within French psychiatry. Paris was the place with maxi-mal prestige and for many the choice would have been to leave Paris for a provincial university post or leave the university setting for a well-remunerated career in private practice.

36. For example, Robert Domenjoz, an innovative pharmacologist at Geigy, the codiscoverer of DDT and creator of phenylbutazone and imipamine, said in a later interview that he knew little about his subordinates' thinking or contributions; see R. Domenjoz, in Healy, *The Psychopharmacologists*, vol. 3, 357–370.

37. P. Simon, "Twenty-First Century Drug Development," in Healy, *The Psychopharmacologists*, vol. 3, 523–542; Broadhurst, personal communication; Paul Janssen, taped nterview with the author, 1997.

38. See J. Delay and J. Thuillier, "Psychiatrie experimentale et psychopharma-cologie," *La Semaine des Hopitaux de Paris* 62 (1956): 1–7, dealing with bio-chemical matters, which Delay knew nothing about.

39. T. Lempérière, "In the Beginning in Paris," in Healy, *The Psychopharmacologists*, vol. 2, 1–16; Thuillier, *Les dix ans qui ont changé la folie*.

40. P. Deniker, "My view of psychopharmacology," *Collegium Internationale Neuro-psychopharmacologium Newsletter*, fall 1998, 18–19.

41. Thuillier, *Les dix ans qui ont changé la folie*; J. Thuillier, "Ten Years Which Changed Psychiatry," in Healy, *The Psychopharmacologists*, vol. 3, 543–559.

42. J. Delay, P. Deniker, and J. M. Harl, "Utilisation en thérapeutique psychiatrique d'une phénothiazine d'action centrale elective," *Annales Medico-Psychoogiques* 110 (1952): 112–131.

43. Thuillier, *Les dix ans qui ont changé la folie*.

44. Thuillier, "Ten Years That Changed Psychiatry," 543–559.

45. Thuillier, *Les dix ans qui ont changé la folie*.

46. CLRTP, "The Birth of Psychopharmacotherapy," 1–54; O. Vinar, "A Psychopharmacology That Nearly Was," in Healy, *The Psychopharmacologists*, vol. 3, 55–79.

47. Thuillier, *Les dix ans qui ont changé la folie*. Phillippe Burg is a pseudonym.

48. CLRTP, "The Birth of Psychopharmacotherapy," 1–54.

49. Ibid.

50. T. Lempérière, "In the Beginning in Paris," 1–16.

51. L. Revol, A. Achaintre, P. Balvet, M. Beaujard, C. Berthier, P. Broussolle, P. Lambert, J. Perrin, and A. Requet, *La thérapeutique par la chlorpromazine en pratique psychiatrique* (Paris: Masson & Cie, 1956); E. Achaintre, "Histoire du Comité Lyonnais de Recherches Thérapeutiques en Psychiatrie (CLRTP)," thesis, L'université Claude Bernard, Lyon, 1985.

52. F. Labhardt, "Die Largactiltherapie bei Schizophrenien und anderen psychotischen Zuständen. Schweiz," *Archiv für Neurologie und Psychiatrie* 73 (1954): 309–338.

53. J. E. Staehelin and F. Labhardt, "Les résultats atteints par les neurologiques dans le traitement des psychoses et des névroses," *L'Encéphale* 4 (1954): 511–517.

54. R. Battegay, "Forty-Four Years of Psychiatry and Psychopharmacology," in Healy, *The Psychopharmacologists*, vol. 3, 371–394.

55. Ibid.

56. N. W. Winkelman, "Chlorpromazine in the treatment of neuropsychiatric disorders," *Journal of the American Medical Association* 155 (1954): 8–21.

57. V. Kinross-Wright, "Chlorpromazine: a major advance in psychiatric treatment," *Postgraduate Medicine* 16 (1954): 297–299; V. Kinross-Wright, "Chlorpromazine treatment of mental disorders," *American Journal of Psychiatry* 111 (1955): 907–917.

58. H. E. Lehmann, "Psychopharmacotherapy," in Healy, *The Psychopharmacologists*, vol. 1, 159–186.

59. H. E. Lehmann and G. E. Hanrahan, "Chlorpromazine, a new inhibiting agent for psychomotor excitement and manic states," *Archives of Neurology and Psychiatry* 71 (1954): 227–237.

60. M. Fink, "Neglected disciplines in psychopharmacology: quantitative EEG and electroshock," in Healy, *The Psychopharmacologists*, vol. 3, 431–458.

61. A. Kurland, "Chlorpromazine in the treatment of schizophrenia," *Journal of Nervous and Mental Disease* 121 (1955): 321.
62. F. Ayd, video interview for the American College of Neuropsychopharmacology Archives, ACNP annual meeting, San Juan, Puerto Rico, December 1999.
63. Swazey, *Chlorpromazine in Psychiatry.*
64. P. Janssen, "From Haloperidol to Risperidone," in Healy, *The Psychopharmacologists,* vol. 2, 39–70.
65. Lehmann, "Psychopharmacotherapy," 159–186.
66. J. O. Cole and R. W. Gerard, *Psychopharmacology: Problems in Evaluation* (Washington, D.C.: National Academy of Sciences/National Research Council, 1959).
67. J. F. Casey et al., "Drug therapy in schizophrenia: a controlled study of the relative effectiveness of chlorpromazine, promazine, phenobarbital, and placebo," *Archives of General Psychiatry* 2 (1961): 210–218; S. Goldberg, J. O. Cole, and G. L. Klerman, "Phenothiazine treatment in acute schizophenia," *Archives of General Psychiatry* 10 (1964): 246–261.
68. H. Hippius, "The Founding of the CINP and the Discovery of Clozapine," in Healy, *The Psychopharmacologists,* vol. 1, 187–214.
69. T. Kobayakawa, "Psychopharmaceuticals in Japan," in Healy, *The Psychopharmacologists,* vol. 3, 281–292.
70. M. Toru, "Neurotransmitter Research in Japan," in Healy, *The Psychopharmacologists,* vol. 3, 293–307.
71. J. Elkes and C. Elkes, "Effect of chlorpromazine on the behaviour of chronically over-active psychotic patients," *British Medical Journal* 1954, 560–565.
72. W. L. Rees, "A controlled study of the value of chlorpromazine in the treatment of anxiety tension states," *L'Encephale* 4 (1956): 547–549.
73. G. Ashcroft, "The Receptor Enters Psychiatry," in Healy, *The Psychopharmacologists,* vol. 3, 189–200.
74. N. S. Kline, "Use of *Rauwolfia serpentina benth* in neuropsychiatric conditions," *Annals of the New York Academy of Sciences* 59 (1954): 107–132.
75. H. J. Bein, "Biological Research in the Pharmaceutical Industry with Reserpine," in F. J. Ayd and B. Blackwell, ed., *Discoveries in Biological Psychiatry* (Philadelphia: Lippincott, 1970), 142–152.
76. G. Sen and K. C. Bose, "*Rauwolfia serpentina,* a new Indian drug for insanity and high blood pressure," *Indian Medical World* 2 (1931): 194.
77. R. N. Chopra and M. Chakravarti, "A preliminary note on the pharmacological action of the alkaloids of *Rauwolfia* " *Indian Journal of Medical Research* 29 (1942): 763; R. N. Chopra, J. C. Gupta, and S. N. Mukherjee, "Hypnotic effect of *Rauwolfia serpentina:* the underlying principle of this action and its probable nature," *Indian Journal of Medical Research* 31 (1943): 71.
78. R. J. Vakil, "A clinical trial of *Rauwolfia serpentina* in essential hypertension," *British Heart Journal* 11 (1949): 350–355.
79. R. W. Wilkins and W. E. Judson, "The use of *Rauwolfia serpentina* in hypertensive patients," *New England Journal of Medicine* 248 (1953): 48–53.

80. J. M. Mueller, E. Schlittler, and H. J. Bein, "Reserpine, the sedative principle of *Rauwolfia serpentina benth*," *Experientia* 8 (1952): 338.
81. R. W. Wilkins, "Clinical usage of rauwolfia alkaloids, including reserpine," *Annals of the New York Academy of Sciences* 59 (1954): 36–44.
82. Bein, "Biological Research in the Pharmaceutical Industry with Reserpine."
83. R. A. Hakim, "Indigenous Drugs in the Treatment of Mental Diseases," paper presented at the Sixth Gujarat and Saurashtra Provincial Medical Conference, Baroda, India, 1953.
84. G. Simpson, "Clinical Psychopharmacology," in Healy, *The Psychopharmacologists*, vol. 2, 285–306.
85. Kline, "Use of *Rauwolfia erpentina enth* in Neuropsychiatric Conditions," 107–132.
86. L. E. Hollister, G. E. Krieger, A. Kringel, and R. H. Roberts, "Treatment of schizophrenic reactions with reserpine," *Annals of the New York Academy of Sciences* 61 (1955): 92–100; L. E. Hollister, "From Hypertension to Psychopharmacology: A Serendipitous Career," in Healy, *The Psychopharmacologists*, vol. 2, 215–236.
87. G. Curzon, "How reserpine and chlorpromazine act: the impact of key discoveries on the history of psychopharmacology," *Trends in Pharmacological Sciences* 11 (1990): 61–63.
88. A. Pletscher, P. A. Shore, and B. B. Brodie, "Serotonin release as a possible mechanism of reserpine action," *Science* 122 (1955): 374–374.
89. F. Sulser, "From the Presynaptic Neurone to the Receptor to the Nucleus," in Healy, *The Psychopharmacologists*, vol. 3, 239–258; L. Iversen, "Neuroscience and Drug Development," in Healy, *The Psychopharmacologists*, vol. 2, 325–350.
90. A. Carlsson, "The Rise of Neuropsychopharmacology: Impact on Basic and Clinical Neuroscience," in Healy, *The Psychopharmacologists*, vol. 1, 51–80.
91. J. Brady, "The Evolution of Behavioural Pharmacology," in Healy, *The Psychopharmacologists*, vol. 2, 71–92.
92. P. B. Bradley, "A technique for recording electrical activity of the brain in the conscious animal," *Electroencephalography and Clinical Neurophysiology* 5 (1953): 451.
93. P. B. Bradley and J. Elkes, "The effects of some drugs on the electrical activity of the brain," *Brain* 80 (1957): 77–117.
94. J. O. Cole and R. W. Gerard, *Psychopharmacology: Problems in Evaluation.*
95. Vinar, "A Psychopharmacology That Nearly Was," 55–79.
96. Hippius, "The Founding of the CINP and the Discovery of Clozapine," 187–214.
97. S. Malitz, *In the Beginning . . . The Origin of the American College of Neuropsychopharmacology* (American College of Neuropsychopharmacology).
98. Ayd, video interview for the American College of Neuropsychopharmacology Archives, December 1999.
99. G. E. Berrios, "Parkinson's Disease," in G. E. Berrios and R. Porter, ed., *A History of Clinical Psychiatry* (London: Athlone Press, 1995), 95–112.

100. See T. Sourkes, "Levodopa and Dopamine Agonists in the Treatment of Parkinson's Disease," in M. J. Parnham and J. Bruinvels, ed., *Discoveries in Pharmacology*, vol. 1 (Amsterdam: Elsevier, 1983), 249–267.

101. CLRTP, "The Birth of Psychopharmacotherapy," 1–54.

102. Ayd, video interview for the American College of Neuropsychopharmacology Archives, December 1999.

103. CLRTP, "The Birth of Psychopharmacotherapy," 1–54.

104. W. L. Rees, "The Randomised Controlled Trial Enters Psychiatry," in Healy, *The Psychopharmacologists*, vol. 2, 167–182.

105. D. Healy, *The Suspended Revolution* (London: Faber & Faber, 1990), chap. 4.

106. D. Healy, *Images of Trauma* (London: Faber & Faber, 1993), chaps. 1 and 2.

107. P. Sachdev, *Akathisia and Restless Legs* (Cambridge: Cambridge University Press, 1995); J. A. Sicard, "Akathisie et tasikinesie," *Presse Medicale* 31 (1923): 265–266.

108. R. W. P. Achor, N. O. Hanson, and R. W. Gifford, "Hypertension treated with *Rauwolfia serpentina* (whole root) and with reserpine: controlled study disclosing occasional severe depression," *Journal of the American Medical Association* 159 (1955): 841–845.

109. R. L. Faucett, E. M. Litin, and R. W. P. Achor, "Neuropharmacologic action of rauwolfia compounds and its psychodynamic implications," *American Medical Association Archives of Neurology and Psychiatry* 77 (1957): 513–518.

110. G. J. Sarwer-Foner and W. Ogle, "Psychosis and enhanced anxiety produced by reserpine and chlorpromazine," *Canadian Medical Association Journal* 74 (1955): 526–532.

111. Ashcroft, "The Receptor Enters Psychiatry"; Kline, "Use of *Rauwolfia erpentina benth* in neuropsychiatric conditions," 107–132.

112. D. L. Davies and M. Shepherd, "Reserpine in the treatment of anxious and depressed patients," *Lancet* 1955, 117–121

113. D. Healy and M. Savage, "Reserpine exhumed," *British Journal of Psychiatry* 172 (1998): 376–378.

114. H. Steck, "Le syndrome extra-pyramidal et diencéphalique au cours des traitements au Largactil et au Serpasil," *Annales Médico-Psychologiques* 112 (1954): 737–743; H.-J. Haase, "Psychiatrische Erfahrungen mit Megaphen und dem Rauwolfiaalkaloid Serpasil unter dem Gesichtspunkt des psychomotorischen Parkinsonsyndroms," *Nervenartz* 26 (1955): 507–510; H. J. Haase, "The Role of Drug-induced Extrapyramidal Syndromes," in N. S. Kline, ed., *Psychopharmacology Frontiers* (Boston: Little Brown, 1958), 197–208. See also Battegay, "Forty-Four Years in Psychopharmacology.

115. C. von Economo, *Encephalitis Lethargica*, trans. K. O. Newman (Oxford: Oxford University Press, 1931).

116. Battegay, "Forty-Four Years in Psychopharmacology."

117. P. Broussolle, J. Perrin, M. Maurel, et al., "La prochlorpémazine en psychiatrie: expérience tirée de 240 cures," *Presse Médicale* 65 (1957): 1628–1631.

118. P. Deniker, "From chlorpromazine to tardive dyskinesia (brief history of the neuroleptics)," *Psychiatric Journal of the University of Ottawa* 14 (1989): 253–259.

119. J. Delay, "In Discussion of Pharmacological Treatment of Schizophrenics," in Kline, ed., *Psychopharmacology Frontiers*, 421–441.

120. Janssen Research Foundation, *Dr Paul: A Chronology of Developments Beerse*, (Beerse, Belgium: Dirk Collier, 1993).

121. Janssen, "From Haloperidol to Risperidone," 39–70. See also P. Janssen, "The Discovery of Haloperidol," in Ayd and Blackwell, ed., *Discoveries in Biological Psychiatry*; P. Janssen, "The Discovery of the Butyrophenones," in Bruinvels and Parnham, ed., *Discoveries in Pharmacology*, vol. 1.

122. T. Okuma, "The Discovery of the Psychotropic Effects of Carbamazepine," in Healy, *The Psychopharmacologists*, vol. 3, 259–280; T. Kobayashi, "The Japanese Psychopharmacology Marketplace," in Healy, *The Psychopharmacologists*, vol. 3, 281–292; M. Toru, "Neurotransmitter Research in Japan," in Healy, *The Psychopharmacologists*, vol. 3, 293–307.

123. S. Tatetsu, A. Goto, and T. Fujiwara, *Kakuseizai chuudoku (Psychostimulant Toxicosis)* (Tokyo: Igaku-shoin, 1956).

124. P. Pichot, "The diagnosis and classification of mental disorders in French speaking countries," *Psychological Medicine* 12 (1982): 475–492.

125. H. Kutchener, *A Cursing Brain: Gilles de la Tourette and His Syndrome* (Cambridge, Mass.: Harvard University Press, 1998).

126. See Waelkens and Bobon in P. Divry, J. Bobon, J. Lopez-Ibor, and P. Pichot, "Symposium international sur le Haloperidol," *Acta Medica Belgica*, suppl. (1960); M. J. Seignot, "Un cas de maladie des tics de Gilles de la Tourette guéri par le R-1625," *Annales Médico-Psychologiques* 119 (1961): 578–579.

127. Pichot, "The Discovery of Chlorpromazine and the Place of Psychopharmacology in the History of Psychiatry," 1–21; Lempérière, "In the Beginning in Paris," 1–17.

128. P. Divry, J. Bobon, J. Lopez-Ibor, and P. Pichot, "Symposium international sur le haloperidol," *Acta Medica Belgica* suppl. (1960).

129. H. C. Denber, P. Rajotte, and D. Kauffman, "Problems in evaluation of R-1625," *American Journal of Psychiatry* 116 (1960): 356–357; H. C. Denber, D. Florio, and P. Rajotte, "Third evaluation of haloperidol," *American Journal of Psychiatry* 119 (1962): 172–173.

130. Janssen, "From Haloperidol to Risperidone."

131. CLRTP, "The Birth of Psychopharmacotherapy," 1–54.

132. Healy, *The Antidepressant Era*.

133. P. Deniker, "Discovery of the Clinical Use of Neuroleptics," in Parnham and Bruinvels, ed., *Discoveries in Pharmacology*, vol. 1, 163–180.

134. P. Deniker, "Qui a inventé les neuroleptiques?" *Confrontations Psychiatriques* 13 (1975): 7–17.

135. J.-P. Olie, D. Ginestet, G. Jolles, and H. Lôo, *Histoire d'une découverte en psychiatrie forty ans de chimiothérapie neuroleptique* (Paris: Doin Editeurs, 1992).

136. Thuillier, *Les dix ans qui ont changé la folie*.

4. PSYCHIATRY OUTSIDE THE WALLS

1. H. S. Sullivan, "Socio-psychiatric research: its implications for the schizo-phrenia problem and for mental hygiene," *American Journal of Psychiatry* 10 (1931): 977–991. See P. Mullahy, "Harry Stack Sullivan's theory of schizo-phrenia," *International Journal of Psychiatry* 4 (1967): 429–521; D. Rioch and A. H. Stanton, "Milieu Therapy," in S. B. Wortis, M. Herman, and C. C. Hare, ed., *Psychiatric Treatment: Proceedings of the Association for Research in Nervous and Mental Disease* (Baltimore: Williams & Wilkins, 1953), 94–103.

2. G. Le Bon, *The Crowd* (1896; London: Benn, 1952).

3. T. Harrison, *Bion, Rickman, Foulkes, and the Northfield Experiments* (London: Jessica Kingsley, 2000).

4. Unpublished interview with David Clark.

5. T. F. Maine, "The hospital as a therapeutic institution," *Bulletin of the Menninger Clinic* 10 (1946): 77–80; T. F. Main, "The concept of a therapeutic community," *Group Analysis* 10 (1977): 2–16.

6. M. Jones, "Maxwell Jones," in G. Wilkinson, ed., *Talking about Psychiatry* (London: Gaskell, 1993), 50–59.

7. A. Sareyan, *The Turning Point: How Men of Conscience Brought about Major Change in the Care of America's Mentally Ill* (Washington, D.C.: American Psychiatric Association Press, 1994).

8. A. Q. Maizel, "Bedlam 1946: Most U.S. Mental Hospitals Are a Shame and Disgrace" *Life*, 6 May 1946.

9. Cited in A. Sareyan, *The Shame of the States, 1948* (New York: Harcourt, 1994), 70.

10. See CLRTP, "The Birth of Pyschopharmacotherapy: Explorations in a New World, 1952–1968," in D. Healy, *The Psychopharmacologists*, vol. 3 (London: Arnold, 2000); and D. Clark, *The Story of a Mental Hospital* (Cambridge: Polity Press, 1996).

11. A. Lewis, "Response to H. Brill," in P. Bradley, P. Deniker, and C. Radouco-Thomas, ed., *Neuropsychopharmacology* (Amsterdam: Elsevier Press, 1959), 211.

12. CLRTP, "The Birth of Psychopharmacotherapy," 1–54. See Clark, *The Story of a Mental Hospital.*

13. H. Y. Meltzer, "A Career in Biological Psychiatry," in D. Healy, *The Psychopharmacologists*, vol. 1 (London: Arnold, 1996), 483–508.

14. L. Hollister, "From Hypertension to Psychopharmacology: A Serendipitous Career," in D. Healy, *The Psychopharmacologists*, vol. 2 (London: Arnold, 1998), 215–236.

15. R. Battegay, "Forty-Four Years in Psychiatry and Psychopharmacology," in Healy, *The Psychopharmacologists*, vol. 3, 371–393.

16. CLRTP, "The Birth of Psychopharmacotherapy," 1–54.

17. D. Healy, *The Antidepressant Era* (Cambridge, Mass.: Harvard University Press, 1997).

18. D. H. Clark, *Mental Health Advisory Services, Japan* (World Health Organization, Western Pacific Regional Office, WPR/210/68, 1968).

19. J. H. Masserman, "Experimental and Clinical Vectors in Pharmacology," in J. H. Masserman, ed., *Current Psychiatric Therapies*, vol. 6 (New York: Grune & Stratton, 1976), 113. See also A. Mandell, *Coming of Middle Age* (New York: Summit Books, 1975); and CLRTP, "The Birth of Psychopharmacotherapy," 1–54.

20. H. E. Lehmann, "Psychopharmacotherapy," in Healy, *The Psychopharmacologists*, vol. 1, 159–186.

21. N. Tomes, *The Gospel of Germs: Men, Women, and the Microbe in American Life* (Cambridge, Mass.: Harvard University Press, 1996).

22. L. Eisenberg, "A very British kind of social psychiatry," *British Journal of Psychiatry* 171 (1997): 309–313.

23. T. McKeown, *The Role of Medicine: Dream, Mirage, or Nemesis?* (London: Nuffield Hospitals Trust, 1976).

24. G. Rosen, "What is social medicine?" *Bulletin of the History of Medicine*, 21 (1947): 674–733; G. Rosen, "Social stress and mental disease from the eighteenth century to the present: some origins of social psychiatry" *Milbank Memorial Fund Quarterly* 37 (1959): 5–32. The term social psychiatry may have been introduced to the United States by Horace Dunham, who in 1948 claimed that it was coined by sociologists to designate a research interest in personality disorders. Used this way, the term clearly means something quite different from epidemiological psychiatry. H. W. Dunham, "The field of social psychiatry," *American Sociological Review* 13 (1948): 183–197.

25. Such efforts led, for instance ,to the first mass X-ray screening programs to detect tuberculosis.

26. M. Jones, *Social Psychiatry and Practice* (Harmondsworth, Eng.: Penguin Books, 1968).

27. E. H. Hare, "Relation between Social Psychiatry and Psychotherapy," in S. H. Foulkes and G. S. Prince, ed., *Psychiatry in a Changing Society* (London: Tavistock, 1969), 3–16.

28. M. Shepherd, "Psychopharmacology: Specific and Non-specific," in Healy, *The Psychopharmacologists*, vol. 2, 237–258.

29. G. W. Brown, E. M. Monck, G. M. Carstairs, et al., "Influence of family life in the course of schizophrenic illness," *British Journal of Preventative and Social Medicine* 1 (1962): 55–68; G. W. Brown, J. L. T. Burley, and J. K. Wing, "Influence of family life in the course of schizophrenic disorders: a replication," *British Journal of Psychiatry* 121 (1972): 241–258.

30. G. E. Hogarty and S. C. Goldberg, "Drugs and sociotherapy in the post hospital maintenance of schizophrenic patients: 1 year relapse rates," *Archives of General Psychiatry* 30 (1973): 90–96; M. Argyle, *The Psychology of Interpersonal Behaviour* (Harmondsworth, Eng.: Penguin Books, 1967).

31. J. K. Wing and G. W. Brown, *Institutionalism and Schizophrenia* (London: Cambridge University Press, 1970); J. K. Wing, "Innovations and social psychiatry," *Psychological Medicine* 10 (1980): 219–230.

32. J. Ryle, "Social medicine: its meaning and its scope" *British Medical Journal* 2 (1943): 633–636.

33. B. Wootton, "Social Psychiatry and Psychopathology: A Layman's Comments on Contemporary Developments," in J. Zubin and F. Freyhan, ed., *Social Psychiatry* (New York: Grune & Stratton, 1968), 283–299. See also M. Shepherd, "From social medicine to social psychiatry," *Psychological Medicine* 10 (1980): 211–218.

34. G. N. Grob, *The Mad among Us: A History of the Care of America's Mentally Ill* (Cambridge, Mass.: Harvard University Press, 1994).

35. N. G. Hale, *The Rise and Crisis of Psychoanalysis in the United States: Freud and the Americans, 1917–1985* (New York: Oxford University Press, 1995).

36. W. Menninger, "Hope," *American Journal of Psychiatry* 116 (1959): 481–491.

37. E. Shorter, *A History of Psychiatry: From the Era of the Asylum to the Age of Prozac* (New York: John Wiley, 1996).

38. B. S. Brown, "The life of psychiatry," *American Journal of Psychiatry* 133 (1976): 489–495.

39. F. Fromm-Reichman, "Some Aspects of Psychoanalytic Therapy with Schizophrenics," in E. B. Brody and S. Redlich, ed., *In Psychotherapy with Schizophrenics* (New York: International Universities Press, 1952), 89.

40. See Hale, *The Rise and Crisis of Psychoanalysis in the United States:* E. Dolnick, *Madness on the Couch: Blaming the Victim in the Heyday of Psychoanalysis* (New York: Simon & Schuster, 1998).

41. S. Arieti, ed., *American Handbook of Psychiatry* (New York: Basic Books, 1959).

42. E. D. Semrad, "Long Term Therapy of Schizophrenia: Formulation of the Clinical Approach," in G. E. Usdin, ed., *Psychoneurosis and Schizophrenia* (Philadelphia: Lippincott, 1966), 155.

43. See J. N. Rosen, "Intervention in the treatment of schizophrenics," *International Journal of Psychiatry* 4 (1968): 545–548.

44. J. M. Masson, *Against Therapy* (London: Collins, 1989).

45. R. Noll, *The Jung Cult* (Princeton: Princeton University Press, 1995).

46. Dolnick, *Madness on the Couch.*

47. P. May, *Treatment of Schizophrenia: A Comparative Study of Five Treatment Methods* (New York: Science House, 1968); J. O. Cole, "The Evaluation of Psychotropic Drugs," in Healy, *The Psychopharmacologists,* vol. 1, 239–264.

48. M. Greenblatt, H. C. Solomon, A. S. Evans, and G. W. Brooks, *Drug and Social Therapy in Chronic Schizophrenia* (Springfield, Ill.: Charles C Thomas, 1965); L. Grinspoon, J. R. Ewalt, and R. I. Shader, *Schizophrenia: Pharmacotherapy and Psychotherapy* (Baltimore: Williams & Wilkins, 1972).

49. See G. Simpson, "Clinical Psychopharmacology," in Healy, *The Psychopharmacologists,* vol. 2, (285–306. It should not be thought that this situation has changed. Today with all the chairs of psychiatry in most of the Western world occupied by neuroscientists, the most difficult patients have migrated to the public hospitals or to rehabilitation facilities, and practicing

clinicians are usually not inclined to refer patients to department heads or other senior figures within the academic world, whose clinical skills they may not trust.

50. See J. Schildkraut, "The Catecholamine Hypotheses," in Healy, *The Psychopharmacologists*, vol. 3, 111–134; H. Y. Meltzer, "A Career in Biological Psychiatry," in Healy, *The Psychopharmacologists*, vol. 1, 483–508.

51. L. L. Judd, "Historical highlights of the National Institute of Mental Health from 1946 to the present," *American Journal of Psychiatry* 155, suppl. (1998): 3–8.

52. G. N. Grob, "The Severely and Chronically Mentally Ill in America: A Historical Perspective," in S. M. Soreff, ed., *Handbook for the Treatment of the Seriously Mentally Ill* (Seattle: Hogrefe & Huber, 1996), 27–44.

53. In other European countries, many psychotic patients had been killed during the war.

54. J. Postel and D. F. Allen, "History and Anti-Psychiatry in France," in M. S. Micale and R. Porter, *Discovering the History of Psychiatry* (New York: Oxford University Press, 1994), 384–414; P. A. Lambert and M. Vacher-Lambert, "Sur un essai de psychiatrie de secteur en milieu rural a partir d'un service mixte," *L'Information Psychiatrique* June (1957): 330–340; CLRTP, "The Birth of Psychopharmacotherapy."

55. D. R. Bennett, "The Drive towards the Community," in G. E. Berrios and H. F. Freeman, ed., *150 Years of British Psychiatry* (London: Gaskell Press, 1991), 321–332.

56. Ibid.

57. B. Mahendra, "Where have all the catatonics gone?" *Psychological Medicine* 11 (1981): 669–671. A reduced number of infections may have played some part, given that catatonia could be induced in animals by tubercular and coliform infections; see "La catatonie expérimentale bulbocapnique," in H. Baruk, *Précis de psychiatrie* (Paris: Masson et Cie, 1950), 190–222.

58. Postel and Allen, "History and Anti-Psychiatry in France," 384–414; N. Dain, "Psychiatry and Antipsychiatry in the United States," in Micale and Porter, ed., *Discovering the History of Psychiatry*, 415–444.

59. D. Burston, *The Wing of Madness: The Life and Work of R. D. Laing* (Cambridge, Mass.: Harvard University Press, 1996).

60. R. D. Laing, *The Divided Self: A Study of Sanity and Madness.* (London: Tavistock, 1960).)

61. R. D. Laing, *The Self and Others* (Harmondsworth, Eng.: Penguin Books, 1971); R. D. Laing, *The Politics of Experience* (Harmondsworth, Eng.: Penguin Books, 1967); R. D. Laing and D. Cooper, *Reason and Violence* (London: Tavistock, 1964); R. D. Laing and A. Esterson, *Sanity, Madness, and the Family* (Harmondsworth, Eng.: Penguin Books, 1970).

62. D. Cooper, *Psychiatry and Anti-Psychiatry* (London: Tavistock, 1967).

63. E. Goffman, *Asylums: Essays on the Social Situation of Mental Patients and Other Inmates* (New York, Anchor Books, 1961).

64. T. Scheff, *Being Mentally Ill: A Sociological Theory* (London, Weidenfield & Nicolson, 1966); T. Scheff, *Labeling Madness* (New York, Prentice-Hall, 1975).

65. T. Szasz, *The Myth of Mental Illness: Foundations of a Theory of Personal Conduct* (New York, Hober-Harper, 1961).

66. Grob, "The Severely and Chronically Mentally Ill in America," 27–44.

67. D. Healy, M. Savage, P. Michael, M. Harris, D. Hirst, D. Cattell, M. Carter, T. McMonagle, N. Sohler, and E. Susser, "Psychiatric service utilization: 1896 and 1996 compared," *Psychological Medicine* 31 (2001): 779–790.

68. J.-P. Sartre, foreword to Laing, *The Politics of Experience*.

69. Postel and Allen, "History and Anti-Psychiatry in France," 384–414.

70. D. Macey, "Frantz Fanon, 1925–1961," *History of Psychiatry* 7 (1996): 489–497; C. L. Razanajao, J. Postel, and D. F. Allen, "The life and psychiatric work of Frantz Fanon," *History of Psychiatry* 7 (1996): 499–524; H. A. Youssef and S. A. Fadl, "Frantz Fanon and political psychiatry," *History of Psychiatry* 7 (1996): 525–532.

71. F. Fanon, *Les damnés de la terre* (Paris: F. Maspero, 1961), trans. by C. Farrington as *The Wretched of the Earth* (Harmondsworth, Eng.: Penguin Books, 1967).

72. M. Foucault, *Madness and Civilization: A History of Insanity in the Age of Reason*, trans. R. Howard (New York: Random House, 1965). The original is M. Foucault, *Histoire de la folie à l'âge classique* (Paris: Plon, 1961).

73. E. F. Torrey, *Schizophrenia and Civilisation* (London: Aronson, 1980); E. Hare, "Was insanity on the increase?" *British Journal of Psychiatry* 142 (1983): 439–455.

74. A. Scull, *Museums of Madness* (London: Allen Lane, 1979); A. Scull, "Was insanity increasing? A response to Edward Hare," *British Journal of Psychiatry* 144 (1984): 432–436. See T. H. Turner, "Schizophrenia as a permanent problem," *History of Psychiatry* 3 (1993): 413–429.

75. A. H. Maslow, *Toward a Psychology of Being* (Princeton: Van Nostrand, 1964); C. R. Rogers, *Encounter Groups* (London: Allen Lane, 1969).

76. J. R. Stevens, *Storming Heaven: LSD and The American Dream* (London: Heinemann, 1988).

77. H. Marcuse, *One-Dimensional Man* (Boston: Beacon Press, 1964).

78. J. K. Galbraith, *The Affluent Society* (London: Hamish Hamilton, 1958).

79. S. Plant, *Writings on Drugs* (London: Faber & Faber, 1999).

80. R. Carson, *Silent Spring* (Boston: Houghton Mifflin, 1962).

81. K. Kesey, *One Flew over the Cuckoo's Nest* (London: Methuen, 1962).

82. M. Fink, "Neglected Disciplines in Psychopharmacology: Pharmaco-EEG and Electroshock," in Healy, *The Psychopharmacologists*, vol. 3, 431–458; G. N. Peterson, "Regulation of Electroconvulsive Therapy: The California Experience," in H. Schwartz, ed., *Psychiatric Practice under Fire: The Influence of the Government, the Media, and Special Interests on Somatic Therapies* (Washington D.C.: American Psychiatric Association Press, 1994), 29–62.

83. L. R. Frank, *The History of Shock Treatment* (San Francisco: Leonard Roy Frank, 1978).

84. M. Burleigh, *Death and Deliverance: Euthanasia in Germany, 1900–1945* (Cambridge: Cambridge University Press, 1994); M. Lafont, *L'extermination douce* (Nantes: Areppi, 1987).

85. CLRTP, "The Birth of Psychopharmacotherapy," 1–54.
86. E. Hobsbawm, "The Year the Prophets Failed," in E. Hobsbawm and M. Weitzmann, ed., *1968: Magnum throughout the World* (Paris: Hazan, 1998); C. Fink, P. Gassert, and D. Junker, "Introduction," in C. Fink, P. Gassert, D. Junker, *The World Transformed* (New York: Cambridge University Press, 1998).
87. C. Bernard, *An Introduction to the Study of Experimental Medicine*, trans. H. C. Greene (New York: MacMillan, 1927).
88. M. S. Pernick, *A Calculus of Suffering: Pain, Professionalism, and Anesthesia in Nineteenth Century America* (New York: Columbia University Press, 1985).
89. D. J. Rothman, *Strangers at the Bedside: A History of How Law and Bioethics Transformed Medical Decision Making* (New York: Basic Books, 1991).
90. Healy, *The Antidepressant Era*.
91. H. K. Beecher, "Ethics and clinical research" *New England Journal of Medicine* 74 (1966): 1354–1360.
92. Rothman, *Strangers at the Bedside*.
93. E. Kubler-Ross, *On Death and Dying* (New York: MacMillan, 1969).
94. S. Alexander, "They Decide Who Lives, Who Dies," *Life*, 9 November 1962, 103.
95. P. McCullagh, *Brain Dead, Brain Absent, Brain Donors: Human Subjects or Human Objects* (Chichester: John Wiley, 1993).
96. I. Illich, *Medical Nemesis: The Expropriation of Health* (London: Marion Boyars, 1976).
97. R. Porter, *The Greatest Benefit to Mankind* (London: HarperCollins, 1997); see chap. 21, "Medicine and the People."
98. E. Haikan, *Venus Envy: A History of Cosmetic Surgery* (Baltimore: Johns Hopkins University Press, 1997).
99. A. Scull, "Mental patients and the community: a critical note," *International Journal of Law and Psychiatry* 9 (1986): 383–392.
100. Hollister, "From Hypertension to Psychopharmacology," 215–235.
101. S. Snelders, "Paradigms of hallucinogenic drug use in psychiatry: some Dutch examples." *Medical History, forthcoming July 2002*; A. Hofmann, *LSD: My Problem Child* (Los Angeles: Jeremy P. Tarcher, 1983).
102. "Six Youths on LSD 'Trip' Blinded by Sun," *New York Times*, 13 January 1968; "Governor Shafer Calls LSD Blindings a Hoax," *New York Times*, 19 January 1968.
103. S. R. Belenko, ed., *Drugs and Drug Policy in America: A Documentary History* (Westport Conn.: Greenwood Press,), 278–284.
104. P. L. Gilbert, J. Harris, L. A. McAdams, and D. V. Jeste, "Neuroleptic withdrawal in schizophrenic patients," *Archives of General Psychiatry* 52 (1995): 173–188, with commentaries by R. Baldessarini and A. Viguera, W. Carpenter and C. Taminga, J. Greden and R. Tandon, H. Meltzer, K. Nuechterlein et al., and R. Wyatt.
105. L. E. Hollister, D. T. Eikenberry, and S. Raffel, "Chlorpromazine in nonpsychotic patients with pulmonary tuberculosis," *American Review of Respiratory Diseases* 81 (1960): 562–566.

106. Hollister, "From Hypertension to Psychopharmacology."
107. V. Berridge and G. Edwards, *Opium and the People: Opiate Use in Nineteenth-Century England* (New Haven: Yale University Press, 1987).
108. E. Levinstein, *Morbid Craving for Morphine* (London: Smith & Elder, 1878).
109. C. C. Mann and M. L. Plummer, *The Aspirin Wars: Money, Medicine, and 100 Years of Rampant Competition* (New York: Alfred A. Knopf, 1991).
110. S. B. Karch, *A Brief History of Cocaine* (Boca Raton: CRC Press, 1998).
111. Healy, *The Antidepressant Era*, chap 1.
112. A. Wikler, *The Relation of Pharmacology to Psychiatry* (Baltimore: Williams & Wilkins, 1957); Hollister, "From Hypertension to Psychopharmacology," 215–236.
113. D. F. Klein, "Reaction Patterns to Psychotropic Drugs and the Discovery of Panic Disorder," in Healy, *The Psychopharmacologists*, vol. 1, 329–352.
114. L. E. Hollister, F. P. Motzenbecker, and R. O. Degan, "Withdrawal reactions from chlordiazepoxide (Librium)," *Psychopharmacologia* 2 (1961): 63–68.
115. M. C. Smith, *A Social History of the Minor Tranquillisers* (New York: Haworth Press, 1991); M. Bury and J. Gabe, "Tranquillisers and health care in crisis," *Social Science and Medicine* 32 (1991): 449–454.
116. D. Sheehan, "Angles on Panic," in Healy, *The Psychopharmacologists*, vol. 3, 479–504.
117. Bury and J. Gabe, "Tranquillisers and health care in crisis," 449–454.
118. D. Healy and R. Tranter, "Pharmacopsychiatric stress syndromes," *Journal of Psychopharmacology* 13 (1999): 287–290, with commentaries by H. Ashton, R. Baldessarini, P. Haddad, I. Anderson, L. Hollister, and P. Tyrer.
119. J. Olds, "Mapping the Mind onto the Brain," in F. G. Worden, J. P. Swazey, and G. Adelman, ed., *The Neurosciences: Paths of Discovery* (Cambridge, Mass.: MIT Press, 1975), 375–400.
120. Taped interview with James Woods at the American College of Neuropsychopharmacology meeting in San Juan, Puerto Rico, December 1998; L. Cook, "Pharmacology, behaviour, and chlorpromazine," in Healy, *The Psychopharmacologists*, vol. 2, 39–70.
121. R. DeGrandpre and E. White, "Drugs in the care of the self," *Common Knowledge* 4 (2000): 27–48.
122. J. Woods, J. L. Katz, and G. Winger, "Abuse liability of benzodiazepines," *Pharmacological Reviews* 39 (1987): 251–414.
123. D. Healy, "The three faces of the antidepressants: critical comments on the clinical-economic framework of diagnosis," *Journal of Nervous and Mental Disease* 187 (1999): 174–180.
124. N. J. Coupland, C. J. Bell, and J. P. Potokar, "Serotonin reuptake inhibitor withdrawal," *Journal of Clinical Psychopharmacology* 16 (1996): 356–362.
125. J. F. Rosenbaum, M. Fava, S. L. Hoog, R. C. Ashcroft, and W. Krebs, "Selective serotonin reuptake inhibitor discontinuation syndrome: a randomised clinical study," *Biological Psychiatry* 44 (1998): 77–87; see C. Medawar, "The antidepressant web," *International Journal of Risk and Safety in Medicine* 10 (1997): 75–126, and see <www.socialaudit.org> for a documentary record of the evolution of the issue.

126. Sheehan, "Angles on Panic."

127. C. Medawar, *Power and Dependence* (London: Social Audit, 1992); Smith, *A Social History of the Minor Tranquillisers.*

128. R. Tranter and D. Healy, "Neuroleptic discontinuation syndromes," *Journal of Psychopharmacology* 12 (1998): 306–311.

129. R. Battegay, "Forty-Four Years in Psychopharmacology," in Healy, *The Psychopharmacologists*, vol. 3, 371–394.

130. R. J. Baldessarini and A. C. Viguera, "Neuroleptic withdrawal in schizophrenic patients," *Archives of General Psychiatry* 52 (1995): 189–192; A. C. Viguera, R. J. Baldessarini, J. D. Hegarty, D. P. van Kammen, and M. Tohen, "Clinical risk following abrupt and gradual withdrawal of maintenance neuroleptic treatment," *Archives of General Psychiatry* 54 (1997): 49–55.

131. Healy and Tranter, "Pharmacopsychiatric stress syndromes," 287–299.

132. R. Battegay and A. Gehring, "Influences of the Course of the Disease in schizophrenic Patients," in A. Cerletti and F. J. Bove, ed., *The Present Status of Psychotropic Drugs* (Amsterdam: Excerpta Medica, 1968), 460–463; see also R. Battegay, "At the Threshold to New Dimensions," in T. Ban, D. Healy, and E. Shorter, ed., *The Triumph of Psychopharmacology* (Budapest: Animula, 2000), 221–223.

133. D. Gaskell, "Drugs against drugs," *Chemistry in Britain* 34 (1998), 12, 27–32.

134. American Psychiatric Association, *Diagnostic and Statistical Manual*, 4th ed. (Washington D.C.: American Psychiatric Association Press, 1994), 263.

135. F. J. Ayd, "The Discovery of Amitriptyline," in Healy, *The Psychopharmacologists*, vol. 1, 81–110.

136. H. Weinstein, "Psychiatry and the CIA," *Journal of Psychopharmacology* 13 (1990): 287–299.

137. T. Ban, "They Used to Call It Psychiatry," in Healy, *The Psychopharmacologists*, vol. 1, 587–620; G. Simpson, "Clinical Psychopharmacology," in Healy, *The Psychopharmacologists*, vol. 2, 285–306.

138. T. Okuma, "The Discovery of the Psychotropic Effects of Carbamazepine," in Healy, *The Psychopharmacologists*, vol. 3, 259–280.

139. M. Toru, "Schizophrenia Research in Japan," in Healy, *The Psychopharmacologists*, vol. 3, 293–308.

140. CLRTP, "The Birth of Psychopharmacotherapy"; P. Simon, "Psychopharmacology in the Twenty-First Century," in Healy, *The Psychopharmacologists*, vol. 3, 523–542; J. Thuillier, "Ten Years That Changed the Face of Psychiatry," in Healy, *The Psychopharmacologists*, vol. 3, 543–560.

141. I got these details from Heinz Lehmann and Pierre Pichot. The restructured department solved the succession problem by creating chairs for both Pichot and Deniker.

5. TWISTED THOUGHTS AND TWISTED MOLECULES

1. S. Finger, *The Origins of Neuroscience* (New York: Oxford University Press, 1994), chap. 16. See also B. J. Clark, "The Versatile Ergot of Rye," in M. J. Parnham and J. Bruinvels, ed., *Discoveries in Pharmacology*, vol. 2 (Amsterdam: Elsevier, 1983), 3–35.
2. T. McKenna, *Food of the Gods: A Radical History of Plants, Drugs, and Human Evolution* (New York: Bantam Books, 1992).
3. G. Ginzburg, *Exstasies* (New York: Pantheon Books, 1991).
4. K. F. Kriple, "Ergotism and Erysipelas: St Anthony's Fire," in K. F. Kriple, ed., *Plagues, Pox, and Pestilence: Disease in History* (London: Weidenfield and Nicholson, 1997), 32–37; M. K. Matossian, *Poisons of the Past* (New Haven: Yale University Press, 1989); S. Plant, *Writing on Drugs* (London; Faber & Faber, 1999).
5. A. Hoffmann, "The Discovery of LSD," in F. J. Ayd and B. Blackwell, ed., *Discoveries in Biological Psychiatry* (Philadelphia: Lippincott, 1970); A. Hofmann, *LSD: My Problem Child* (Los Angeles: Jeremy P. Tarcher, 1983).
6. J.-J. Moreau de Tours, *Du haschisch et de 'aliénation mentale: études psycholigiques* (Paris: Fortin and Masson, 1845).
7. W. James, *The Varieties of Religious Experience: A Study in Human Nature* (1902; Harmondsworth, Eng.: Penguin Books, 1986).
8. K. Jaspers, *Algemeine Psychopathologie* (1912), trans. by M. Hamilton and J. Hoenig as *General Psychopathology*, 2nd ed., (Baltimore: Johns Hopkins University Press, 1965).
9. J. Thuillier, "Ten Years Which Changed Psychiatry," in D. Healy, *The Psychopharmacologists*, vol. 3 (London: Arnold, 2000).
10. J. Thuillier, *Les dix ans qui on changé la folie* (1980), trans. by G. Hickish and D. Healy as *Ten Years Which Changed the Face Of Mental Illness* (London: Martin Dunitz, 1999).
11. Ibid.
12. R. A. Sandison, A. M. Spencer, and J. D. Whitelaw, "The therapeutic value of lysergic acid diethylamide in mental illness," *Journal of Mental Science* 100 (1954): 491–507; R. A. Sandison, "Psychological aspects of the LSD treatment of the neuroses," *Journal of Mental Science* 100 (1954): 508–515; R. A. Sandison and J. D. Whitelaw, "Further studies in the therapeutic value of lysergic acid diethylamide in mental illness," *Journal of Mental Science* 103 (1957): 332–343.
13. H. H. de Jong, "Die experimentelle Katatonie," *Zentralblatt für die Gesamte Neurologie und Psychiatrie* 139 (1932): 468 ff.; also in H. H. de Jong, *Experimental Catatonia: A General Reaction Form of the Central Nervous System and Its Implications for Human Pathology* (Baltimore: Williams & Wilkins, 1945). L. Noteboom, "Experimental catatonia by means of derivatives of mescaline and epinephrine," *Proceedings of the Academy of Sciences* 37 (1934): 562.
14. D. Healy, *The Antidepressant Era* (Cambridge, Mass.: Harvard University Press, 1997), chap. 2; monoamine oxidase had been discovered earlier by Molly Hare but Richter's work gave it prominence. D. Richter, *A Life in*

Research (London: Stuart Phillips, 1987); D. Richter and D. Healy, "The origins of mental health neurosciences in Britain" *Journal of Psychopharmacology* 9 (1995): 392–399.

15. H. Osmond and J. R. Smythies, "Schizophrenia: a new approach," *Journal of Mental Science* 98 (1952): 309–315; A. Hoffer, H. Osmond, and J. R. Smythies, "Schizophrenia: a new approach: result of a year's research," *Journal of Mental Science* 100 (1954): 29–42.

16. Hoffer, Osmond, and Smythies, "Schizophrenia: a new approach: result of a year's research," 29–42; J. Smythies, "From Transmethylation to Oxidative Mechanisms," in T. Ban, D. Healy, and E. Shorter, *The Rise of Psychopharmacology and the Story of the CINP* (Budapest: Animula, 1998), 348–350; A. Hoffer, "The introduction of megavitamin therapy for treating schizophrenia," in T. Ban, D. Healy, and D. Shorter, *The Rise of Psychopharmacology and the Story of the CINP* (Budapest: Animula, 1998), 26–30.

17. W. L. Rees and G. N. King, "Desoxycortisone acetate and ascorbic acid treatment of schizophrenia," *Journal of Mental Science* 97 (1951): 376–380; W. L. Rees and G. N. King, "Cortisone in the treatment of schizophrenia," *Journal of Mental Science* 98 (1952): 408–413.

18. M. Vogt, communication to the British Pharmacological Society, 5 January 1952; M. Vogt, "The concentration of sympathin in different parts of the central nervous system under normal conditions and after the administration of drugs," *Journal of Physiology* 123 (1954): 451–481.

19. I. Page, "Neurochemistry as I Have Known It," in Ayd and Blackwell, ed., *Discoveries in Biological Psychiatry*, 53-58.

20. A. H. Amin, T. B. Crawford, and J. H. Gaddum, "The distribution of substance P and 5-hydroxytryptamine in the central nervous system of the dog," *Journal of Physiology* 126 (1954): 596–618.

21. A. Hoffer, "The Introduction of Megavitamin Therapy for Treating Schizophrenia," in Ban, Healy, and Shorter, *The Rise of Psychopharmacology and the Story of the CINP*, 26–30.

22. J. Stevens, *Storming Heaven: LSD and the American Dream* (London: Heinemann, 1988).

23. A. Huxley, *Brave New World* (London: Harper & Brothers, 1946).

24. A. Huxley, *The Doors of Perception* (London: Chatto and Windus, 1954); A. Huxley, *Heaven and Hell* (London: Chatto and Windus, 1956).

25. T. A. Ban and H. E. Lehmann, *Nicotinic Acid in the Treatment of Schizophrenias*, Canadian Mental Health Association Collaborative Study, Progress Report 1 (Montreal: Canadian Mental Health Association, 1970).

26. Healy, *The Antidepressant Era*, chap. 5.

27. See G. Ashcroft, "The Receptor Enters Psychiatry," in Healy, *The Psychopharmacologists*, vol. 3, 189–200, for a sense of the excitement of the period and an account of the discovery of HVA.

28. M. Sandler, "The place of chemical pathology in the development of psychopharmacology," *Journal of Psychopharmacology* 8 (1994): 124–133.

29. A. Jenner, "Catatonia, pink spots, and antipsychiatry," in Healy, *The Psychopharmacologists*, vol. 3, 135–156.

30. R. Baldessarini, "Biological transmethylation involving S-adenosylmethio-nine: development of assay methods and implications for neuropsychiatry," *International Review of Neuropsychiatry* 18 (1975): 41–67; Ban and Lehmann, *Nicotinic Acid in the Treatment of Schizophrenias.*

31. A. J. Friedhoff and E. Van Winkle, "Characteristics of amine found in the urine of schizophrenic patients," *Journal of Nervous and Mental Disease* 135 (1962): 550–555; A. J. Friedhoff and E. Van Winkle, "Conversion of dopamine to 3,4-dimethoxyphenylacetic acid in schizophrenic patients," *Nature* 199 (1963): 1271.

32. Ban and H. Lehmann, *Nicotinic Acid in the Treatment of Schizophrenias.*

33. R. E. Bourdillon, C. A. Clarke, P. Ridges, P. M. Sheppard, P. Harper, and S. A. Leslie, "Pink spot in urine of schizophrenics," *Nature* 208 (1965): 453–455.

34. S. Szara, "Hallucinogenic effects and metabolism of tryptamine derivatives in man," *Federation Proceedings* 20 (1961): 885–888.

35. E. Fischer, T. A. F. Lagravere, A. J. Vazquez, and A. O. DiStefano, "A bufotenine like substance in the urine of schizophrenics," *Journal of Nervous and Mental Disease* 133 (1961): 441–444.

36. Ban and Lehmann, *Nicotinic Acid in the Treatment of Schizophrenias.*

37. D. F. Efron, "Biochemistry of the psychoses," *Experimental Medicine and Surgery* 124, suppl. (1965): 8–12.

38. K. Smith, G. F. Thompson, and H. Koster, "Sweat in schizophrenic patients: identification of the odorous substance," *Science* 166 (1969): 398. See Cornelius van Rhyn in T. A. Ban and O. S. Ray, *A History of CINP* (Brentwood, Tenn.: J. M Productions, 1996), 230–234.

39. A. Jenner, "Catatonia, pink spots, and antipsychiatry," in Healy, *The Psychopharmacologists,* vol. 3, 135–156.

40. A. Hoffer, "Adrenochrome in blood plasma," *American Journal of Psychiatry* 114 (1958): 752.

41. S. Kety, "Current biochemical approaches to schizophrenia," *New England Journal of Medicine* 276 (1967): 325–331.

42. J. R. Smythies, "From Transmethylation to Oxidative Mechanisms," in Ban, Healy, and Shorter, *The Rise of Psychopharmacology and the Story of the CINP,* 348–350.

43. R. Baldessarini, interview at the American College of Neuropsychophar-macology annual meeting in San Juan, Puerto Rico, December 1998; H. A. Friedel, K. L. Goa, and P. Benfield, "S-adenosyl-L-methionine: a review of its pharmacological properties and therapeutic potential in liver dysfunc-tion and affective disorders in relation to its physiological role in cell me-tabolism," *Drugs* 38 (1989): 389–416.

44. R. Baldessarini, G. Stramentinoli, and J. F. Lipinski, "Methylation hypoth-esis," *Archives of General Psychiatry* 36 (1979): 303–307.

45. Ban and Lehmann, *Nicotinic Acid in the Treatment of Schizophrenias.*

46. Smythies, "From Transmethylation to Oxidative Mechanisms," 348–350.

47. H. M. Weinstein, *Psychiatry and the CIA: Victims of Mind Control* (Washing-ton D.C.: American Psychiatric Association Press, 1990).

48. D. Healy, *Images of Trauma* (London: Faber & Faber, 1993).

49. R. Crockett, R. A. Sandison, and A. Walk, "Hallucinogenic Drugs and Their Psychotherapeutic Use," in *Proceedings of the Quarterly Meeting of the Royal Medico-Psychological Association* (London, February 1961) (London: H. K. Lewis, 1963).; L. E. Hollister, "From Hypertension to Psychopharmacology: A Serendipitous Career," in D. Healy, *The Psychopharmacologists*, vol. 2 (London: Arnold, 1998), 215–235.

50. L. Grinspoon and J. B. Bakalar, *Psychedelic Drugs Reconsidered* (New York: the Lindesmith Center, 1997).

51. Thuillier, *Ten Years Which Changed the Face of Mental Illness*.

52. Weinstein, *Psychiatry and the CIA*.

53. D. Healy and F. Watson, "Human Volunteers in Psychopharmacology: Problems and Opportunities," in I. Hindmarch and P. Stonier, ed., *Human Psychopharmacology: Materials and Methods*, vol. 5 (Chichester, Eng.: John Wiley, 1995), 63–87.

54. Healy, *Images of Trauma*; R. Darnton, *Mesmerism and the End of the Enlightenment in France* (Cambridge, Mass.: Harvard University Press, 1968).

55. Healy, *Images of Trauma*.

56. L. Wright, *Twins: Genes, Environment, and the Mystery of Identity* (London: Weidenfeld and Nicolson, 1997).

57. D. Rosenthal and S. Kety, "The transmission of schizophrenia," *Journal of Psychiatric Research* 6, suppl.(1968): 1.

58. I. Gottesman, "Predisposed to Predispositions," in Healy, *The Psychopharmacologists*, vol. 2, 377–408.

59. This collapse seems to have been variously interpreted. Leon Eisenberg thought Wynne had had a heart attack; others thought he had become hysterical.

60. E. Slater, as reported by Rosenthal in Rosenthal and Kety, "The transmission of schizophrenia."

61. E. Kringlen, "Twin studies in schizophrenia with special emphasis on concordance figures," *American Journal of Medical Genetics* 97 (2000): 4–11.

62. See E. Kringlen, "Twins: still our best method," *Schizophrenia Bulletin* 2 (1976): 429–433; and E. Kringlen, "Schizophrenia: research in the Nordic countries," *Schizophrenia Bulletin* 6 (1980): 566–578.

63. E. Kringlen, "Twin studies in schizophrenia with special emphasis on concordance figures," *American Journal of Medical Genetics* 97 (2000): 4–11.

64. A. G. Debus, *The French Paracelsians* (Cambridge: Cambridge University Press, 1991).

65. Sometimes they are called the R and S forms of the molecule.

66. D. Barlow, "Receptors and the Chemist," in Healy, *The Psychopharmacologists*, vol. 3, 157–174. See also CLRTP, "The Birth of Psychopharmacotherapy: Explorations in a New World, 1952–1968," in Healy, *The Psychopharmacologists*, vol. 3, for an example of the different effects of l- and d-trimipramine.

67. R. Stephenson, "Receptors and Classical Pharmacology," in Healy, *The Psychopharmacologists*, vol. 3, 175–188; Parascandola, "The Development of

Receptor Theory," in Parnham and Bruinvels, ed., *Discoveries in Pharmacology*, vol. 3, 129–155.

68. G. Barger and H. H. Dale, "β-lmidazolylethylamine, a depressor constituent of intestinal mucosa," *Journal of Physiology* 41 (1910): 499–503.
69. See P. Mazumdar, *Species and Specificity* (Cambridge: Cambridge University Press, 1996).
70. Richter, *A Life in Research*.
71. A. J. Clark, *The Mode of Action of Drugs on Cells* (London: Arnold, 1933); A. J. Clark, "General Pharmacology," in *Heffter's Handbuch der experimentellen Pharmakologie* (Berlin: Springer, 1937).
72. Stephenson, "Receptors and Classical Pharmacology," 175–188.
73. Parascandola, "The Development of Receptor Theory," 129–155.
74. G. O. Carrier, "Evolution of the Dual Adrenergic Receptor Concept: Key to Past Mysteries and Modern Therapy," in Parnham and Bruinvels, ed., *Discoveries in Pharmacology*, vol. 3, 203–221.
75. D. Barlow, "Receptors and the Chemists."
76. Quotation from R. W. Gerard, "Biological roots of psychiatry," *Science* 122 (1955): 255; see also R. W. Gerard, "Physiology and psychiatry," *American Journal of Psychiatry* 105 (1949): 161–173.
77. For example, John Eccles was one of the key proponents of the electrophysiological view, and although he "came over" to the neurotransmitter view in 1950, he remained to the end of his life very concerned about the implications of neuroscientific research for our views of ourselves. See K. Popper and J. Eccles, *The Self and Its Brain* (London: Routledge, 1979).
78. See J. Watkins, "Excitatory Amino Acids: From Basic Science to Therapeutic Applications," in Healy, *The Psychopharmacologists*, vol. 2, 351–375.
79. D. R. Curtis, J. W. Phillis, and J. C. Watkins, "Actions of amino-acids on the isolated hemisected spinal cord of the toad," *British Journal of Pharmacology* 16: (1961), 262–283.
80. Watkins, "Excitatory amino acids," 351–375.
81. Stephenson, "Receptors and Classical Pharmacology," 175–188.
82. Recognition of the role norepinephrine played in the brain was delayed by a belief that it came in with blood and was not intrinsic to the brain. Vogt showed a disparity between the distribution of blood vessels and NE (sympathin) in dog brains, and this finding opened up the possibility of endogenous norepinephrine transmission.
83. M. Vialli and V. Erpsamer, "Cellule enterocromaffini e cellule basigranulose acidofile nei vertebrati," *Zischrift Zellforsch und Mikroscopie Anatomie* 19 (1933): 743. See also V. Erpsamer, "The Search for and Discovery of Biogenic Amines and Neuropeptides in Unexpected Places, in *The Neurosciences: Paths of Discovery*, vol. 2, ed. F. Samson and G. Adelman (Boston: Birkhäuser, 1989), 65–80.
84. M. Rapoport, A. Green, and I. H. Page, "Purification of the substance which is responsible for vasoconstrictor activity of serum," *Federation Proceedings* 6 (1949): 184.

85. Page, "Neurochemistry as I Have Known It," 53–58.
86. A. H. Amin, T. B. Crawford, and J. H. Gaddum, "The distribution of substance P and 5-hydroxytryptamine in the central nervous system of the dog," *Journal of Physiology* 126 (1954): 596–618.
87. S. Garattini and D. Healy, "The Role of Independent Science in Psychopharmacology D. Healy, *The Psychopharmacologists*," vol. 1 (London: Chapman & Hall, 1996), 135–157.
88. I owe these details to a conversation with Gaddum's daughter; see J. A. Gaddum, "Antagonism between lysergic acid-dieythlamide and 5-hydroxytryptamine," *Journal of Physiology* 121 (1953): 15.
89. E. Shaw and D. W. Woolley, "Yohimbine and ergot alkaloids as naturally occurring antimetabolites of serotonin," *Journal of Biological Chemistry* 203 (1953): 979–989; D. W. Woolley and E. Shaw, "A biochemical and pharmacological suggestion about certain mental disorders," *Science* 119 (1954): 587–588; D. W. Woolley and E. Shaw, "Some neurophysiological aspects of serotonin," *British Medical Journal* 2 (1954): 122–126; J. Thuillier, "La sérotonine," *Concours Médical* 7 (1956): 3177; J. Delay and J. Thuillier, "Psychiatrie expérimentale et psychopharmacologie," *La Semaine des Hôpitaux de Paris* 62 (1956): 1–7.
90. J. H. Gaddum and K. A. Hameed, "Drugs which antagonise 5-hydroxytryptamine," *British Journal of Pharmacology* 9 (1954): 240–248; J. H. Gaddum and Z. P. Piccarelli, "Two kinds of trypamine receptor," *British Journal of Pharmacology* 12 (1957): 323–328.
91. D. Richter, M. Reiss, and J. Elkes, "Ignorances in Biochemistry, Endocrinology, and Pharmacology," in J. M. Tanner, ed., *Prospects in Psychiatric Research* (Oxford: Blackwell Scientific Publications, 1953), 109–155; P. B. Bradley and J. Elkes, "The effects of some drugs on electrical activity of the brain," *Brain* 80 (1957): 77–117.
92. Ciba Foundation symposium in London in 1960: see Healy, *The Antidepressant Era*, chap. 5.
93. A. Carlsson, "The Rise of Neuropsychopharmacology: Impact on basic and Clinical Neuroscience," in Healy, *The Psychopharmacologists*, vol. 1, 51–80; J. Elkes, "Towards Footings in a New Science: Psychopharmacology, Receptors, and the Pharmacy within," in Healy, *The Psychopharmacologists*, vol. 2, 183–214.
94. A. Pletscher, P. A. Shore, and B. B. Brodie, "Serotonin release as a possible mechanism of reserpine action," *Science* 122 (1955): 374–375.
95. F. Sulser, "My Early Years with Tricyclics," in Ban, Healy, and Shorter, ed., *The Rise of Psychopharmacology and the Story of the CINP*, 81–83; M. Bickel, "From Imipramine to Desipramine," in Ban, Healy, and Shorter, ed., *The Rise of Psychopharmacology and the Story of the CINP*, 84–86.
96. See Healy, *The Antidepressant Era*; Sulser, "My Early Years with Tricyclics," 81–83; Bickel, "From Imipramine to Desipramine," 84–86; and F. Sulser "From the Presynaptic Neurone to the Receptor and the Nucleus," in Healy, *The Psychopharmacologists*, vol. 3.

97. A. Carlsson and M. Lindqvist, "Effect of chlorpromazine or haloperidol on the formation of 3-methoxytyramine and normetanephrine in mouse brain," *Acta Pharmacologica* (Kobenhavn) 20 (1963): 140–144.

98. J. M. van Rossum, "The significance of dopamine receptor blockade in the mechanism of action of neuroleptic drugs," *Archives of International Pharmacodynamics and Therapeutics* 60 (1966): 492–494.

99. A. Carlsson, "Arvid Carlsson," in L. R. Squire, ed., *The History of Neuroscience in Autobiography*, vol. 2 (San Diego: Academic Press, 1998), 28–66; Carlsson, "The Rise of Neuropsychopharmacology," 51–80.

100. A. Bertler and E. Rosengren, "Occurrence and distribution of dopamine in brain and other tissues," *Experientia* 15 (1959): 10–20; A. Carlsson, M. Lindqvist, T. Magnusson, and B. Waldeck, "On the presence of 3-hydroxytryptamine in brain," *Science* 127 (1958): 471. See A. Carlsson, "The occurrence, distribution, and physiological role of catecholamines in the nervous system," *Pharmacological Reviews* 11 (1959): 490–493. This work led Carlsson to a share of the 2000 Nobel Prize for medicine.

101. H. Ehringer and O. Hornykiewicz, "Veteilung von Noradrenalin und Dopamin im Gehirn des Menschen und ihr Verhalten bei Erkrankungen des extrapyramidalen Systems," *Klinische Wochenschrift* 38 (1960): 1236–1239; W. Birkmaier and O. Hornykiewicz, "Der L-3-4-Dihydroxyphenylalanin (= DOPA): Effekt beim Parkinson-Syndrom des Menschen: Zur Pathogenese und Behandlung der Parkinson-Akinese," *Archiv für Psychiatrie und Nervenkrantz* 203 (1961): 560–574; O. Hornykiewicz, "From Dopamine to Parkinson's Disease: A Personal Research Record," in F. Samson and G. Adelman, ed., *The Neurosciences: Paths of Discovery*, vol. 2 (Boston: Birkhauser, 1992), 125–148.

102. G. Curzon, "From Neurochemistry to Neuroscience," in Healy, *The Psychopharmacologists*, vol. 2, 307–323.

103. G. C. Cotzias, M. H. Van Woert, and I. M. Schiffer, "Aromatic amino acids and modification of Parkinsonism," *New England Journal of Medicine* 276 (1967): 374–379.

104. Carlsson, "Arvid Carlsson," 28–66.

105. J. J. Schildkraut, "The catecholamine hypothesis of affective disorders: a review of supporting evidence," *American Journal of Psychiatry* 122 (1965): 519–522; J. J. Schildkraut, "The Catecholamine Hypothesis," in Healy, *The Psychopharmacologists*, vol. 3, 111–134; See Healy, *The Antidepressant Era*, chap 5.

106. The problems with this position were discussed in Chapter 2; briefly, reserpine in clinical trials has been shown to be an antidepressant but in practice it can cause akathisia and dysphoria that may precipitate suicide.

107. Arvid Carlsson and Hans Corrodi developed the first of the SSRIs, zimelidine; see Healy, *The Antidepressant Era*, chap. 5.

108. Carlsson and Lindqvist, "Effect of chlorpromazine or haloperidol on the formation of 3-methoxytyramine and normetanephrine in mouse brain," 140–144.

109. Van Rossum, "The significance of dopamine receptor blockade in the mechanism of action of neuroleptic drugs," 492–494.

110. S. Snyder, "Visualising Receptors and Beyond," in Healy, *The Psychopharmacologists*, vol. 3, 213–238.

111. B. H. Kelves, *Naked to the Bone: Medical Imaging in the Twentieth Century* (New Brunswick: Rutgers University Press, 1997).

112. Snyder, "Visualising Receptors and Beyond," 213–238; C. Pert, *Molecules of Emotion* (New York: Simon & Schuster, 1998).

113. J. Hughes, "The Discovery of the Opioid Peptides," in Healy, *The Psychopharmacologists*, vol. 1, 539–564.

114. S. Snyder, S. P. Banerjee, H. I. Yamamura, and A. Greenberg, "Drugs, neurotoxins, and schizophrenia," *Science* 188 (1974): 1243–1245; I. Creese, D. R. Burt, and S. Snyder, "Dopamine receptor binding predicts clinical and pharmacological potencies of antischizophrenic drugs," *Science* 192 (1976): 481–483; P. Seeman, T. Lee, M. Chau-Wong, and K. Wong, "Antipsychotic drug doses and neuroleptic/dopamine receptors," *Nature* 261 (1976): 717–719.

115. D. Tarsy and R. J. Baldessarini, "Pharmacologically induced behavioral sensitivity to apomorphine," *Nature* 245 (1973): 262–263.

116. L. I. Iversen, "Neuroscience and Drug Development," in Healy, *The Psychopharmacologists*, vol. 2, 325–350; S. Snyder, "The dopamine hypothesis of schizophrenia: focus on the dopamine receptor," *American Journal of Psychiatry* 133 (1976): 197–202; H. Y. Meltzer and S. Stahl, "The dopamine hypothesis of schizophrenia: a review," *Schizophrenia Bulletin* 2 (1976): 19–.

117. S. H. Snyder, "Schizophrenia," *Lancet* 2 (1982): 970–973.

118. A. Carlsson, "The current status of the dopamine hypothesis," *Neuropsychopharmacology* 1 (1988): 179–186.

119. Iversen, "Neuroscience and Drug Development," 325–350.

120. H. N. Wagner, H. D. Burns, R. F. Daniels, D. F. Wong, B. Langstrom, T. Duelfer, J. J. Frost, H. T. Raesrt, J. M. Links, S. B. Rosenbloom, S. E. Lukas, A. V. Kramer, and M. J. Kuhar, "Imaging dopamine receptors in the human brain by positron emission tomography," *Science* 221 (1983): 1264–1266.

121. D. F. Wong, H. N. Wagner, L. E. Tune, R. F. Dannals, G. D. Pearlsson, J. M. Links, C. A. Tamminga, E. P. Broussolle, H. T. Ravert, A. A. Wilson, J. K. Toung, J. Malat, F. A. Williams, L. A. O'Tuama, S. H. Snyder, M. J. Kuhar, and A. Gjedde, "Positron emission tomography reveals elevated D-2 dopamine receptors in drug-naïve schizophrenics," *Science* 234 (1986): 1558–1563.

122. L. Farde, F.-A. Wiesel, S. S. Elander, C. Halldin, A.-L. Nordstrom, H. Hall, and G. Sedvall, "D2-dopamine receptors in neuroleptic-naïve schizophrenic patients," *Archives of General Psychiatry* 47 (1988): 213–219.

123. D. L. Rosenhan, "On being sane in insane places," *Science* 179 (1973): 250–258.

124. M. Roth, "Psychiatry and its critics," *British Journal of Psychiatry* 122 (1973): 373–378.

125. F. Sulser, "From Presynaptic Neurone to the Receptor and the Nucleus," in Healy, *The Psychopharmacologists*, vol. 3, 239–258.

126. P. Simon, "Twenty-First Century Drug Development," in Healy, *The Psychopharmacologists*. vol. 3, 543–542.

127. G. Chouinard and B. D. Jones, "Neuroleptic-induced supersensitivity psychosis," *American Journal of Psychiatry* 135 (1978): 1409–1410.

128. J. Pressman, *Last Resort: Psychosurgery and the Limits of Medicine* (Cambridge: Cambridge University Press, 1998).

129. S. Peroutka and S. H. Snyder, "Multiple serotonin receptors: differential binding of 3H.5-hydroxytryptamine, 3H.lysergic acid diethylamide, and 3H.spiroperidol," *Molecular Pharmacology* 16 (1979): 687–699.

130. D. Healy, "D1 and D2 and D3," *British Journal of Psychiatry* 159 (1991): 319–324.

131. Iversen, "Neuroscience and Drug Development," 325–350.

132. H. Y. Meltzer, "The mechanism of action of novel antipsychotic drugs," *Schizophrenia Bulletin* 17 (1992): 263–287.

133. M. Carlsson and A. Carlsson, "Interactions between glutamatergic and monoaminergic systems within the basal ganglia: implications for schizophrenia and Parkinson's disease," *Trends in Neuroscience* 13 (1994): 272–276.

134. D. Rushton and H. Steinberg, "Mutual potentiation of amphetamine and amylobarbitone measured by activity in rats," *British Journal of Pharmacology* 21 (1963): 295—305.; H. Steinberg, "Bridging the Gap: Psychology, Pharmacology, and after," in Healy, *The Psychopharmacologists*, vol. 1, 215–238.

135. H. Steinberg, "Drugs and animal behaviour," *British Medical Bulletin* 20 (1964): 75–80; H. Steinberg, C. Davies, C. Stanford, E. Sykes, and P. Terry, "Immobility and backward walking induced by co-administration of clenbuterol, amitriptyline, or imipramine with chlordiazepoxide in mice," *Pharmacopsychoecologia* 1 (1988): 15–22; M. Hughes, E. Sykes, and H. Steinberg, "Drug interactions represented by high resolution computer graphics," *Neuropharmacology and Neurotoxicology* 3 (1992): 625–628.

136. M. Taeschler, "Pharmacological Aspects," in D. Bente and P. B. Bradley, ed., *Neuropsychopharmacology*, vol. 4 (Amsterdam: Elsevier, 1965), 201. See D. Healy, "Drugs and Industry," in Ban, Healy, and Shorter, *The Rise of Psychopharmacology and the Story of the CINP*, 51–55.

137. V. Pedersen and K. Bøgesø, "Drug Hunting," in Healy, *The Psychopharmacologists*, vol. 2, 561–579.

138. Snyder, "Visualising Receptors and beyond," 213–238.

139. E. Warawa, "From Neuroleptics to Antipsychotics," in Healy, *The Psychopharmacologists*, vol. 3, 505–522.

140. J. Watkins, "Excitatory Amino Acids: From Basic Science to Therapeutic Applications," in Healy, *The Psychopharmacologists*, vol. 2, 351–375.

6. POSITIVE AND NEGATIVE

1. J. F. Brady, "The Evolution of Behavioural Pharmacology," in D. Healy, *The Psychopharmacologists*, vol. 2 (London: Arnold, 1998), 71–92.

2. J. Thuillier, *Les dix ans qui ont changé la folie*, trans. by G. Hickish and D. Healy as *Ten Years That Changed the Face of Mental Illness* (London: Martin Dunitz, 2000); see the case of Philippe Burg.

3. R. Battegay, "Forty-Four Years in Psychiatry and Psychopharmacology," in D. Healy, *The Psychopharmacologists*, vol. 3 (London: Arnold, 2000), 371–397.

4. D. Klein, "Reaction Patterns to Psychotropic Drugs and the Birth of Panic Disorder," in D. Healy, *The Psychopharmacologists*, vol. 1 (London: Arnold, 1996), 329–352.

5. H. Lehmann, "Psychopharmacotherapy," in Healy, *The Psychopharmacologists*, vol.1, 159–186.

6. L. Hollister, "From Hypertension to Psychopharmacology: A Serendipitous Career," in Healy, *The Psychopharmacologists*, vol. 2, 215–236.

7. CLRTP, "The Birth of Psychopharmacotherapy: Explorations in a New World, 1952–1968," in Healy, *The Psychopharmacologists*, vol. 3, 1–54.

8. S. Goldberg, J. O. Cole, and G. L. Klerman, "Phenothiazine treatment in acute schizophrenia," *Archives of General Psychiatry* 10 (1964): 246–261; S. C. Goldberg, G. L. Klerman, and J. O. Cole, "Changes in schizophrenic psychopathology and ward behaviour as a function of phenothiazine treatment," *British Journal of Psychiatry* 111 (1965): 120–133.

9. A. Broadhurst, "Before and after Imipramine," in Healy, *The Psychopharmacologist*, vol. 1, 111–134; R. Domenjoz, "From DDT to Imipramine," in Healy, *The Psychopharmacologists*, vol. 3, 357–370.

10. D. Healy, *The Antidepressant Era* (Cambridge, Mass.: Harvard University Press, 1997), chap 2.

11. T. Kobayakawa, "The Japanese Psychopharmacology Marketplace," in Healy, *The Psychopharmacologists*, vol. 3, 281–292.

12. CLRTP, "The Birth of Psychopharmacotherapy," 1–54. J. Guyotat and P. A. Lambert, "Un nouvel antidepressif derive de l'iminodibenzyl: la Trimeprimine," in P. Bradley et al., *Neuropsychopharmacology* (Amsterdam: Elsevier, 1963), 290–294.

13. See Chapter 4 and see also D. Healy, "D-1, D-2, and D-3," *British Journal of Psychiatry* 159 (1991): 319–324.

14. G. Eikmeier, M. Berger, E. Lodemann, K. Muszynski, S. Kaumeier, and M. Gastpar, "Trimipramine: an aytpical neuroleptic?" *International Clinical Psychopharmacology* 6 (1991): 147–153.

15. L. L. Iversen, "From Neuroscience to Drug Development," in Healy, *The Psychopharmacologists*, vol. 2, 325–350.

16. M. Uchiyama, K. Tanaka, K. Isse, and M. Toru, "Efficacy of mianserin on symptoms of delirium in the aged," *Progress in Neuro-Psychopharmacology and Biological Psychiatry* 20 (1996): 651–656

17. CLRTP, "The Birth of Psychopharmacotherapy," 1–54.

18. "Science Notes: Mental Drug Shows Promise," *New York Times*, 7 April 1957.

19. See Healy, *The Antidepressant Era*.

20. V. Pedersen and K. Bøgesø, "Drug Hunting," in Healy, *The Psychopharmacologists*, vol. 2, 561–580.

21. F. Ayd, video interview for American College of Neuropsychopharmacology Archives, ACNP annual meeting, December 1998.

22. CLRTP, "The Birth of Psychopharmacotherapy," 1–54.

23. R. de Alarcon and M. W. P. Carney, "Severe depressive mood changes following slow-release intramuscular fluphenazine injection," *British Medical Journal* 1969, 564–567.

24. V. Pedersen and K. Bøgesø, "Drug Hunting," in D. Healy, *The Psychopharmacologists*, vol. 2, 561–579.

25. Pedersen and Bøgesø, "Drug Hunting," 561–579.

26. M. Toru and M. Takashima, "Haloperidol in large doses reduces the cataleptic response and increases noradrenaline metabolism in the brain of the rat," *Neuropharmacology* 24 (1981): 231–236.

27. C. Thompson, "The use of high dose antipsychotic medication," *British Journal of Psychiatry* 164 (1994): 448–458.

28. Pedersen and Bøgesø, "Drug Hunting," 561–579.

29. R. J. Baldessarini, B. M. Cohen, and M. H. Teicher, "Significance of neuroleptic doses and plasma levels in the pharmacological management of the psychoses," *Archives of General Psychiatry* 45 (1988): 79–91.

30. L. Farde, F.-A. Wiesel, C. Halldin, and G. Sedvall, "Central D-2 dopamine receptor occupancy in schizophrenic patients treated with antipsychotic drugs," *Archives of General Psychiatry* 45 (1988): 71–76.

31. H. Coppens, C. J. Sloof, A. M. Paans, T. Wiegman, W. Vaalburg, and J. Korf, "High central D2 dopamine receptor occupancy as assessed with positron emission tomography in medicated but therapy resistant schizophrenic patients," *Biological Psychiatry* 29 (1991): 629–634.

32. T. van Putten, S. R. Marder, and J. Mintz, "A controlled dose comparison of haloperidol in newly admitted schizophrenic patients," *Archives of General Psychiatry* 47 (1989): 754–758; A. Rifkind, S. Doddi, B. Karagigi, M. Borenstein, and M. Washspress, "Dosage of haloperidol for schizophrenia," *Archives of General Psychiatry* 48 (1991): 166–170.

33. Healy, *The Antidepressant Era*.

34. J. Schmutz and E. Eichenberger, "Clozapine," in J. S. Bindra and D. Lednicer, ed., *Chronicles of Drug Discovery*, vol. 1 (New York: John Wiley, 1982), 39–59.

35. H. Heimann and G. Stille, "Clozapin: Ein historischer Ruckblick und eine Laudatio," in D. Naber and F. Muller-Spahn, ed., *Clozapin: Pharmakologie und Klinik eines atypischen Neuroleptikums* (Berlin: Springer-Verlag, 1994), 1–4.

36. G. I. Gessa and G. U. Corsini, *Apomorphine and Other Dopaminomimetics*, vol. 1: *Basic Pharmacology* (New York: Raven Press, 1981).

37. Schmutz and Eichenberger, "Clozapine," 39–59.

38. Heimann and Stille, "Clozapin," 1–4.

39. P. Simon, "Twenty-First Century Drug Development," in Healy, *The Psychopharmacologists*, vol. 3, 523–542.

40. G. Stille and K. Fischer-Cornelssen, "Die Entwicklung von Clozapin (Leponex): ein Mysterium?" in O. Linde, ed., *Pharmakopsychologie im Wandel der Zeit* (Berlin: Springer-Verlag, 1988), 333–348.

41. H. Hippius, "The Foundation of the CINP and the Discovery of Clozapine," in Healy, *The Psychopharmacologists*, vol. 1, 187–214. See Battegay, "Forty-Four Years of Psychiatry and Psychopharmacology," 371–394.

42. J. Angst, D. Bente, P. Berner, H. Heimann, H. Helmchen, and H. Hippius, "Das klinische Wirkungsbild von Clozapin," *Pharmakopsychiatrie* 4 (1971): 201–221; J. Angst, U. Jaenicke, A. Padrutt, and C. Scharfetter, "Ergebnis eines Doppelblindversuches von HF 1854 im vergleich zu Levomepromazin," *Pharmakopsychiatrie Neuro-Psychopharmakologie* 4 (1971): 192–200; J. Angst, "The Myths of Psychopharmacology," in Healy, *The Psychopharmacologists*, vol. 1, 287–308.

43. R. J. Baldessarini, "Clozapine: a novel antipsychotic agent," *New England Journal of Medicine* 324 (1990): 746–754; D. Healy, "Psychopharmacology and the ethics of resource allocation," *British Journal of Psychiatry* 162 (1993): 23–29.

44. Hippius, "The Foundation of the CINP and the Discovery of Clozapine," 187–214.

45. Angst, "The Myths of Psychopharmacology," 287–308.

46. J. Idanpaan-Heikkila, E. Alhava, M. Olkinuora, and I. Pavla, "Clozapine and agranulocytosis," *Lancet* 2 (1975): 657; H. A. Amsler, L. Teerenhovi, E. Barth, K. Harjula, and P. Vuopio, "Agranulocytosis in patients treated with clozapine: a study of the Finnish epidemic," *Acta Psychiatrica Scandinavia* 56 (1977): 241–248; P. Wyden, *Conquering Schizophrenia* (New York: Basic Books, 1997).

47. H. Hippius, "Dynamic Action of Phenothiazines and Reserpine," in N. S. Kline, ed., *Psychopharmacology Frontiers* (Boston: Little Brown, 1957).

48. Clozapine was, in fact, later to become the most widely used antipsychotic in China.

49. The clinical trial program was too small to establish for certain that it did not cause agranulocytosis.

50. E. Warawa, "From Neuroleptics to Antipsychotics," in Healy, *The Psychopharmacologists*, vol. 3, 505–522.

51. The trade name Leponex can be read as a combination of "lepus," Latin for a hare, and "ex," meaning former or out. One of the main proponents of the neuroleptics as opposed to the antipsychotics was Hans Haase, whose name also means hare. The name Leponex was widely taken as a rebuff to the ideas advocated by Janssen, Haase, and Deniker.

52. R. Battegay, "At the Threshold to New Dimensions," in T. Ban, D. Healy, and E. Shorter, ed., *The Triumph of Psychopharmacology* (Budapest: Animula, 2000), 221–223.

53. H. Hippius, unpublished manuscript on Hanns Bühlmann.

54. G. Simpson, "Clinical Psychopharmacology," in Healy, *The Psychopharmacologists*, vol. 2, 285–306.

55. The evidence on clozapine and tardive dyskinesia is reviewed in J. A. Lieberman, B. L. Saltz, C. A. Johns, S. Pollack, M. Borenstein, and J. Kane, "The effects of clozapine on tardive dyskinesia," *British Journal of Psychiatry* 158 (1991): 503–510. See also G. Honigfeld, J. Parin, and J. Singer, "Clozapine: antipsychotic activity in treatment resistant schizophrenics," *Advances in Therapy* 1 (1984): 77–97.

56. P. Leber, unpublished interview conducted at the CINP meeting in Washington, D.C., June 1994.

57. J. Kane, G. Honigfeld, J. Singer, and H. Meltzer, "Clozapine for the treatment-resistant schizophrenic," *Archives of General Psychiatry* 45 (1988): 789–796; H. Meltzer, "A Career in Biological Psychiatry," in Healy, *The Psychopharmacologists*, vol. 1, 483–508.

58. Meltzer, "A Career in Biological Psychiatry," 483–508; Wyden, *Conquering Schizophrenia*.

59. Healy, "Psychopharmacology and the ethics of resource allocation," 23–29.

60. J. Sigwald, D. Bouttier, C. Raymond, and C. Piot, "Quatre cas de dykinésie facio-bucco-linguo-masticatrice a évolution prolongée secondaire a un traitement par les neuroleptiques," *Revue Neurologique* 100 (1959): 751–755.

61. L. Uhrbrand and A. Faurbye, "Reversible and irreversible dyskinesia after treatment with perphenazine, chlorpromazine, reserpine, and ECT," *Psychopharmacologia* 1 (1960): 408–418.

62. F. J. Ayd, "A survey of drug induced extrapyramidal reactions," *Journal of the American Medical Association* 175 (1961): 1054–1060.

63. Ayd, video interview for American College of Neuropsychopharmacology Archives, December 1998.

64. R. Hunter, C. J. Earl, and S. Thornicroft, "An apparently irreversible syndrome of abnormal movements following phenothiazine medication," *Proceedings of the Royal Society of Medicine* 57 (1964): 758–762.

65. Battegay, "Forty-Four Years of Psychiatry and Psychopharmacology."

66. Ayd, video interview for American College of Neuropsychopharmacology Archives, December 1998.

67. O. Vinar, "My Memories of Early Psychotropic Drug Development," in Ban, Healy, and Shorter, ed., *The Rise of Psychopharmacology and the Story of the CINP,* 229–235.

68. A. Faurbye, P. J. Rasch, P. B. Peterson, G. Brandborg, and G. Pakkenberg, "Neurological symptoms in pharmacotherapy of the psychoses," *Acta Psychiatrica Scandinavia* 40 (1964): 10–27.

69. F. J. Ayd, "Persistent dyskinesia," *Medical Science* 18 (1967): 32–40.

70. G. E. Crane and G. Paulson, "Dyskinesia and neuroleptics," *Archives of General Psychiatry* 19 (1968): 700–703.

71. G. E. Crane, "Persistent dyskinesia," *British Journal of Psychiatry* 122 (1997): 395–405. See D. G. C. Owen, *A Guide to the Extrapyramidal Side-Effects of Antipsychotic Drugs* (Cambridge: Cambridge University Press, 1999).

72. S. Gelman, *Medicating Schizophrenia: A History* (New Brunswick: Rutgers University Press, 1999); Owen, *A Guide to the Extrapyramidal Side-Effects of Antipsychotic Drugs.*

73. H.-J. Haase, "The therapeutic axial syndrome of neuroleptic drugs and its relationship with extrapyramidal symptoms," *Fortschrift für Neurologie und Psychiatrie,* 5 (1961): 245–268.

74. Gelman, *Medicating Schizophrenia.*

75. G. Crane, N. Kline, et al., *American Journal of Psychiatry* 124 (1968): February supplement.

76. Healy, *The Antidepressant Era,* chap 3.

77. D. Tarsy and R. J. Baldessarini, "Pharmacologically induced behavioral sensitivity to apomorphine," *Nature* 245 (1973): 262–263; D. Tarsy, "History and definition of tardive dyskinesia," *Clinical Neuropharmacology* 6 (1983): 91–99. Some years earlier, a dopamine hypothesis of tardive dyskinesia had been proposed by a Russian psychiatrist, E. L. Schelkunov; see Schelkunov, *Nature* 214 (1967): 1210–1212. See G. Oxenkrug, "Psychopharmacology behind the Iron Curtain," in Ban, Healy, and Shorter, ed., *The Rise of Psychopharmacology and the Story of the CINP* 330–333. Harold Klawans had also put forward a dopamine hypothesis of tardive dyskinesia; see R. J. Baldessarini and D. Tarsy, "Relationship of the actions of neuroleptic drugs to the pathophysiology of tardive dyskinesia," *International Review of Neurobiology* 21 (1979): 1–45. See also P. Deniker, "From chlorpromazine to tardive dyskinesia (brief history of the neuroleptics)," *Psychiatric Journal of the University of Ottawa* 14 (1989): 253–259.

78. American College of Neuropsychopharmacology Task Force, "Neurological syndromes associated with antipsychotic drug use: a special report" *Archives of General Psychiatry* 28 (1973): 465 ff.

79. H. L. Lennard and A. Bernstein, "Perspectives on the new psychoactive drug technology," in R. Cooperstock, *Social Aspects of the Medical Use of Psychotropic Drugs* (Toronto: Addiction Research Foundation, 1974), 149–161; P. Brown and S. Funk, "Tardive dyskinesia: barriers to the professional recognition of an iatrogenic disease," *Journal of Health and Social Behavior* 27 (1986): 116.

80. R. J. Baldessarini, J. O. Cole, J. M. Davis, G. Gardos, G. Simpson, D. Tarsy, et al., *Tardive Dykinesia: Task Force Report* (Washington, D.C.: American Psychiatric Association, 1980).

81. R. Baldessarini, video interview at the American College of Neuropsychopharmacology annual meeting, San Juan, Puerto Rico, December 1998.

82. M. Fink, "Neglected Disciplines in Psychopharmacology: Pharmaco-EEG and Electroshock," in Healy, *The Psychopharmacologists,* vol. 3, 431–458.

83. A. Sugerman, "Remembrance of Drugs Past," in Ban, Healy, and Shorter, ed., *The Triumph of Psychopharmacology,* 78–81.

84. P. Waldmeier, "From Mental Illness to Neurodegeneration," in Healy, *The Psychopharmacologists,* vol. 1, 565–586.

85. P. Breggin, *Toxic Psychiatry* (New York: St. Martin's Press, 1990).

86. B. H. Kevles, *Naked to the Bone: Medical Imaging in the Twentieth Century* (New Brunswick: Rutgers University Press, 1997).

87. P. Janssen, "From Haloperidol to Risperidone," in Healy, *The Psychopharmacologists*, vol. 2, 39–70.

88. A. A. Sugerman, "A pilot study of fluoropipamide (Dipiperone)," *Diseases of the Nervous System* 25 (1964): 355–358.

89. Janssen, "From Haloperidol to Risperidone," 39–70.

90. S. Snyder, "Visualising Receptors and More," in Healy, *The Psychopharmacologists*, vol. 3, 213–238.

91. M. Davis, "Mescaline: excitatory effects on acoustic startle are blocked by serotonin-2 antagonists," *Psychopharmacology* 93 (1987): 286–291.

92. P. Janssen, "From Haloperidol to Risperidone in the CINP Times," in Ban, Healy, and Shorter, ed., *The Triumph of Psychopharmacology*, 359–362.

93. These drugs are useful in treating delirious states and are antipsychotic in that sense.

94. Janssen, "From Haloperidol to Risperidone," 39–70.

95. Meltzer, "A Career in Biological Psychiatry," 483–508.

96. Healy, *The Antidepressant Era*.

97. J. L. Neumeyer, S. Lal, and R. J. Baldessarini, "Historical Highlights of the Chemistry, Pharmacology, and Early Clinical Uses of Apomorphine," in Gessa and Copsini, *Apomorphine and Other Dopaminomimetics*, vol. 1: *Basic Pharmacology*, 4–17.

98. S. Gee, *Transactions of the Clinical Society of London* 2 (1869): 166–169; E. Bleuler, *Dementia Praecox of a Group of Schizophrenias*, trans. J. Zinkin and N. Lewis (New York: International Universities Press, 1950), 486.

99. A. Carlsson, "Dopamine Autoreceptors," in O. Almgren, A. Carlsson, and J. Engel, ed., *Chemical Tools in Catecholamine Research*, vol. 2 (Amsterdam: North-Holland, 1975), 219–225.

100. C. A. Tamminga, M. H. Schaffer, R. C. Smith, and J. M. Davis, "Schizophrenic symptoms improve with apomorphine," *Science* 200 (1978): 567–568.

101. A. Carlsson, "Arvid Carlsson," in L. Squire, ed., *A History of Neuroscience in Autobiography* (San Diego: Academic Press, 1998), 28–66.

102. M. Ruffat, *175 Years of French Pharmaceutical Industry: History of Synthélabo* (Paris: La Découverte, 1998).

103. M. T. Nourissier, "Delagrange sur le divan de Marie-Thérèse," *L'Archer 21* (1990): 1–11.

104. P. Borenstein, C. Champion, Ph. Cujo, F. Gekiere, C. Olivenstein, and P. Kramarz, "Un psychotrope original: le sulpiride," *La Semaine des Hopitaux* 45 (1969): 1301–1314.

105. M. Toru, "Neurotransmitter research in Japan," in Healy, *The Psychopharmacologists*, vol. 3, 293–307.

106. M. Da Prada, R. Kettler, H. H. Keller, M. Cesura, J. G. Richards, J. Saura Marti, E. D. Muggli-Maniglio, P. C. Wyss, E. Kyburz, and R. Imhof, "From Moclobemide to Ro-10–6327 and Ro 41–1049: the development of

a new class of reversible, selective MAO-A and MAO-B inhibitors," *Journal of Neural Transmission* 29, suppl. (1990): 279–292.

107. G. Sedvall, "Development of the new antipsychotic Remoxipride," *Acta Psychiatrica Scandinavia* 82, suppl. (1990): 358.

108. D. J. King, "Atypical antipsychotics and the negative symptoms of schizophrenia," *Advances in Psychiatric Treatment* 4 (1998): 53–61.

109. J. Ravn, "The Discovery of the Thioxanthenes," in F. J. Ayd and B. Blackwell, *Discoveries in Biological Psychiatry* (Philadelphia: Lippincott, 1970).

110. Pedersen and Bøgesø, "Drug Hunting," 561–580.

111. P. Leber, "Managing Uncertainty," in Healy, *The Psychopharmacologists*, vol. 3, 607–622.

112. Wyden, *Conquering Schizophrenia*.

113. C. M. Beasley, B. E. Dornseif, J. C. Bosomworth, M. E. Sayler, A. H. Rampey, J. H. Heiligenstein, et al., "Fluoxetine and suicide: a meta-analysis of controlled trials of treatment for depression," *British Medical Journal* 303 (1991): 685–692.

114. See the preface in Healy, *The Psychopharmacologists*, vol. 3.

115. Warawa, "From Neuroleptics to Antipsychotics," 505–522.

116. K. Dewhurst, *Hughlings Jackson on Psychiatry* (Oxford: Sandford Publications, 1982); D. Healy, "Schizophrenia: basic, release, reactive, and defect processes," *Human Psychopharmacology* 5 (1990): 105—121; G. E. Berrios, "Positive and negative symptoms and Jackson," *Archives of General Psychiatry* 42 (1985): 95–97

117. Bleuler, *Dementia Praecox or the Group of Schizophrenias*.

118. Healy, "Schizophrenia: basic, reactive, release, and defect processes," 105–121.

119. J. K. Wing and G. W. Brown, *Institutionalism and Schizophrenia* (London: Cambridge University Press, 1970).

120. A. McGhie and J. Chapman, "Disorders of attention and perception in early schizophrenia," *British Journal of Medical Psychology* 34 (1961): 103–116; A. McGhie, *Pathology of Attention* (Harmondsworth, Eng.: Penguin Books, 1969); J. Chapman and A. McGhie, "An approach to the psychotherapy of cognitive dysfunction in schizophrenia," *British Journal of Medical Psychology* 36 (1963): 253–260; J. Chapman, "The early symptoms of schizophrenia," *British Journal of Psychiatry* 112 (1996): 225–251.

121. T. J. Crow, "Molecular pathology of schizophrenia: more than one disease process?" *British Medical Journal* 280 (1980): 66–68; T. J. Crow, "Positive and negative schizophrenic symptoms and the role of dopamine," *British Journal of Psychiatry* 137 (1980): 383–386; T. J. Crow, "The dopamine hypothesis survives but there must be a way ahead," *British Journal of Psychiatry* 151 (1987): 460–465.

122. M. Bleuler, *The Schizophrenic Disorders: Long-Term Patient and Family Studies* (New Haven: Yale University Press, 1978); L. Ciompi, "The natural history of schizophrenia in the long-term," *British Journal of Psychiatry* 136 (1980): 413—420; G. Huber, G. Gross, R. Schuttla, and M. Lanz, "Longitudinal studies of schizophrenia patients," *Schizophrenia Bulletin* 6 (1980): 592–605.

123. CLRTP, "The Birth of Psychopharmacotherapy," 1–54.

124. O. Vinar, "A Psychopharmacology That Nearly Was," in Healy, *The Psychopharmacologists*, vol. 3, 55–79.

125. Breggin, *Toxic Psychiatry*.

126. F. J. Fish, "The influence of the tranquilizers on the Leonhard schizophrenic syndromes," *Encéphale* 53 (1963): 245–249.

127. Janssen, "From Haloperidol to Risperidone," 39–70.

128. H. Baruk, J. Launay, and J. Berges, "Experimental catatonia and psychopathology of neuroleptics," *Journal of Clinical and Experimental Psychopathology* 19 (1958): 277–291.

129. H. Baruk, "Henri Baruk," in T. Ban and O Ray, ed., *The History of the CINP* (Brentwood, Tenn.: J. M. Productions, 1996), 195–196.

130. J. Delay, P. Pichot, T. Lempérière, et al., "L'emploi des butyrophenones en psychiatrie," in *Symposium Internazionale sull'Haloperidol e Triperidol* (Milan: Instituto Luso Farmaco d'Italia, 1962), 305–319.

131. S. N. Caroff, "Neuroleptic malignant syndrome," *Journal of Clinical Psychiatry* 41 (1980): 79–83.

132. A. Lazarus, S. C. Mann, and S. N. Caroff, *The Neuroleptic Malignant Syndrome and Related Conditions* (Washington, D.C.: American Psychiatric Press, 1989).

133. G. L. Fricchione, E. Cassem, et al, "Intravenous lorazepam in neuroleptic induced catatonia," *Journal of Clinical Psychopharmacology* 3 (1983): 338–342.

134. Cassem was a Jesuit priest. After the patient had responded, he was asked when leaving the ward what he had given the patient, and Cassem replied, "Holy Water." These details were reported by Frichione at an APA meeting in Washington, D.C., in May 1999.

135. Fink, "Neglected Disciplines in Psychopharmacology: Pharmaco-EEG and Electroshock."

136. W. J. Bleckwenn, "Production of sleep and rest in psychotic cases," *Archives of Neurology and Psychiatry* 24 (1930): 365–375.

137. G. Bush, M. Fink, G. Petrides, F. Dowling, and A. Francis, "Catatonia: rating scale and standardised examination," *Acta Psychiatrica Scandinavia* 93 (1996): 129–136.

138. See J. B. Lohr and A. A. Wisniewski, *Movement Disorders: A Neuropsychiatric Approach* (New York: John Wiley, 1987); D. Rogers, *Motor Disorder in Psychiatry: Toward a Neurological Psychiatry* (Chichester, Eng.: John Wiley, 1993).

139. Baruk, "Henri Baruk," 195–196.

140. Bush, Fink, Petrides, Dowling, and Francis, "Catatonia: rating scale and standardised examination," 129–136.

141. S. N. Caruff, S. C. Mann, and E. C. Campbell, "Atypical Antipsychotics and neuroleptic malignant syndrome," *Psychiatric Annals* 30 (2000): 314–324.

142. T. Van Putten, "Why do schizophrenic patients refuse to take their drugs?" *Archives of General Psychiatry* 31 (1974): 67–72; T. Van Putten, L. R. Mutalipassi, and S. R. Marder, "Phenothiazine induced decompensation," *Archives of General Psychiatry* 30 (1974): 13–19; T. Van Putten, "The many

faces of akathisia," *Comprehensive Psychiatry* 16 (1975): 43–47; Daniel Tarsy and David Marsden also drew attention to the problem.

143. M. R. Munetz and C. L. Cornes, "Distinguishing akathisia and tardive dyskinesia: a review of the literature," *Journal of Clinical Psychopharmacology* 3: (1983) 343–347.

7. THE SORCERER'S APPRENTICE

1. I. P. Pavlov, *Lectures on Conditioned Reflexes*, trans. W. H. Gantt (New York: International Publishers, 1928).
2. T. Ban, *Conditioning and Psychiatry* (Chicago: Aldine Press, 1964).
3. S. Freud, "Letter to Maria Bonaparte, 15th January 1930," in E. Jones, ed., *The Life and Work of Sigmund Freud*, vol. 3 (New York: Basic Books, 1930), 480.
4. S. Guze, "Psychotherapy and managed care," *Archives of General Psychiatry* 55 (1998): 561–562; R. Michels, "The role of psychotherapy: psychiatry's resistance to managed care," *Archives of General Psychiatry* 55 (1998): 563.
5. S. Guze, "Biological psychiatry: is there any other kind?" *Psychological Medicine* 90: (1989) 315–323.
6. R. Michels and P. M Marzuk, "Progress in psychiatry (1) & (2)," *New England Journal of Medicine* 329 (1993): 552–560 and 628–638.
7. American Psychiatric Association, "Practice guidelines for the treatment of patients with schizophrenia," *American Journal of Psychiatry* 154, suppl. (1997): 1–63.
8. D. Healy, *The Antidepressant Era* (Cambridge, Mass.: Harvard University Press, 1997), chap. 1.
9. P. Mazumdar, *Species and Specificity* (Cambridge: Cambridge University Press, 1995); N. Tomes, *The Gospel of Germs: Men, Women, and the Microbe in American Life* (Cambridge, Mass.: Harvard University Press, 1998).
10. J. Pressman, *Last Resort: Psychosurgery and the Limits of Medicine* (New York: Cambridge University Press, 1998).
11. Healy, *The Antidepressant Era*, chap. 3.
12. J. O. Cole, "The Evaluation of Psychotropic Drugs," in D. Healy, *The Psychopharmacologists*, vol. 1 (London: Arnold, 1996), 239–263; J. D. Cole and R. W. Gerard, *Psychopharmacology: Problems in Evaluation* (Washington, D.C.: National Academy of Sciences/National Research Council, 1956).
13. J. O. Cole, "The ECDEU program: a view from both sides of the table," *Psychopharmacology Bulletin* 6 (1970): 74–81.
14. F. Bernstein, "A ten-year history of the Early Clinical Drug Evaluation Unit (ECDEU) program," *Psychopharmacology Bulletin* 6 (1970): 1–21; M. Fink, "The Early Clinical Drug Evaluation Unit," in T. Ban, D. Healy, and E. Shorter, ed., *The Triumph of Psychopharmacology* (Budapest: Animula, 2000), 441–462.
15. D. F. Klein and M. Fink, "Psychiatric reaction patterns to imipramine," *American Journal of Psychiatry* 119 (1962): 432–438; D. F. Klein and

M. Fink, "Behavioral reaction patterns with phenothiazines," *Archives of General Psychiatry* 7 (1962): 449–459.

16. C. D. Burrell, "The foresight saga: ECDEU from the point of view of one member of industry," *Psychopharmacology Bulletin* 6 (1970): 64–73.

17. R. R. Bonato, W. Guy, P. Cleary, and K. Yang, "BLIPS: the information processing system for the ECDEU program," *Psychopharmacology Bulletin* 6 (1970): 22–47.

18. A. A. Sugerman, "Remembrance of Drugs Past," in Ban, Healy, and Shorter, ed., *The Triumph of Psychopharmacology*, 78–81.

19. Healy, *The Antidepressant Era*, chap. 3.

20. L. M. Dub and L. Lurie, "Use of Benzedrine in the depressed phase of the psychotic state," *Ohio State Medical Journal* 35 (1939: 39–45. Louis Lurie was the father of Max Lurie, the discoverer of the antidepressants.

21. Healy, *The Antidepressant Era*, chap. 3.

22. W. L. Rees, "The place of controlled trials in the development of psychopharmacology," *History of Psychiatry* 8 (1997): 1–20.

23. D. Davies and M. Shepherd, "Reserpine in the treatment of anxious and depressed patients," *Lancet* 2 (1955): 117–120; J. Elkes and C. Elkes, "Effects of chlorpromazine on the behaviour of chronically overactive psychotic patients," *British Medical Journal* 2 (1954): 560–565; L. E. Hollister, G. E. Krieger, A. Kringel, and R. H. Roberts, "Treatment of schizophrenic reactions with reserpine," *Annals of the New York Academy of Sciences* 61 (1955): 92–100; W. L. Rees and C. Lambert, "The value and limitations of chlorpromazine in the treatment of anxiety states," *Journal of Mental Science* 101 (1955): 834–840.

24. A. F. Frank and J. G. Gunderson, "The role of the therapeutic alliance in the treatment of schizophrenia," *Archives of General Psychiatry* 47 (1990): 228–236; J. Day, R. Bentall, F. Randall, D. Healy, and A. Rogers, "Therapeutic alliances and compliance," in press.

25. T. V. Moore, "A Century of Psychology in Its Relationship to American Psychiatry," in J. Hall, ed., *One Hundred Years of American Psychiatry* (New York: Columbia University Press, 1944), 462.

26. J. H. Masserman, *Behavior and Neurosis: An Experimental Psychoanalytic Approach to Psychobiologic Principles* (Chicago: University of Chicago Press, 1943). See also J. H. Masserman, "Experimental and Clinical Vectors in Pharmacology," in J. H. Masserman, ed., *Current Psychiatric Therapies*, vol. 6 (New York: Grune & Stratton, 1976), 107–116.

27. Moore, "A Century of Psychology in Its Relationship to American Psychiatry," 462.

28. H. J. Eysenck, "The effects of psychotherapy: an evaluation," *Journal of Consulting and Clinical Psychology* 16 (1952): 319–324.

29. J. Wolpe, *Psychotherapy by Reciprocal Inhibition* (Stanford: Stanford University Press, 1958); I. Marks, "Marketing the Evidence," in D. Healy, *The Psychopharmacologists*, vol. 2 (London: Arnold, 1998), 543–560.

30. H. J. Eysenck, ed., *Behaviour Therapy and the Neuroses* (Oxford: Pergamon Press, 1960).

31. H. J. Eysenck, *Rebel with a Cause* (London: W. H. Allen, 1990).
32. T. Ayllon and N. Azin, *The Token Economy* (New York: John Wiley, 1968).
33. S. Rachman, "The Evolution of Cognitive Behaviour Therapy," in D. N. Clarke and C. H. Fairburn, ed., *The Science and Practice of Cognitive Behaviour Therapy* (Oxford: Oxford University Press, 1997), 3–26.
34. H. J. Eysenck, *The Structure of Human Personality* (London: Methuen, 1960); Eysenck, *Rebel with a Cause*; G. Claridge, "The psychopharmacology of individual differences," in Healy, *The Psychopharmacologists*, vol. 1, 441–462.
35. J. M. Reisman, *A History of Clinical Psychology* (New York: Hemisphere Publishing Corporation, 1991); E. Miller, "Twentieth Century British Clinical Psychology and Psychiatry: Their Historical Relationship," in H. Freeman and G. E. Berrios, ed., *150 Years of British Psychiatry*, vol. 2 (London: Athlone Press, 1996), 156–168.
36. M. Argyle, *The Psychology of Interpersonal Behaviour* (Harmondsworth, Eng.: Penguin Books, 1980).
37. M. Weissman, "Gerald Klerman and Psychopharmacotherapy," in Healy, *The Psychopharmacologists*, vol. 2, 521–542.
38. A. Ellis, "Rational psychotherapy," *Journal of General Psychology* 59 (1958): 35–49; A. Ellis, *Reason and Emotion in Psychotherapy* (New York: Lyle Stuart, 1962).
39. A. T. Beck, *Depression* (New York: Harper & Row, 1967).
40. Healy, *The Antidepressant Era*, chap. 7.
41. A. T. Beck, *Cognitive Therapy and the Emotional Disorders* (New York: International Universities Press, 1976).
42. D. Healy, *Images of Trauma* (London: Faber and Faber, 1993).
43. J. Brady, "The Evolution of Behavioural Pharmacology," in Healy, *The Psychopharmacologists*, vol. 2, 71–92.
44. A. Meyer, "The nature and conception of dementia praecox," *Journal of Abnormal Psychology* 1911: 274–285.
45. E. Kraepelin, "Die Erscheinungsformen des Irreseins" (1920), trans. as "The manifestations of insanity," *History of Psychiatry* 3 (1992): 499–529.
46. 8 March 1907. I owe these details to a telephone conversation with Dr. Cohen on 1 September 1999.
47. The link with Paul Dudley White provided Cohen with a political base when White became Eisenhower's cardiologist. See E. O. Wheeler, P. D. White, E. W. Reed, and M. E. Cohen, "Neurocirculatory asthenia (anxiety neurosis, effort syndrome, neurasthenia): a 20 year follow-up of 173 patients," *Journal of the American Medical Association* 142 (1950): 878–888.
48. M. Cohen and D. Healy, "The origins of DSM-III," *History of Psychiatry*, submitted.
49. P. W. Bridgman, *The Logic of Modern Physics* (New York: MacMillan, 1928). See also G. Bergman, "The logic of psychological concepts," *Philosophy of Science* 18 (1951): 93–110.
50. *Neurocirculatory Asthenia, Anxiety Neurosis, and Allied States* (Washington, D.C.: Office of the Surgeon General, Department of the Army, 1951).

51. W. L. Cassidy, N. B. Flanagan, M. Spellman, and M. E. Cohen, "Clinical observations in manic-depressive disease: a quantitative study of 100 manic-depressive patients and 50 medically sick controls," *Journal of the American Medical Association* 164 (1962): 1535–1546.

52. J. Purtell, E. Robins, and M. Cohen, "Prospective observations on clinical aspects of hysteria: a quantitative study of 50 hysteria patients and 156 control subjects," *Journal of the American Medical Association* 146 (1951): 902–909; E. Robins, J. J. Putell, M. Altmann, D. E. Reid, and M. E. Cohen, "Excessive surgery in hysteria: study of surgical procedures in 50 women with hysteria and 190 controls," *Journal of the American Medical Association* 151 (1953): 977–986.

53. E. Robins, J. Purtell, and M. Cohen, "'Hysteria' in men: a study of 38 patients so diagnosed and 194 control subjects," *New England Journal of Medicine* 246 (1951): 677–684.

54. S. Guze, "The Neo-Kraepelinian Revolution," in D. Healy, *The Psychopharmacologists*, vol. 3 (London: Arnold, 2000), 395–414.

55. G. Winokur, "Obituary," *Archives of General Psychiatry* 54 (1996): 374–375.

56. S. B. Guze, "The diagnosis of hysteria: what are we trying to do?" *American Journal of Psychiatry* 124 (1967): 491–498; E. Robins and S. B. Guze, "Establishment of diagnostic validity in psychiatric illness: its application to schizophrenia," *American Journal of Psychiatry* 126 (1970): 983–987.

57. S. B. Guze, "The need for toughmindedness in psychiatric thinking," *Southern Medical Journal* 63 (1970): 662–671.

58. R. Woodruffe, D. Goodwin, and S. B. Guze, *Psychiatric Diagnosis* (Oxford: Oxford University Press, 1975).

59. S. B. Guze, "The Neo-Kraepelinian Revolution," 395–414.

60. M. Kramer, "Some Problems for International Research Suggested by Observations on Differences at First Admissions to the Mental Hospitals of England and Wales," in *Proceedings of the Third World Congress of Psychiatry*, vol. 3 (Toronto: University of Toronto Press, 1963).

61. J. E. Cooper, R. E. Kendal, B. J. Gurland, L. Sharpe, J. R. Copeland, and R. Simon, *Psychiatric Diagnosis in New York and London* (London: Oxford University Press, 1972).

62. M. M. Katz, J. O. Cole, and H. A. Lowery, "Studies of the diagnostic process: the influence of symptom perception, past experience, and ethnic background on diagnostic decisions," *American Journal of Psychiatry* 125 (1969): 937–947.

63. R. E. Kendell et al., "Diagnostic criteria of American and British Psychiatrists," *Archives of General Psychiatry* 25 (1971): 123–130.

64. R. Spitzer, "A Manual for Diagnosis and Statistics," in Healy, *The Psychopharmacologists*, vol. 3, 415–430.

65. M. Shepherd, E. M. Brook, J. E. Cooper, et al., "An experimental approach to psychiatric diagnosis," *Acta Psychiatrica Scandinavia* 00, suppl. (1968); 201.

66. World Health Organization, *The International Pilot Study of Schizophrenia* (Geneva: World Health Organization, 1973).

67. World Health Organization, *Schizophrenia: A Multi-National Study* (Geneva: World Health Organization, 1975); World Health Organization, *Schizophrenia: An International Follow-up Study* (New York, John Wiley, 1979).

68. D. Rosenhan, "On being sane in insane places," *Science*, 179 (1973), 250–258.

69. M. M. Katz and G. L. Klerman, "Introduction: overview of the clinical studies programme (Psychobiology of Depression Study)," *American Journal of Psychiatry* 136 (1979): 49–51.

70. J. Schildkraut, "The catecholamine hypothesis of depression: a review of supporting evidence," *American Journal of Psychiatry* 122 (1965): 509–522.

71. T. A. Williams, M. M. Katz, and J. A. Shields, *Recent Advances in the Psychobiology of Depressive Illness*, Proceedings of the Williamsburg Conference in Virginia, 1969 (Washington, D.C.: Government Printing Office, 1972).

72. Katz and Klerman, "Introduction: overview of the clinical studies programme," 49–51.

73. M. M. Katz, J. O. Cole, and W. E. Barton, ed., *The Role and Methodology of Classification in Psychiatry and Psychopharmacology* (Washington, D.C.: Government Printing Office, 1968).

74. J. P. Feighner, E. Robins, S. B. Guze, R. Woodruffe, G. Winokur, and R. Munoz, "Diagnostic criteria for use in psychiatric research," *Archives of General Psychiatry* 26 (1972): 57–63.

75. R. L. Spitzer, J. Endicott, and E. Robins, *Research Diagnostic Criteria (RDC) for a Selected Group of Functional Disorders"* (New York: New York State Department of Mental Hygiene, Biometics Branch, 1975).

76. G. L. Klerman, "The neo-Kraepelinian Revival in American Psychiatry: Its History, Promise, and Prospect," paper given at a scientific symposium in honor of the retirement of Eli Robins, St. Louis, Missouri, 27 May 1977.

77. R. Michels, "First rebuttal," *American Journal of Psychiatry* 141 (1984): 548–560.

78. Ibid.

79. Interview with Ross Baldessarini, American College of Neuropsychopharmacology meeting, San Juan, Puerto Rico, December 1998.

80. Spitzer, "A Manual for Diagnosis and Statistics," 415–430; R. Bayer, *Homosexuality and American Psychiatry: The Politics of Diagnosis* (New York: Basic Books, 1981).

81. At the APA meeting in New Orleans in May 2001, Bob Spitzer ended up at the center of a media storm after delivering a paper widely reported as titled something like "Gays Have a Mental Illness That Can Be Cured." See R. L. Spitzer, "Subjects Who Claim to Have Benefited from Sexual Reorientation Therapy," Abstract 67B in *Proceedings of the American Psychiatric Association* (Washington, D.C.: American Psychiatric Press, 2001).

82. R. Bayer and R. L. Spitzer, "Neurosis, psychodynamics, and DSMIII," *Archives of General Psychiatry* 42 (1985): 187–196. The core group was Endicott, Spitzer, Klein, and Gittelman-Klein from Columbia, and Andreasen, Cantwell, Clayton, Goodwin, Saslow, and Woodruffe, all of

whom had links with Washington University in St. Louis, and Robert Arnstein, William Frosch, Morton Kramer, Zbigniew Lipowski, Michael L. Mavroidis, Theodore Millon, Henry Pinsker, Michael Sheehy, and Lyman Wynne.

83. J. P. Feighner, E. Robins, S. B. Guze, R. Woodruffe, G. Winokur, and R. Munoz, "Diagnostic criteria for use in psychiatric research," 57–63; R. K. Blashfield, "Feighner et al.: invisible colleges and the Matthew Effect," *Schizophrenia Bulletin* 8 (1982): 1–12; R. Blashfield, *The Classification of Psychopathology* (New York: Plenum Books, 1984).

84. F. M. Quitkin and D. F. Klein, "Follow-up of treatment failure, psychosis, and character disorder," *American Journal of Psychiatry* 144 (1967): 499–505.

85. R. Bayer and R. L. Spitzer, "Neurosis, psychodynamics and DSMIII," 187–196; Healy, *The Antidepressant Era*, chap. 7.

86. See D. Sheahan, "Angles on Panic," in Healy, *The Psychopharmacologists*, vol. 3, 479–504; J. J. Lopez-Ibor, "Personality, Disease, and Psychopharmacology," in Healy, *The Psychopharmacologists*, vol. 2, 409–434.

87. G. L. Klerman, "The Advantages of DSM-III," *American Journal of Psychiatry* 141 (1984): 539–542; G. E. Vaillant, "The disadvantages of DSM-III outweigh its advantages," *American Journal of Psychiatry* 141 (1984): 542–543; R. L. Spitzer, " DSM-III: first defense," *American Journal of Psychiatry* 141 (1984): 545–548; Michels, "First rebuttal," 548–560.

88. M. Wilson, "DSM-III and the transformation of American psychiatry," *American Journal of Psychiatry* 150 (1993): 339–410.

89. Bayer, and Spitzer, "Neurosis, psychodynamics, and DSMIII," 187–196.

90. J. Cole, "The Evaluation of Psychotropic Drugs," in Healy, *The Psychopharmacologists*, vol. 1, 239–264.

91. H. Pardes, "The Demise of a Major Innovation: Carter's 1980 Community Mental Health System Act in Reagan's Hands," in I. Marks and R. Scott, ed., *Mental Health Care Delivery* (Cambridge: Cambridge University Press, 1989), 189–200.

92. P. Leber, "The Role of the Regulator in the Evaluation of the Acceptability of New Drug Products," in D. Healy and D. Doogan, ed., *Psychotropic Drug Development* (London: Arnold, 1996), 69–77; P. Leber, "Managing Uncertainty," in Healy, *The Psychopharmacologists*, vol. 2, 607–622.

93. D. Healy, "A failure to warn," *International Journal of Risk and Safety in Medicine* 12 (1999): 156–159.

94. N. S. Kline, "Scales and Checklists," in J. O. Cole and R. W. Gerard, ed., *Psychopharmacology: Problems in Evaluation* (Washington, D.C.: National Academy of Sciences and National Research Council, 1959,) 475.

95. B. A. Baruch, *Ethical Issues in Drug Testing, Approval, and Pricing* (New York: Oxford University Press, 1995).

96. The first article in a major journal entirely written by company personnel was probably C. M. Beasley, B. E. Dornseif, J. C. Bosomworth, M. E. Sayler, A. H. Rampey, J. H. Heiligenstein, et al., "Fluoxetine and suicide: a meta-analysis of controlled trials of treatment for depression," *British Medical Journal* 303 (1991): 685–692.

97. L. E. Hollister, "From Hypertension to Psychopharmacology: A Serendipitous Career," in Healy, *The Psychopharmacologists*, vol. 2, 215–236.
98. S. Stecklow and L. Johannes, "Questions Arise on New Drug Testing: Drug Makers Relied on Clinical Researchers Who Now Await Trial," *Wall Street Journal*, 15 August 1997, 1–3; K. Eichenwald and G. Kolata, "Drug Trials Hide Conflict for Doctors," *New York Times*, 16 May 1999, 1, 28, 29; "A Doctor's Drug Studies Turn into Fraud," *New York Times*, 17 May 1999, 1, 16, 17; S. Boseley, "Trial and Error Puts Patients at Risk," *Guardian*, 27 July 1999, 8.
99. D. A. Kessler, "Drug promotion and scientific exchange," *New England Journal of Medicine* 325 (1991): 201–203.
100. All of the material in the first part of this paragraph is based on practices I have not only witnessed but engaged in.
101. D. Rennie, "Fair conduct and fair reporting of clinical trials," *Journal of the American Medical Association* 282 (1999): 1766–1768; P. Huston and D. Moher, "Redundancy, disaggregation, and the integrity of medical research," *Lancet* 347 (1996): 1024–1026.
102. S. M. Gilbody and F. Song, "Publication bias and the integrity of psychiatry research," *Psychological Medicine* 30 (2000): 253–258; N. Freemantle, I. M. Anderson, and P. Young, "Predictive value of pharmacological activity for the relative efficacy of antidepressant drugs: meta-regression analysis," *British Journal of Psychiatry* 177 (2000): 292–302.
103. I. Chalmers, "Under-reporting research is scientific misconduct," *Journal of the American Medical Association* 263 (1990): 1405–1408.
104. D. Healy, "The assessment of outcome in depression: measures of social functioning," *Reviews in Contemporary Pharmacotherapy* 11 (2000): 295–301.
105. See Healy, *The Antidepressant Era*, chap. 6.
106. D. Healy, "The three faces of the antidepressants," *Journal of Nervous and Mental Disease* 187 (1999): 174–180.
107. R. K. Fuller, L. Branchey, and D. R. Brightwell, "Disulfiram treatment of alcoholism: a Veterans Administration cooperative study," *Journal of the American Medical Association* 256 (1986): 1449–1455.
108. P. R. Joyce, R. T. Mulder, and C. R. Cloninger, "Temperament predicts clomipramine and desipramine response in major depression," *Journal of Affective Disorders* 30 (1994): 35–46; R. Tranter, H. Healy, D. Cattell, and D. Healy, "Differential functional effects of agents selective to monoamine systems," *Psychological Medicine*, submitted.
109. P. Janssen, "From haloperidol to risperidone," in Healy, *The Psychopharmacologists*, vol. 2, 39–70.
110. L. Lasagna, "Back to the Future," in Healy, *The Psychopharmacologists*, vol. 2, 135–166.
111. P. Slade and R. Bentall, *Sensory Deception: Towards a Scientific Analysis of Hallucinations* (London: Croom Helm, 1988). See also I. Leudar and P. Thomas, *Voices of Reason, Voices of Insanity: Studies of Verbal Hallucinations* (London: Routledge, 2000).

112. See H. M. Sharp, C. F. Fear, J. M. G. Williams, D. Healy, C. F. Lowe, H. Yeaden, and R. Holden, "Delusional phenomenology: dimensions of change," *Behaviour Research and Therapy* 34: (1996) 123–142.

113. R. E. Kendell, "The next 25 years," *British Journal of Psychiatry* 176 (2000): 6–9.

114. C. H. Kemp, F. N. Silverman, B. F. Steele, W. Droegmueller, and H. K. Silver, "The battered child syndrome," *Journal of the American Medical Association* 181 (1962): 17–25.

115. J. C. Nemiah, "Hysterical Neurosis: Dissociative Type," in A. M. Freedman, H. I. Caplan, and B. J. Saddock, ed., *Comprehensive Textbook of Psychiatry* (Baltimore: William and Wilkins, 1975), 1220–1230.

116. E. L. Bliss, *Multiple Personality, Allied Disorders, and Hypnosis* (Oxford: Oxford University Press, 1986).

117. D. Healy, "Altered states of consciousness; phenomenology and pharmacology," *Journal of Psychopharmacology* 6 (1992): 425–435.

118. H. Kind, "The psychogenesis of schizophrenia," *International Journal of Psychiatry* 3 (1967): 383–413.

119. J. L. Herman, *Father-Daughter Incest* (Cambridge, Mass.: Harvard University Press, 1987).

120. E. Bass and L. Davies, *The Courage to Heal: A Guide to Women Survivors of Child Sexual Abuse* (New York: Harper & Row, 1988).

121. S. Brandon, J. Boakes, and D. Glaser, "Recovered memories of childhood sexual abuse: implications for clinical practice," *British Journal of Psychiatry* 172 (1998): 296–307; S. Brandon, "Recovered memory syndrome: fact or fiction?" *Primary Care Psychiatry* 5 (1999): 13–17; E. Showalter, *Hystories: Hysterical Epidemics and Modern Culture* (New York: Columbia University Press, 1997).

122. American Psychiatric Association, *Statement on Memories of Sexual Abuse* (Washington, D.C.: APA Press, 1993).

123. M. A. J. Romme, and A. D. Escher, "Hearing voices," *Schizophrenia Bulletin* 15 (1989): 209–216.

124. E. Shorter, *A History of Psychiatry: From the Age of the Asylum to the Era of Prozac* (New York: John Wiley, 1996).

125. U. Osby, N. Correia, L. Brandt, A. Ekbom, and P. Sparen, "Time trends in schizophrenia mortality in Stockholm County, Sweden: a cohort study," *British Medical Journal* 321 (2000): 483–484.

126. V. Pedersen and K. Bøgesø, "Drug Hunting," in Healy, *The Psychopharmacologists*, vol. 2, 561–580.

127. N. S. Jacobson, K. S. Dobson, P. A. Truax, M. E. Addis, K. Koerner, J. K Gollan, E. Gortner, and S. E. Prince, "A component analysis of cognitive behavioral treatment for depression," *Journal of Consulting and Clinical Psychology* 64 (1996): 295–304.

128. I. Marks, "Computer aids to mental health care," *Canadian Journal of Psychiatry* 44 (1999): 548–555. History suggests that this therapy is doomed, but not for lack of either evidence or efficacy. Pfizer put $6 million into the

development before it pulled out, not because the product did not work but because it would not be sufficiently profitable.

129. M. D. Waldinger, M. H. Hengeveld, and A. H. Zwinderman, "Paroxetine treatment of premature ejaculation: a double-blind randomized placebo-controlled study," *American Journal of Psychiatry* 151 (1994): 1377–1379.

130. Healy, *The Antidepressant Era*, chap. 6; D. Healy and D. Nutt, "Prescriptions, licenses, and evidence," *Psychiatric Bulletin* 22 (1998): 680–684.

131. J. L. Bisson, P. L. Jenkins, J. Alexander, and C. Bannister, "Randomised controlled trial of psychological debriefing for victims of acute burn trauma," *British Journal of Psychiatry* 171 (1997): 78–81. See B. Raphael, L. Meldrum, and A. C. McFarlane, "Does debriefing after psychological trauma work? time for randomised controlled trials," *British Medical Journal* 310 (1995): 1479–1480.

132. W. Reich, "American psycho-ideology," *Psychiatric Bulletin* (1982): 43; D. Healy, "A dance to the music of the century," *Psychiatric Bulletin* 24 (2000): 1–3.

133. M. Shepherd, "Review: *Diagnostic and Statistical Manual,* 3rd edition," *Psychological Medicine* 11 (1981): 215.

134. D. Healy, M. Savage, P. Michael, M. Harris, D. Hirst, M. Carter, D. Cattell, T. McMonagle, N. Sohler, and E. Susser, "Psychiatric service utilization: 1896 and 1996 compared," *Psychological Medicine* 31 (2001): 779–790.

135. T. Detre and M. C. McDonald, "Managed care and the future of psychiatry," *Archives of General Psychiatry* 54 (1997): 201–204.

136. E. S. Valenstein, *Blaming the Brain* (New York: Free Press, 1998).

137. Mimi Hall, "You Have to Get Help: Frightening Experience Now a Tool to Help Others," *USA Today,* 7 May 1999, B1.

138. *Guardian,* "Oh No! We're Not Really Getting More Depressed Are We?" 15 September 1997, G2 section, 1–3.

139. D. Healy, "A failure to warn," *International Journal of Risk and Safety in Medicine* 12 (1999): 151–156.

140. American Psychiatric Association, Online News Stand, release no. 99–19, 28 April 1999.

141. G. L. Klerman, "Psychiatric Research at the MGH," in T. P. Hackett, A. Weisman, and A. Kucharsky, ed., *General Hospital Psychiatry: The First Fifty Years* (Littleton, Mass.: PSG Publishing Co., 1987).

142. Interview with Mandell Cohen, 28 March 2000. Cohen died on 19 November 2000.

143. J. A. Lieberman and A. J. Rush, "Redefining the role of psychiatry in medicine," *American Journal of Psychiatry* 153 (1996): 1388–1397.

144. E. Evarts, "A Discussion of the Relevance of Effects of Drugs on Animal Behavior to the Possible Effects of Drugs on Psychopathological Processes in Man," in Cole and Gerard, ed.,. *Psychopharmacology,* 284–306, especially 302.

8. DEMOCRACY

1. S. Kety, in U.S. Senate Committee on Government Operations, Report to the Senate Subcommittee on Government Research, "Hearings of the National Commission on Health Sciences and Society," 90th Congress, 2nd. Session, 1968, 292.
2. J.-J. Rousseau, *The Social Contract*, trans. M. Cranston (1762; Harmondsworth, Eng.: Penguin Books, 1968).
3. I. Hacking, *The Emergence of Probability* (Cambridge: Cambridge University Press, 1975); G. Gigerenzer, Z. Swijtink, T. Porter, L. Daston, J. Beatty, and L. Krüger, *The Empire of Chance* (Cambridge: Cambridge University Press, 1989); L. Krüger, L. Daston, and M. Heidelberger, *The Probabilistic Revolution*, vol. 1 (Cambridge Mass.: MIT Press, 1987), and L. Krüger, G. Gigerenzer, and M. Morgan, *The Probabilistic Revolution*, vol. 2 (Cambridge Mass.: MIT Press, 1987).
4. D. Healy, *The Antidepressant Era* (Cambridge, Mass.: Harvard University Press, 1997), chap. 3.
5. See C. E. Rosenberg, *No Other Gods: On Science and American Social Thought* (Baltimore: Johns Hopkins University Press, 1997).
6. J. Kagan, *Three Seductive Ideas* (Cambridge Mass.: Harvard University Press, 1998).
7. U. Beck, *Risk Society: Towards a New Modernity* (London: Sage, 1992).
8. E. Haikan, *Venus Envy: A History of Cosmetic Surgery* (Baltimore: Johns Hopkins University Press, 1998).
9. D. Healy, *Images of Trauma: From Hysteria to Post-traumatic Stress Disorder* (London: Faber & Faber, 1993); I. Hacking, *Rewriting the Soul: Multiple Personality and the Sciences of Memory* (Princeton: Princeton University Press, 1995).
10. N. Rose, *Governing the Soul: The Shaping of the Private Self* (London: Free Association Books, 1989); N. Rose, *Inventing Our Selves: Psychology, Power, and Personhood* (Cambridge: Cambridge University Press, 1998); N. Rose, *Powers of Freedom* (Cambridge: Cambridge University Press, 1999).
11. Rosenberg, *No Other Gods*.
12. D. Kahneman, P. Slovic, and A. Tversky, *Judgement under Uncertainty: Heuristic and Biases* (Cambridge: Cambridge University Press, 1982). See also D. Healy, *The Suspended Revolution: Psychiatry and Psychotherapy Reexamined* (London: Faber & Faber, 1990).
13. K. F. Kiple, "The History of Disease," in R. Porter, ed., *Cambridge Illustrated History of Medicine* (Cambridge: Cambridge University Press, 1996), 16–51.
14. G. Grob, "The Social History of Medicine and Disease in America: Problems and Possibilities," in P. Branca, ed., *The Medicine Show* (New York: Science History Publications, 1977), 63–68; S. Sontag, *Illness as Metaphor* (New York: Farrar, Strauss & Giroux, 1978).
15. A. Zanca, ed., *Pharmacy through the Ages: Ancient Drugs* (Parma: Astrea Coop.r.l, 1990).

16. Healy, *The Antidepressant Era*, chap. 1.
17. S. Plant, *Writings on Drugs* (London: Faber & Faber, 1999).
18. W. James, *The Varieties of Religious Experience: A Study in Human Nature* (1902; Harmondsworth, Eng.: Penguin Books, 1986).
19. T. McKenna, *Food of the Gods: A Radical History of Plants, Drugs, and Human Evolution* (New York: Bantam Books, 1992).
20. G. Ginzburg, *Exstasies* (New York: Pantheon Books, 1991).
21. J. Stevens, *Storming Heaven: LSD and the American Dream* (London: William Heinemann, 1988).
22. See R. Darnton, *Mesmerism and the End of the Enlightenment in France* (Cambridge Mass.: Harvard University Press, 1968); Healy, *Images of Trauma.*
23. See W. E. Barton, "Trends in community mental health programs," *Hospital and Community Psychiatry* 11 (1966); reprinted in *Psychiatric Services* 51 (2000): 611–615, with commentary by S. S. Sharfstein, "Whatever happened to community mental health?" *Psychiatric Services* 51 (2000): 616–620.
24. D. Martin, *Hospitals in Trouble* (Oxford: Blackwells, 1983).
25. *News of the World*, 20 August 1967, 1.
26. D. Healy, M. Savage, P. Michael, M. Harris, D. Hirst, M. Carter, D. Cattell, T. McMonagle, N. Sohler, and E. Susser, "Psychiatric bed utilization: 1896 and 1996 compared," *Psychological Medicine* 31 (2001): 779–790.
27. O. F. Wahl, *Media Madness: Public Images of Mental Illness* (New Brunswick, N.J.: Rutgers University Press, 1995); S. L. Gilman, *Seeing the Insane* (Lincoln: University of Nebraska Press, 1982).
28. C. E. Koop and G. D. Lundberg, "Violence in America: a public health emergency," *Journal of the American Medical Association* 267 (1992): 3075–3076; M. L. Rosenberg, P. W. O'Carroll, and K. E. Powell, "Let's be clear: violence is a public health problem," *Journal of the American Medical Association* 267 (1992): 3071–3072; A. H. Flitcraft, "Violence, values, and gender," *Journal of the American Medical Association* 267 (1992): 3194–3195.
29. P. Bech, "Methodology and Organisation in Psychopharmacology," in D. Healy, *The Psychopharmacologists*, vol. 2 (London: Arnold, 1998), 499–520.
30. Healy, Savage, Michael, Harris, Hirst, Carter, Cattell, McMonagle, Sohler, and Susser, "Psychiatric bed utilization."
31. N. Rose, "The biology of culpability: pathological identity and crime control in a biological culture," *Theoretical Criminology* 4 (2000): 5–34.
32. D. Wasserman, "Research into genetics and crime: consensus and controversy," *Politics and the Life Sciences* 15 (1996): 107–109. See also D. Wasserman, "Science and social harm: genetic research into crime and violence," *Report from the Institute of Philosophy and Public Policy* 15 (1995): 14–19.
33. I. Gottesman, "Predisposed to Predispositions," in Healy, *The Psychopharmacologists*, vol. 2, 377–408.
34. N. Rose, "The biology of culpability," 5–34.

35. See R. DeGrandpre, "Constructing the Pharmacological," *Capitalism, Nature, Socialism* 13 (2002); R. DeGrandpre, *The Cult of Pharmacology* (Durham: Duke University Press, forthcoming).

36. R. E. Meyer, "The disease called addiction: emerging evidence in a 200-year debate," *Lancet* 347 (1996): 162–166; C. P. O'Brien and T. McLellan, "Myths about the treatment of addiction," *Lancet* 347 (1996): 227–231; N. A. Sievewright and J. Greenwood, "What is important in drug misuse treatment," *Lancet* 347 (1996): 373–376.

37. J. M. Zito, D. J. Safer, S. dos Reis, J. F. Gardner, M. Boles, and F. Lynch, "Trends in the prescribing of psychotropic medications to preschoolers," *Journal of the American Medical Association* 283 (2000): 1025–1030.

38. L. Johnston, "Paxil, Prozac, Ritalin . . . Are These Drugs Safe for Kids? Many Parents Are Using Powerful Pills to Control Behavior," *U.S. News & World Report*, 6 March 2000,

39. Rose, *Inventing Our Selves*.

40. S. J. Gould, *The Mismeasure of Man* (New York: W. W Norton, 1981).

41. A. B. Hill, "Reflections on the controlled trial," *Annals of the Rheumatic Diseases* 25 (1966): 107–113.

42. M. Hamilton, "Rating Scales in Depression," in P. Kielholz, ed., *Depressive Illness, Diagnosis, Assessment, Treatment* (Bern: Hanns Huber Publishers, 1972), 100.

43. CLRTP, "The Birth of Psychopharmacotherapy:. Explorations in a New World, 1952–1968," in D. Healy, *The Psychopharmacologists*, vol. 3 (London: Arnold, 2000), 1–54; A. Mandell, *Coming of Middle Age* (New York: Summit Books, 1977); A. Mandell, video interview at the American College of Neuropsychopharmacology Annual Meeting, San Juan, Puerto Rico, December 1998.

44. Healy, *The Antidepressant Era*.

45. P. Kramer, *Listening to Prozac* (New York: Viking Press, 1993).

46. C. Elliott, "Lost at the Mall; or The Use of Prozac in a Time of Normal Nihilism," in C. Elliott, *A Philosophical Disease: Bioethics, Culture, and Identity* (New York: Routledge, 1999), 49–74; C. Elliott, "The Tyranny of Happiness: Ethics and Cosmetic Psychopharmacology," in E. Parens, ed., *Enhancing Human Traits: Ethical and Social Implications* (Washington, D.C.: Georgetown University Press, 1999), 177–188. See the following articles in *Hastings Center Report* 30 (2000): C. Elliott, "Pursued by happiness and beaten senseless," 7–12; P. Kramer, "The valorisation of sadness," 13–18; D. Healy, "Good science or good business?" 19–22; J. C. Edwards, "Passion, activity, and 'the care of the self,'" 31–33; D. DeGrazia, "Prozac, enhancement, and self-creation," 34–40.

47. G. L. Klerman, "The efficacy of psychotherapy as the basis for public policy," *American Psychologist*, August 1983, 929–934; P. London and G. L. Klerman, "Evaluating psychotherapy," *American Journal of Psychiatry* 139 (1982): 709–717.

48. Healy, *The Antidepressant Era*, chap. 7.

49. M. Bury and J. Gabe, "A Sociological View of Tranquillizer Dependence: Challenges and Responses," in I. Hindmarch, G. Beaumont, S. Brandon, and B. E. Leonard, ed., *Benzodiazepines: Current Concepts* (Chichester, Eng.: John Wiley, 1990), 211–225; J. Gabe and M. Bury, "Tranquillisers and health care in crisis," *Social Science and Medicine* 32 (1991): 449–454.

50. K. F. Kiple, ed., *Plague, Pox, and Pestilence: Disease in History* (London: Weidenfield and Nicholson, 1997).

51. J. Kagan, *Galen's Prophecy: Temperament in Human Nature* (New York: Basic Books, 1994).

52. Haikan, *Venus Envy.*

53. D. Dickenson, *Moral Luck in Medical Ethics and Practical Politics* (Aldershot, Eng.: Avebury Press, 1991).

54. K. Wellman, *La Mettrie* (Durham: Duke University Press, 1991).

55. R. M. Bell, *Holy Anorexia* (Chicago: University of Chicago Press. 1985); R. Van Deth, and W. Vandereycken, "Continuity and discontinuity in the history of self-starvation," *European Eating Disorders Review* 2 (1994): 47–54; W. Vandereycken and R. Van Deth, *From Fasting Saints to Anorexic Girls: The History of self-Starvation* (London: Athlone Press, 1994).

56. W. Vandereycken and R. Van Deth, "Who was the first to describe anorexia nervosa: Gull or Laségue?" *Psychological Medicine* 19 (1989): 837–845.

57. G. F. M. Russell, "Bulimia nervosa: an ominous variant of anorexia nervosa," *Psychological Medicine* 9 (1979): 429–448; W. Vandereycken, "Emergence of bulimia nervosa as a separate diagnostic entity: review of the literature from 1960–1979," *International Journal of Eating Disorders* 60 (1994): 105–116.

58. P. Janet, *Les obsessions et la psychaesthenie* (Paris: Felix Alcan, 1903).

59. H. B. Richardson, "Simmonds disease and anorexia nervosa," *Archives of Internal Medicine* 63 (1939): 1–8; E. L. Bliss and C. H. Branch, *Anorexia Nervosa: Its History, Psychology, and Biology* (New York: Churchill & Row, 1960).

60. P. J. Cowen, E. M. Clifford, A. E. Walsh, C. Williams, and C. G. Fairburn, "Moderate dieting causes 5HT-2c receptor supersensitivity," *Psychological Medicine* 26 (1996): 1155–1159; L. S. Hsu, "Can dieting cause an eating disorder?" *Psychological Medicine* 27 (1997): 509–513.

61. H. Bruch, "Perceptual and conceptual disturbances in anorexia nervosa," *Psychosomatic Medicine* 24 (1962): 187–194; H. Bruch, "Anorexia nervosa and its differential diagnosis," *Journal of Nervous and Mental Disorders* 141 (1966): 555–561; H. Bruch, *Eating Disorders: Obesity, Anorexia Nervosa, the Person Within* (New York: Basic Books, 1973); H. Thoma, "Some psychoanalytic observations on anorexia nervosa," *British Journal of Medical Psychology*, 36 (1963): 239–246.

62. R. L. Palmer, R. Oppenheimer, A. Dignon, D. A. Chaloner, and K. Howells, "Childhood sexual experiences with adults reported by women with eating disorders: an extended series," *British Journal of Psychiatry* 156 (1990): 699–703.

63. P. E. Garfinkel and D. M. Garner, *Anorexia Nervosa: A Multi-dimensional Perspective* (New York: Brunner-Mazel, 1992).

64. R. Littlewood, "Psychopathology and personal agency: modernity, cultural change, and eating disorders in South Asian societies," *British Journal of Medical Psychology* 68 (1995): 45–63.

65. H. Gremillion, "Psychiatry as social ordering: anorexia nervosa, a paradigm," *Social Science and Medicine* 35 (1992): 57–71.

66. S. Lee, "Self-starvation in context: towards a culturally sensitive understanding of anorexia nervosa," *Social Science and Medicine* 41 (1995): 25–36.

67. See D. B. Mumford, A. M. Whitehouse, and M. Platts, "Sociocultural correlates of eating disorders among Asian schoolgirls in Bradford," *British Journal of Psychiatry* 158 (1991): 222–228; S. K. Khandelwal, P. Sharan, and S. Saxena, "Eating disorders: an Indian perspective," *International Journal of Social Psychiatry* 41 (1995): 132–146.

68. S. Bordo, *Unbearable Weight: Feminism, Western Culture, and the Body* (Berkeley: University of California Press, 1993); S. Orbach, *Hunger Strike: The Anorectic's Struggle as a Metaphor for Our Age* (London: Faber & Faber, 1987); K. Chernin, *The Hungry Self: Women, Eating, and Identity* (New York: Times Books, 1985).

69. H. Schwartz, *Never Satisfied: A Cultural History of Diets, Fantasies, and Fat* (New York: Free Press, 1986).

70. It is, however, difficult to establish with any certainty what the prevalence of anorexia nervosa was before the 1960s. Whatever the prevalence of the disorder in an absolute sense, few sufferers received medical attention. The situation changed dramatically in the 1970s and 1980s; at one point in that period almost all heads of psychiatric departments in London were eating disorder researchers.

71. B. G. Quigley and B. K. Doane, "Anorexia nervosa and visual experience," *Lancet* 2 (1981): 1113; W. Vandereycken, "Anorexia nervosa and visual impairment," *Comprehensive Psychiatry* 27 (1986): 545–548; J. Yager and C. Hatton, "Anorexia nervosa in a woman totally blind since the age of two," *British Journal of Psychiatry* 149 (1986): 506–509.

72. J. H. Masserman, *Behavior and Neurosis: An Experimental Psychoanalytic Approach to Psychobiologic Principles* (Chicago: University of Chicago Press, 1943).

73. J. R. Saul, *The Unconscious Civilization* (Toronto: House of Anansi Press, 1995).

74. J. K. Galbraith, *The New Industrial State* (London: Hamish Hamilton, 1967).

75. Healy, *The Antidepressant Era*.

76. D. Healy, "The three faces of the antidepressants: a critical comment on the clinical-economic context of diagnosis," *Journal of Nervous and Mental Disorders* 187 (1999): 174–180.

77. Kety, "Hearings of the National Commission on Health Sciences and Society," 292.

78. R. Kuhn, "The treatment of depressive states with G22355 (imipramine hydrochloride)," *American Journal of Psychiatry* 115 (1958): 459–464.

79. See Healy, *The Antidepressant Era*, chap. 1.

80. M. Lambert, *Medieval Heresy: Popular Movements from the Gregorian Reform to the Reformation* (Oxford: Blackwell, 1992).

81. Healy, *The Antidepressant Era.*

82. E. Shorter, *The Health Century* (New York: Doubleday, 1987).

83. B. H. Kelves, *Naked to the Bone: Medical Imaging in the Twentieth Century* (New Brunswick, N.J.: Rutgers University Press, 1997).

84. L. Farde, J. P. Gustavsson, and E. Jonsson, "D2 dopamine receptors and personality traits," *Nature* 380 (1997): 590; A. Breier, L. Kestler, C. Adler, I. Elman, N. Wiesenfeld, A. Malhotra, and D. Pickar, "Dopamine D-2 receptor density and personal detachment in healthy subjects," *American Journal of Psychiatry* 155 (1998): 1440–1442.

85. Healy, "The three faces of the antidepressants, 174–180.

86. D. Healy, "The marketing of 5HT: anxiety or depression?" *British Journal of Psychiatry* 158 (1991): 737–742.

87. Healy, *The Antidepressant Era.*

88. D. Healy, "A failure to warn," *International Journal of Risk and Safety in Medicine* 12 (1999): 151–156.

89. Healy, Savage, Michael, Harris, Hirst, Carter, Cattell, McMonagle, Sohler, and Susser, "Psychiatric bed utilization."

90. Healy, *The Antidepressant Era*, chap. 6.

91. O. Ray, "A Psychologist in American Neuropsychopharmacology," in Healy, *The Psychopharmacologists*, vol. 2, 435–454.

92. Examples are cimetidine and ranitidine, used in the management of heartburn and ulcers, respectively.

93. C. R. Cloninger, "A systematic method for clinical description and classification of personality variants: a proposal," *Archives of General Psychiatry* 44 (1987): 573–588.

94. Haikan, *Venus Envy.*

95. Plant, *Writings on Drugs.*

96. See DeGrandpre, "Constructing the Pharmacological"; DeGrandpre, *The Cult of Pharmacology.*

97. T. Bittker, "The industrialization of American psychiatry," *American Journal of Psychiatry* 142 (1985): 149–154.

98. L. Eisenberg, "Whatever happened to the faculty on the way to the agora?" *Archives of Internal Medicine* 159 (1999): 2251–2256.

99. L. Wright, *Twins: Genes, Environment, and the Mystery of Identity* (London: Weidenfeld and Nicolson, 1997).

100. J. A. Lieberman and A. J. Rush, "Redefining the role of psychiatry in medicine," *American Journal of Psychiatry* 153 (1996): 1388–1397.

101. Healy, Savage, Michael, Harris, Hirst, Carter, Cattell, McMonagle, Sohler, and Susser, "Psychiatric bed utilization."

102. See D. Sheahan, "Angles on Panic," in Healy, *The Psychopharmacologists*, vol. 3, 479–504; J. J. Lopez-Ibor, "Personality, Disease, and Psychopharmacology" in Healy, *The Psychopharmacologists*, vol. 2, 409–434.

Acknowledgments

Transport metaphors dominate my acknowledgments. As I finished this book on a train in Britain, another such metaphor pushed its way forward. In the year 2000, the country that introduced the railway, a technological development that led to a new mental disorder—traumatic neurosis—was gripped by a railway crisis. The crisis had twin roots in botched efforts at privatizing public services and a peculiar conversion of hazards into liabilities, both of which lie close to the central themes of this book. All of a sudden, no train journey could be guaranteed. No travelers could be sure of getting to their destination. It took twenty-three hours of travel time for me to go five hundred miles, not to mention an unplanned overnight stay without a change of clothes or any toiletries.

Imagine then if you will a British train in December 2000. I could fill several cars with those to whom I am indebted. Among those who thought the journey was a good idea and who have helped keep the rolling stock on the tracks were Tom Ban, Ross Baldessarini, Elizabeth Knoll of Harvard University Press, and Ned Shorter and Others—German Berrios, Allan Beveridge, Max Fink, Stephanie Krüger, Brian Leonard, Gene Paykel, and

Trevor Turner—told me everything I know about some things. Some, such as Nikolas Rose and Carl Elliott, I met only while I was on the train, but they have been one of the good things about the delays. There are train cars full of psychopharmacologists I have interviewed, almost a hundred at the last count, from my first interview in a train car in 1993 with George Beaumont. Most of these have been published, but the interviews with David Clark and Ross Baldessarini have not. Among the most important published interviews for this book have been those with Frank Ayd, Klaus Bøgesø, Arvid Carlsson, Jonathan Cole, Len Cook, Leo Hollister, Paul Janssen, Pierre Lambert and his colleagues in Lyon, Roger Pinder, Pierre Simon, Jean Thuillier, Peter Waldmeier, and Ed Warawa. Most of these people have worked either in the pharmaceutical industry or very closely with it. In a book like this, this is as it should be. In another railway car are Dinah Cattell, Manikarssa Devakumar, Tony Roberts, Jackie Thomas, and of course Helen, Justin, Sarah, and Rita, who have helped provide me with a base from which to make this and other journeys.

Who knows where we will spend the night? The conductor will tell us that every day is different. Every time one bit of track is repaired another is found to be defective. It feels as if we are traveling back in time—very far back, when travel was an adventure, but one with a strangely hallucinogenic quality, as what should be familiar and predictable grows increasingly strange. We pass slowly enough to notice the herds of cows trying to graze in fields that have not been so flooded in a century. There is time to wonder about a strange new neuropsychiatric disease, BSE (bovine spongiform encephalopathy), caught from cattle, which by the time this book is published may have claimed thousands of lives. There is time to wonder whether global warming or BSE will get our children or us first.

It goes without saying that with the current state of the railways in Britain, none of the above would have undertaken this journey of their own accord and the responsibility accordingly is mine alone.

Index

Index

Prichard, J. C., 14

Prinzmetal, Myron, 61

Prochlorperazine, 98, 111–112, 126–127, 231

Promazine, 81, 227

Promethazine, 77, 78–79, 82, 228

Propranediol drugs, 67

Prozac, 103, 290, 305, 309, 354, 355, 356; discovery of, 2, 4; uses of, 48, 379–380; action and effectiveness of, 50, 114, 219, 353; absence of side effects from, 59; reception of, 68; marketing and promotion of, 170–171, 209, 308; debates about, 247; successors to, 262; suicide issues and, 263, 374; licensing of, 307–308; behavior of patients on, 330; used to treat children, 348; marketing of, 352; development of, 375

Psyche, dynamic, 27, 338

Psychedelics, 153–154, 186, 202

Psychiatric research, 157

Psychiatric survivor groups, 155

Psychiatry, 8, 31, 144, 154, 215, 295, 296, 304, 305; biological, 6, 40, 56, 134, 135, 146, 175, 176, 187, 188, 192, 202, 207, 280, 295, 328, 332, 346, 359; criticism of, 30, 129–130, 155, 173, 174; at turn of twentieth century, 31–36; social, 32, 135, 136, 137, 138, 139, 144, 146, 149, 152, 174; business aspects of, 32–33, 175, 311; transcultural, 66; scientific, 75, 107, 182, 315, 350; psychodynamic, 85; in hospital settings, 96; impact of World War II on, 130–136; epidemiological, 136–139; community, 140, 147, 148, 150, 343; post-war American, 140–144; in Europe, 147–148; alienation of patients by, 149, 218; social changes and, 157, 158; opposition to, 162; illegal treatment regimes, 163; political consequences of, 163; clinical, 175, 188; controlled trials and, 185; metabolic, 188, 222; orthomolecular, 190; genetic, 195, 197; language of, 215; legal liability and, 249; office practice of, 303; pharmaceutical companies/industry and, 312; decline in, 312–315; forensic, 345; pharmacogenetic developments and, 370; future of, 381–390; standards

within, 382; influence of pharmaceutical companies on, 387

Psychic driving, 162

Psychoanalysis, 23, 36, 130, 142, 145, 293; impact of World War II on, 139–144; as public health issue, 140–141; office-based, 144, 146, 150; as treatment for schizophrenia, 144–145; opposition to, 286

Psychobiology, 197, 292–293, 299

Psychodrama, 130

Psychodynamic therapy, 51, 137, 139, 176, 276, 290, 338–339, 343, 352, 353

Psychology, 24, 288, 338–339; clinical, 288–289, 291, 316

Psychometric instruments, 86

Psychoneuroses, 26, 29, 30

Psychopathology, 30, 64, 143, 166, 270, 287, 328, 344, 382

Psychoses, 3, 23, 35, 112, 150; treatment of, 7, 41, 43, 50, 78–79, 93, 116, 141, 145, 312; classification of, 85; medical approach to, 87; chlorpromazine as treatment for, 89, 90, 101, 107, 115, 126; as growth experience, 142; management of, 144, 387; drug-induced, 145, 181–182; psychiatry as treatment for, 146; diagnostic markers for, 187; LSD model of, 193; awakening from, 225; atypical, 228; imipramine as treatment for, 229; drug treatment for, 276; behavior therapy applied to, 287; psychotherapy of, 316–320

Psychosocial measures, 316

Psychosomatic medicines, 36

Psychosurgery, 3, 40, 144, 155, 219, 249, 280

Psychosyndromes, 138, 370, 371, 385

Psychotherapy, 27, 55, 286, 332, 386; to treat psychoses, 7, 316–320; intervention as, 142; role of therapist, 142–143; failure of, 143; long-term effectiveness of, 143, 145; humanistic, 175; specificity and, 286–291

Psychotogens, 180, 186

Psychotomimetic effects, 181, 183, 184, 185

Psychotropic drugs, 7, 60, 66–67, 82, 88, 105–106, 133, 344; used to treat chil-

Index

Index

Index

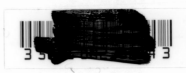
GAYLORD F